VENOUS THROMBOSIS – PRINCIPLES AND PRACTICE

Edited by **Ertugrul Okuyan**

Venous Thrombosis – Principles and Practice
Edited by Ertugrul Okuyan

Published by InTech

Janeza Trdine 9, 51000 Rijeka, Croatia

Publishing Process Manager Masa Vidovic

Technical Editor Teodora Smiljanic

Cover Designer InTech Design Team

Additional hard copies can be obtained from orders@intechopen.com

Venous Thrombosis – Principles and Practice, Edited by Ertugrul Okuyan
p. cm.
ISBN 978-953-307-885-4

For EU product safety concerns:
IN TECH d.o.o., Prolaz Marije Krucifikse Kozulić 3, 51000 Rijeka, Croatia,
info@intechopen.com or visit our website at intechopen.com.

Meet the editor

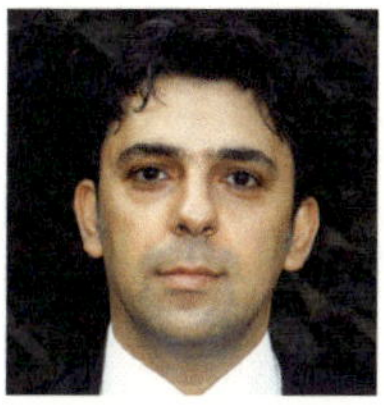

Dr. Ertugrul Okuyan was born in Hatay, Turkey, in 1973. He graduated from Marmara University, Faculty of Medicine in 1997, and obtained the title of Cardiology Specialist from the Istanbul University Institution of Cardiology in September 2003. He works at the Cardiology Clinic of the Istanbul Bagcilar Education and Research Hospital. His main areas of interest are heart failure, atherosclerosis, pulmonary hypertension, venous and arterial thrombosis and arterial hypertension. Having been published in many highly ranked papers, Dr Okuyan is a member of the Turkish Cardiology Association, European Society of Cardiology, American Heart Association, European Atherosclerosis Society, American Society of Hypertension and European Association of Cardiac Rehabilitation and Prevention.

Contents

Preface

The venous thrombosis care and profession has evolved considerably over the past 20 years. This book reflects the current practice, both technical and professional, of physicians from different fields. Venous thromboembolism became treatable with the discovery of heparin at the beginning of the 20th century. The presence of an effective therapy increased the importance of diagnosing venous thromboembolism, fueling a plethora of medical research and technological developments over the next century. Despite the advances made, venous thromboembolism remains an elusive entity because of its atypical presentations and associated diagnostic challenges.

This book is a fresh synthesis of venous thromboembolism care and considers the opinions and studies from different fields of medicine. As venous thrombosis spectrum is wide and can affect many organ systems, from deep veins of the leg to the cerebral venous system, our intent is for this to be a comprehensive, up-to-date and readable book. Section 1 covers the etiology of venous thrombosis and specific disease conditions that are largely associated with venous thrombosis. Section 2 is a review of the current catheter-based therapy and late complications of the venous thrombosis. Section 3 covers all aspects of assessment of the patients with cerebral venous thrombosis and venous thrombosis of the eye. Section 4 focuses on venous thrombosis in general surgery patients and catheter-related venous thrombosis in cancer patients. Section 5 covers special issues about venous thrombosis, clinical experiences and perspectives of the authors about the special topics.

We sought the best contributing authors to write these chapters. Many of them are not only experts in their assigned topics, but also have extensive teaching experience. We encouraged all contributors to present a new synthesis of the existing material infused with new ideas and perspectives, their own clinical studies and even case-reports.

So, we present to you the fruits of our efforts. We all hope that this book will be a significant contribution to the scientific knowledge about venous thrombosis.

Dr. Ertugrul Okuyan
Istanbul Bagcilar Education and
Research Hospital Cardiology Clinic, Istanbul
Turkey

Part 1

Etiology

1

Aetiology of Venous Thrombosis

Mehrez M. Jadaon
Kuwait University
Kuwait

1. Introduction

Blood is a fluid tissue that circulates in the body inside intact blood vessels (veins, arteries and capillaries) to perform several vital functions. For perfect performance, blood should flow smoothly inside blood vessels without interruption. If a blood vessel gets injured or perforated, blood will flow out and be lost, which may be fatal. To prevent this, several natural physiological processes occur to form a "plug", usually called "blood clot", to block the puncture and prevent blood loss. These processes are called "Haemostasis", which involves the blood vessels themselves, specialized blood cells called platelets, as well as specific blood proteins called clotting factors. Haemostasis functions to prevent blood loss from injured blood vessels and ensure the fluidity of blood inside intact (uninjured) blood vessels (Hoffbrand et al., 2001; Escobar et al., 2002; Laffan & Manning, 2002a).

Like any other physiological process in the body, haemostasis may get abnormal due to many reasons. It may not be able to function well and therefore the blood becomes unable to clot, which leads to bleeding problems (haemophilia). On the other hand, haemostasis may happen abnormally inside intact blood vessels, without any injury, forming a blood clot (thrombus) inside the vessel (intravascular thrombosis), which may lead to partial or complete blockage of blood flow through this vessel. This mostly occurs in the deep veins of the lower extremities, and to a less extent in the upper extremities, and this pathological condition is called deep vein thrombosis (DVT). If a thrombus detaches (called embolus), it usually goes up through the circulation and settles in an arterial branch in the lungs causing pulmonary embolism (PE). DVT and PE together are called venous thromboembolic disorders (VTE). VTE are serious vascular conditions that account for high morbidity and mortality rates in many countries with an annual incidence of 1/1000 (Dahlbäck, 1995; Ridker et al., 1997).

Several "genetic" and "acquired" risk factors were identified to cause VTE, and this is why the WHO expert group described VTE in 1996 as being genetically determined, acquired or both (Lane et al., 1996). This chapter describes the different genetic and acquired risk factors for VTE. The chapter is divided into two main sections: genetic factors and acquired factors, and it is concluded by a third section on intersections of risk factors. In order to better understand how these factors cause VTE, a preliminary section is given to explain the major processes of haemostasis, namely the Coagulation and Fibrinolysis processes, and how abnormalities may lead to VTE.

2. Coagulation and Fibrinolysis

As explained above, haemostasis is the normal physiological process by which an injured blood vessel is sealed by a blood clot to prevent blood loss. Haemostasis involves many processes, two of which are "The Coagulation Process" and "The Fibrinolysis Process". In both processes, blood clotting factors are the crucial constituents. Clotting factors are enzymatic proteins that are synthesised mostly in the liver and circulate in the blood in an inactive form. When a blood vessel gets injured, these factors get activated and start a cascade of chemical reactions leading to the formation of a fibrin "clot" which blocks the site of injury and therefore prevents blood loss and allows for wound healing. Although the clotting factors have specific names, they are usually given Roman numerals. Figure 1 gives a schematic drawing of the process of Coagulation showing the participation of each clotting factor.

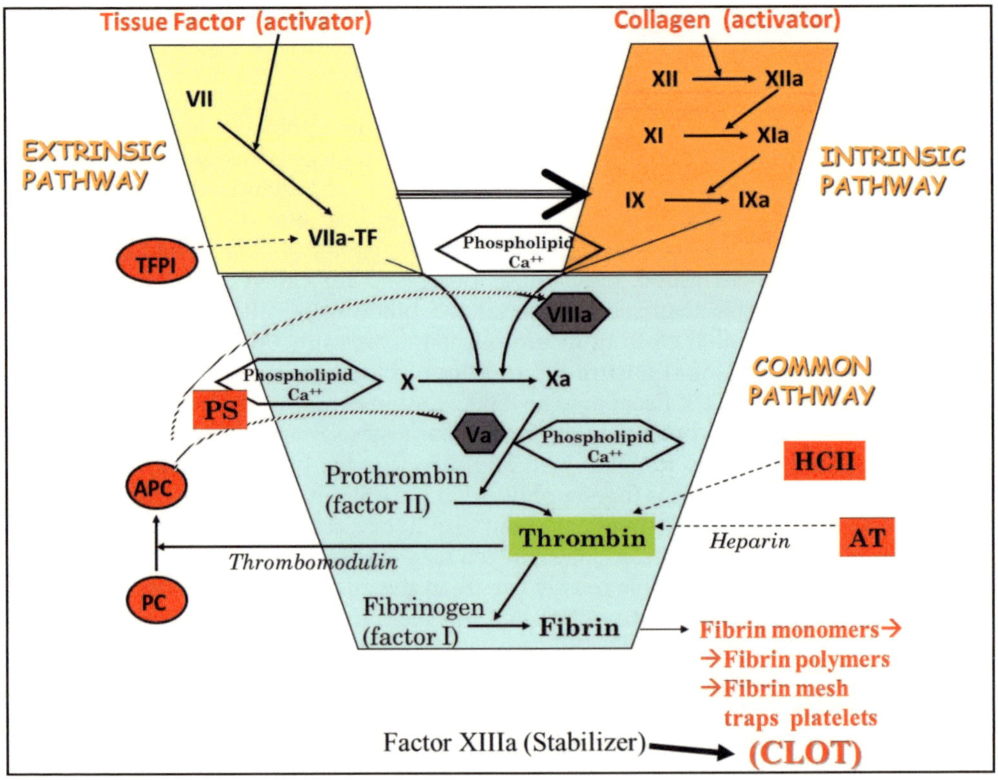

Fig. 1. The Coagulation process and its control elements. Solid arrows indicate activation; dotted arrows indicate inactivation (prepared and drawn by the author).

The Coagulation process maybe virtually divided into three pathways: Extrinsic, Intrinsic and Common pathways. When a blood vessel is injured, the components of the blood vessels start to activate the clotting factors by two methods. Firstly, the injured tissues release a membrane protein called thromboplastin (tissue factor [TF] or clotting factor III) which is capable of activating clotting factor VII in the Extrinsic pathway. Activated clotting factor VII (VIIa) forms a complex with TF, and this tends to activate clotting factor X in the Common pathway. On the other hand, the subendothelial layers of blood vessels have abundant amounts of collagen embedded inside them. This collagen gets exposed in injured vessels, and collagen is capable of activating clotting factor XII in the Intrinsic pathway. Activated factor XII (XIIa) in turn activates clotting factor XI, which in turn activates clotting factor IX. Activated clotting factor IX, with the help of clotting co-factor VIII, is capable of activating clotting factor X in the Common pathway. So, both the Extrinsic and Intrinsic pathways team up to activate the Common pathway. In the Common pathway, activated clotting factor X, with the help of clotting co-factor V, continues the process by activating clotting factor II (prothrombin) into thrombin. The main function of thrombin is the conversion of fibrinogen (clotting factor I) into fibrin. Fibrin molecules then polymerize to form thread-like structures which form a mesh that gives the basis of blood clot. Finally, clotting factor XIII crosslinks fibrin polymers to form a stable fibrin mesh which traps activated platelets and other blood cells to form the final blood clot which eventually blocks the injured blood vessel. In addition to co-factors V and VIII, phospholipids and calcium ions (factor IV) act as co-factors in the process of Coagulation (Kane & Davie, 1988; Furie & Furie, 1988; Walker & Fay, 1992; Davie, 1995; Hoffbrand et al., 2001; Escobar et al., 2002; Laffan & Manning, 2002a).

After clot formation, wound healing starts and the injured blood vessel regenerates and becomes intact again. When the healing process is complete, the fibrin clot will no longer be needed and therefore it has to be removed. This occurs by the process of Fibrinolysis (figure 2). The key enzyme in this process is plasmin, which normally circulates in the blood in an inactive form called plasminogen. Plasminogen is usually activated into plasmin by tissue plasminogen activator (tPA) produced by the endothelial cells in the healing blood vessels. Plasmin breaks down fibrin threads into smaller pieces called fibrin degradation products (FDP) which are excreted from the circulation, and therefore the clot dissolves and the blood flow recovers normally (Rock & Wells, 1997; Hoffbrand et al., 2001; Escobar et al., 2002; Laffan & Manning, 2002a).

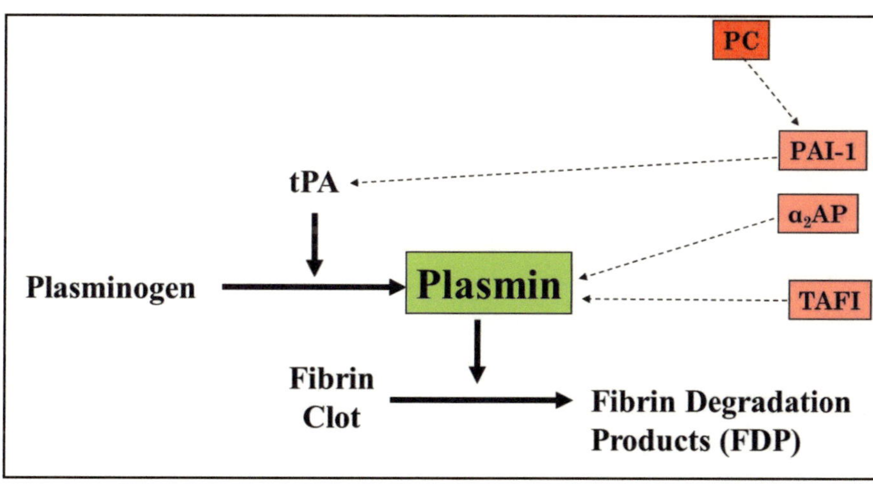

Fig. 2. Fibrinolysis process and its control elements. Solid arrows indicate activation; dotted arrows indicate inactivation (prepared and drawn by the author).

The processes of Coagulation and Fibrinolysis are carefully monitored and supervised by several control systems. This is important to prevent excessive or unnecessary coagulation or fibrinolysis. In the Coagulation process, thrombin is a very robust enzyme which exerts many coagulation functions. It can activate other clotting factors and form many positive feedback loops in the Coagulation process. Therefore, the clotting process may continue forever and the clot may enlarge until it blocks the whole lumen of the blood vessel. Therefore, the Coagulation process should be limited to the area of blood vessel injury and should be prevented from extending abroad. This is achieved by three main proteins that circulate normally in the blood, namely protein C (PC), protein S (PS) and antithrombin (AT). Together they are called "natural anticoagulants" since they function as antagonists to clotting. They exert their function after a blood clot is formed to prevent excessive clotting. They also interfere with the Coagulation process if it starts working accidently inside intact blood vessels. To explain more, AT, as its name indicates, inactivates thrombin, and therefore stops the process of Coagulation. PC, which is first activated into activated protein C (APC), tends to breakdown co-factors V and VIII and therefore slows down the Coagulation process. For APC to function normally, PS is involved as a cofactor. Phospholipids and calcium ions also assist in this process. Another inhibitor specific for the Extrinsic pathway, namely Tissue Factor Pathway Inhibitor (TFPI), limits the action of TF in activating factor VII (Kalafatis et al., 1994; Novotny, 1994; Davie, 1995; Esmon et al., 1997; Rosing & Tans, 1997; Cella et al., 1997; Hoffbrand et al., 2001; Escobar et al., 2002; Laffan & Manning, 2002a).

Regarding the control of the Fibrinolysis process, there are many proteins involved. For example, plasminogen activator inhibitors (PAI) prevent tPA from activating plasminogen and therefore stop the initiation of fibrinolysis. This is important to avoid early removal of blood clot before the completion of blood vessel healing. Another anti-fibrinolysis protein is α2-antiplasmin (AP) which is a major inhibitor of plasmin. Thrombin-Activatable Fibrinolysis Inhibitor (TAFI) is a protein that is activated by thrombin to prevent the binding of plasmin to fibrin and therefore stops plasmin from breaking down the clot. The control actions of these fibrinolysis antagonists are illustrated in figure 2 (Hoffbrand et al., 2001; Escobar et al., 2002; Laffan & Manning, 2002a).

For normal healthy clotting/anticlotting results, the Coagulation and Fibrinolysis processes, with their control systems, should work in a highly balanced manner. Any abnormalities may disturb this balance leading to serious consequences. Abnormalities can be quantitative (deficiency or increase in quantity) or qualitative (abnormal structure or function [loss, lowering or gain]) that may affect any of the proteins involved. For example, abnormalities in clotting factors may lead to bleeding problems (termed haemophilia), while abnormalities in the natural anticoagulants may lead to increased clotting tendency (termed hypercoagulability) leading to thrombosis, with certain exceptions in both (figure 3).

In the following sections, different genetic and acquired abnormalities affecting the Coagulation and Fibrinolysis processes are discussed. Only those leading to thrombosis are included in accordance with the scope of this chapter. These abnormalities are usually referred to as "risk factors" since they put forth clinical manifestations in patients suffering from these abnormalities.

3. Genetic risk factors for venous thrombosis

Like all proteins produced in the body, clotting factors and other proteins of the Coagulation and Fibrinolysis processes are encoded by genes in the DNA of human cells. Any genetic abnormalities may lead to lower or no production of these proteins, or the production of molecules with abnormal structure and/or functions, although the quantity of which may be normal. Many of these abnormalities were found to cause venous thrombosis. For example, genetic defects in the genes of the natural anticoagulants may lead to lower

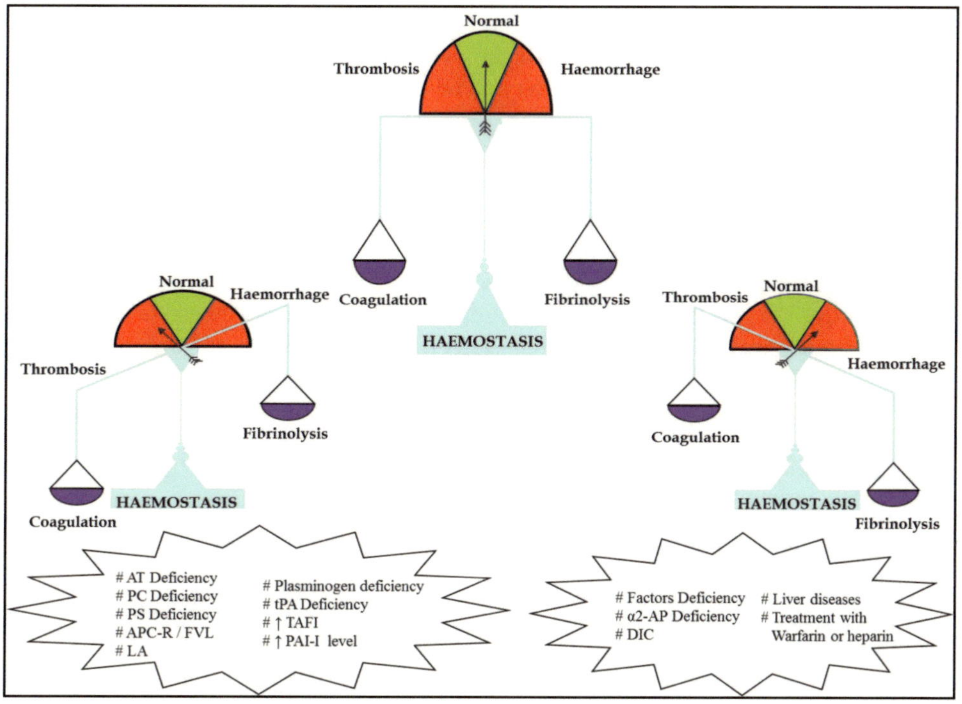

Fig. 3. Balance between the Coagulation and Fibrinolysis processes, in health and disease (prepared and drawn by the author).

production of these proteins and therefore lower control over the Coagulation process. This usually leads to an increase in the rate of coagulation, a phenomenon called "hypercoagulability", which is usually manifested clinically in patients as VTE. On the other hand, the natural anticoagulants may be produced normally, but they can not exert their function normally on their targets, and therefore hypercoagulability and VTE are expected too. Also, certain genetic defect may affect the clotting factors themselves leading to overproduction of such factors causing hypercoagulability. Moreover, abnormalities in the Fibrinolysis process may lower the efficiency of removal of clot, which leads to accumulation of clots and formation of thrombosis. In the following lines, several genetic abnormalities (risk factors) leading to venous thrombosis are discussed. These usually cause VTE at relatively earlier ages (less than 40 years-old) and may be referred to as "familial or hereditary thrombophilia". Although the condition known as "Activated Protein C Resistance" is the most common genetic defect associated with VTE, this defect will be left till the end because it was discovered relatively more recently and it was found to be the most common and important genetic risk factor for VTE.

3.1 Antithrombin (AT) deficiency

Historically, Egeberg (1965) was the first to associate cases of venous thrombosis with a hereditary defect in the Coagulation system; namely AT deficiency. AT is an inhibitor for thrombin, and its inhibition action is largely enhanced by heparin as a co-factor. AT deficiency causes lower control over thrombin, and therefore the Coagulation process becomes overactive (hypercoagulability) leading to VTE. Also, decreased control over

thrombin in cases with AT deficiency may have a positive effect on an inhibitor of fibrinolysis called thrombin-activatable fibrinolysis inhibitor (TAFI), which may add to the hypercoagulable status in these patients, as will be explained later.
Hereditary AT deficiency has been found in 1-5 % of thrombotic cases, with a prevalence of one in 500-5000 in different populations (Tait et al., 1991; Koster et al., 1995a; Koeleman et al., 1997; Bertina, 1997; Laffan & Manning, 2002b; Ehsan & Plumbley, 2002; Dahlbäck, 2008; Patnaik & Moll, 2008). It has an autosomal dominant mode of inheritance, and it accounts for a 10-fold increased risk of developing VTE (Dahlbäck, 2008). AT deficiency maybe divided into two types: Type I (quantitative; lower amount) and Type II (qualitative; abnormal function). Type II AT deficiency is also subdivided into three subtypes based on the kind of abnormality in function it has: affecting inhibition of thrombin, affecting the binding to heparin, or affecting both. More than 80 genetic abnormalities (missense, nonsense, deletions) were reported to cause AT deficiency (Bertina, 1997; Hoffbrand et al., 2001; Ehsan & Plumbley, 2002; Dahlbäck, 2008). More than half of the patients with hereditary AT deficiency have been reported to suffer from VTE at an age less than 40 years (Finazzi et al., 1987; van Boven et al., 1996). No reports are present on cases of homozygous AT deficiency, suggesting it is incompatible with life to have complete absence of AT in the blood (Dahlbäck, 2008).

3.2 Protein C (PC) deficiency

PC and its active form APC inactivate clotting co-factors V and VIII and therefore down-regulates the Coagulation process. Hence, any abnormality in PC may lead to continuous running of co-factors V and VIII causing VTE. Another method by which PC deficiency may cause VTE is through its interaction with the Fibrinolysis process. PC usually inhibits plasminogen activator inhibitor-1 (PAI-1), which is an inhibitor of tissue plasminogen activator (tPA) responsible for the presence of active plasmin (figure 2). Therefore, PC deficiency causes an impaired control over PAI-1, and this interferes with the normal function of the Fibrinolysis process, and hence may lead to accumulation of clots and eventually VTE.
Several cases of VTE were reported to have genetic deficiency of PC, which was first described in 1981 (Griffin et al, 1981). Hereditary PC deficiency has an autosomal dominant mode of inheritance, but many reports also claimed autosomal recessive mode (Mohanty et al., 1995; Ehsan & Plumbley, 2002; Bereczky et al., 2010). Almost 250 different genetic defects have been reported so far to be associated with PC deficiency (Bertina, 1997; D'Ursi et al., 2007; Bereczky et al., 2010). The prevalence of PC deficiency has been reported to be one in 200 to 16,000 normal individuals in different studies (Miletich et al., 1987; Tait et al., 1995; Mohanty et al., 1995; Koster et al., 1995b; Ehsan & Plumbley, 2002). The prevalence in patients with first episode of VTE is 2-5% (Bertina, 1997; Laffan & Manning, 2002b; Dahlbäck, 2008;). Heterozygous carriers of PC deficiency have 50% reduction in PC level, and they have an increased risk of developing thrombosis (Svensson & Dahlbäck, 1994; Hoffbrand et al., 2001). Homozygotes for PC deficiency may suffer from recurrent VTE episodes and from skin necrosis especially when treated with Warfarin, which is a vitamin K antagonist commonly used for treatment of VTE (Heeb et al., 1989; Svensson & Dahlbäck, 1994; Bennett, 1997; Hoffbrand et al., 2001; Dahlbäck, 2008). Infants with homozygous PC deficiency usually have fatal multiple microvascular thrombosis known as neonatal purpura fulminans (Ehsan & Plumbley, 2002; Dahlbäck, 2008). Two types of PC deficiency are present: Type I PC deficiency in which the level and function of PC are abnormal; and type II deficiency in which the level of PC is normal but the function is

defective. Type I is more common and has been found to be present in 1 to 14 % of cases having recurrent thrombosis. Type II is present in 10-15% of PC deficiency cases (Mohanty et al., 1995, Ehsan & Plumbley, 2002; Bereczky et al., 2010).

3.3 Protein S (PS) deficiency

PS acts as a co-factor in the process of inactivation of clotting co-factors V and VIII by APC, enhancing the process by 10-fold (ten Kate & van der Meer, 2008). PS has a very high affinity towards complement 4b binding protein (C4bBP). PS bound to C4bBP becomes inactive, and only free PS is active. Normally, the concentration of PS is more than C4bBP, and therefore only 60% of PS is present in an inactive form bound to C4bBP, while 40% remain as free active PS (Simmonds et al, 1998; Ehsan & Plumbley, 2002; Laffan & Manning, 2002b; Dahlbäck, 2008). First cases with hereditary PS deficiency were reported in 1984 (Comp & Esmon, 1984; Comp et al, 1984). Hereditary PS deficiency is an autosomal dominant disorder that has been associated with a 3- to 11-fold increased risk of venous thrombosis (Svensson and Dahlbäck, 1994; Hoffbrand et al, 2001; Ehsan & Plumbley, 2002; ten Kate & van der Meer, 2008; Bereczky et al., 2010). Similar to PC deficiency, homozygous cases with PS deficiency have tendency towards developing neonatal purpura fulminans and Warfarin-associated skin necrosis (Hoffbrand et al, 2001; Ehsan & Plumbley, 2002). In addition, PS deficiency has been linked to foetal loss (ten Kate & van der Meer, 2008). More than 200 genetic abnormalities in the PS gene were identified to cause PS deficiency, half of which were missense mutations and one-fifth were deletions or insertions (Bertina, 1997; ten Kate & van der Meer, 2008; Bereczky et al., 2010). The prevalence of PS deficiency is 0.03-2% in the general population and 1-13% in patients with VTE (Lane et al., 1996; Bertina, 1997; Seligsohn & Lubetsky, 2001; Dykes et al., 2001; Ehsan & Plumbley, 2002; Beauchamp et al., 2004; ten Kate & van der Meer, 2008; Bereczky et al., 2010). There are three types of hereditary PS deficiency. In Type I, total and free PS levels are lower than normal. Type II PS deficiency is the dysfunctional type of PS deficiency, in which the level of PS remains normal. A third type (Type III) is characterized by a mild deficiency in PS, and this is reflected in lower free PS level (Ehsan & Plumbley, 2002; ten Kate & van der Meer, 2008; Bereczky et al., 2010). Type I and III are the quantitative types of PS deficiency while Type II is the qualitative type. Certain sources refer to Type II as Type IIb and Type III as Type IIa (Ehsan & Plumbley, 2002). The majority of hereditary PS deficiency are Type I while 5-15% of cases are Type II (Bertina, 1997; Bereczky et al., 2010).

3.4 Tissue Factor Pathway Inhibitor (TFPI) deficiency

TFPI is a protease that inhibits TF-VIIa complex in the presence of factor Xa, thereby regulating the Extrinsic pathway of coagulation. Only 10% of TFPI is present as a free active form in the blood while the majority is in combination with lipoproteins. Deficiency in TFPI may lead to a hypercoagulable state and hence VTE (Novotny et al., 1989; Novotny, 1994; Samama et al, 1996; Cella et al, 1997; Ehsan & Plumbley, 2002). TFPI decreased activity was noticed to contribute in developing thrombosis in women using oral contraceptives, and in patients with paroxysmal nocturnal haemoglobinuria (Maroney & Mast; 2008). Experiments on genetically modified mice with TFPI gene disruption showed that they die prematurely in embryonic stage and before birth due to haemorrhagic and intravascular thrombi. Human embryos with TFPI deficiency may suffer a similar problem and this may explain why no cases with TFPI deficiency has been identified so far (Broze, 1998; Chan, 2001; Maroney & Mast; 2008).

3.5 Heparin Cofactor II (HCII) deficiency

HCII was first detected and isolated in the early 80s (Tollefsen & Blank, 1981, Tollefsen et al., 1982). It specifically inhibits thrombin with less affinity than AT and therefore it may be considered as a second line inhibitor of thrombin (Ehsan & Plumbley, 2002). A number of cases with HCII deficiency were reported to have VTE, but many cases remained asymptomatic (Ehsan & Plumbley, 2002; Laffan & Manning, 2002b). More studies are needed on larger number of cases to determine any significant effect of this defect in causing VTE.

3.6 Dysfibrinogenaemia

As explained earlier, the main aim of the Coagulation system is to convert fibrinogen (clotting factor I) into fibrin clot. Fibrinogen is encoded by three genes on chromosome 4 (Acharya & Dimichele, 2008; Miesbach et al., 2010). Genetic abnormalities in the fibrinogen genes may lead to lower or no production of fibrinogen (quantitative defects), causing bleeding problems in patients. On the other hand, other genetic abnormalities may lead to the production of fibrinogen molecules with abnormal structure and/or function (qualitative defects). Such abnormalities may negatively affect the binding of fibrinogen with thrombin, the polymerization of fibrin molecules, or the fibrinolytic inactivation by plasmin. This is the condition known as "Dysfibrinogenaemia", which has an autosomal dominant or recessive mode of inheritance (Dahlbäck, 1995; Koeleman et al, 1997; Ehsan & Plumbley, 2002; Laffan & Manning, 2002b; Acharya & Dimichele; 2008). Dysfibrinogenaemia was first reported in 1965 (Beck et al., 1965). Around 60% of cases show no clinical manifestations, while 20% show bleeding problems and 20% show thrombosis (Ehsan & Plumbley, 2002; Miesbach et al., 2010). There are at least 15 different genetic defects affecting the fibrinogen gene that were associated with Dysfibrinogenaemia (Bertina, 1997; Miesbach et al., 2010;). Still, Dysfibrinogenaemia remains a very rare disorder (1% of VTE cases) and more cases should be studied to fully understand the disease (Manucci, 2000; Acharya & Dimichele; 2008).

3.7 Elevated clotting factors

Several cases with VTE were found to be associated with elevated levels of clotting factors such as VIII, IX, XI, XII, fibrinogen and prothrombin. Elevated prothrombin is mostly associated with a genetic mutation in the prothrombin gene, which will be discussed in the next section. Elevated fibrinogen (hyperfibrinogenaemia) was found to promote faster fibrin formation and increased thrombus fibrin content, density, strength and stability. Hyperfibrinogenaemia was also found to have increased thrombolysis resistance, which explains more the association with VTE (Koster et al., 1995a; Poort et al, 1996; O'Donnell et al., 1997; Meijers et al., 2000; Kamphuisen et al., 2001; de Visser et al., 2001; Bertina et al., 2005; Machlus et al., 2011).

3.8 Prothrombin G20210A mutation

In 1996, Poort et al performed extensive DNA sequencing on the prothrombin gene located on chromosome 11 for patients with unexplained VTE. They discovered a single missense mutation (guanine to adenine; G→A) at nucleotide position 20210 in the 3' untranslated region of the prothrombin gene. Since the mutation is present outside the coding region for prothrombin, it does not affect the structure of the prothrombin molecule. However, the

Prothrombin G20210A mutation was found to be associated with elevated levels of plasma prothrombin (elevation by one-third above normal; 133%), and therefore accounts for hypercoagulability and an increased risk of developing VTE (2 to 4-fold) (Poort et al, 1996; Bertina, 1997; Koeleman et al, 1997; Hillarp et al, 1997; Alhenc-Gelas et al. 1997; Hoffbrand et al., 2001; Ehsan & Plumbley, 2002; Laffan & Manning, 2002b; Dahlbäck, 2008). In fact, it has been demonstrated that prothrombin levels more than 115% have 2-fold increased risk of developing VTE (Poort et al, 1996). A study by Ceelie et al (2004) has proven that Prothrombin G20210A mutation leads to increased mRNA and protein expression. Another point worth mentioning here is that increased prothrombin levels may lead to an increase in the inhibitor of fibrinolysis called TAFI. This increase in TAFI disturbs the Fibrinolysis process and therefore may add to the hypercoagulable status in these patients, as will be explained later (Ehsan & Plumbley, 2002).

Several studies reported the prevalence of Prothrombin G20210A mutation to be 1-4% in healthy populations and 6-8% in patients with VTE. However, that was true when populations of Caucasian origin were studied. The Prothrombin G20210A mutation was very rare or absent in populations of East Asia and Africa, and in native populations of America and Australia (Franco et al., 1998; Dilley et al., 1998; Lin et al., 1998; Isshiki et al., 1998; Ruiz-Argüelles et al., 1999; Angelopoulou et al, 2000; Ghosh et al., 2001; Ruiz-Argüelles, 2001; Bennett et al, 2001; Lee, 2002; El-Karaksy et al, 2004; Eid & Rihani, 2004; Erber et al, 2004; Gibson et al., 2005; Dahlbäck, 2008). This brought speculations that Prothrombin G20210A mutation might have occurred as a single event in a single Caucasian ancestor. This hypothesis was strengthened by a molecular study that estimated the occurrence of the mutation around 24 thousand years ago (Zivelin et al., 2006).

Another mutation in the prothrombin gene was later discovered in 2002 at a neighbour position to the Prothrombin G20210A mutation, namely Prothrombin C20209T mutation. Unlike the Prothrombin G20210A mutation, this newer mutation was found in non-Caucasians in addition to Caucasians (Warshawsky et al, 2002; Arya, 2005; Danckwardt et al, 2006). Still, clear-cut association with VTE has to be established.

3.9 Defects of fibrinolysis

Fibrinolysis is the process responsible for the removal of intravascular clots. Therefore, one may expect that defects in this process can provide an environment suitable for the development of thrombosis. However, there is yet no final or definite proof of that in spite of the fact that reduced fibrinolysis efficacy (hypofibrinolysis) was observed in many patients with VTE with higher risk values (Laffan & Manning, 2002b; Lisman et al., 2005; Meltzer et al., 2008). For example, defects in plasminogen may cause defective fibrinolysis and impaired removal of fibrin clots, and hence might lead to accumulation of thrombi. There are two types of hereditary plasminogen deficiency: Type I hypoplasminogenaemia (quantitative) and Type II dysplasminogenaemia (qualitative), which are caused by many mutations and thought to be inherited as autosomal dominant defects. Hypoplasminogenaemia is associated with abnormal fibrin removal during wound healing, leading to pseudomembrane diseases in the mucous membranes, while dysplasminogenaemia is probably only a silent polymorphism without clinical manifestations (Aoki et al., 1978; Song et al., 2003; Schuster et al., 2007; Mehta & Shapiro, 2008; Klammt et al., 2011). At the same time, hereditary plasminogen deficiency was found in 2-8% of patients with thrombosis (Aoki et al., 1978; Dolan et al., 1988; Heijboer et al., 1990; Brandt, 2002; Song et al., 2003). Thus, more studied maybe needed before definitely

linking plasminogen deficiency with VTE, and establishing Plasminogen Deficiency Registry databases may help to determine the prevalence and risk of this defect.
Another member of the Fibrinolysis process is tissue plasminogen activator (tPA) which is the main activator of plasmin in the Fibrinolysis process. Therefore, tPA deficiency may also lead to thrombosis. However, there is paucity in reports on cases with hereditary tPA deficiency to justify that (Patrassi et al., 1991; Brandt, 2002). The main inhibitor of tPA is the plasminogen activator inhibitor-1 (PAI-1). In this context, one should expect thrombosis to develop in cases having higher levels of PAI-1, rather than PAI-1 deficiency. This has been shown in different human cases and in transgenic mouse models. At least 5 polymorphisms were found in the PAI-1 gene, two of which were associated with thrombosis. In fact, this encouraged trials to use inhibitors of PAI-1 as anti-thrombotic treatments (Carmeliet et al., 1993; Huber, 2001; Wu & Zhao, 2002; Meltzer et al., 2010a; Jankun & Skrzypczak-Jankun, 2011). Trials were also conducted on inhibitors of another regulator of the Fibrinolysis process, namely Thrombin-Activatable Fibrinolysis Inhibitor (TAFI). TAFI, which was discovered in 1988, circulates as an inactive form, and is activated into its active form (TAFIa) by thrombin. TAFIa inhibits binding of plasmin to fibrinogen and therefore down-regulates the Fibrinolysis process. AT deficiency, previously described, causes elevated levels of thrombin, and therefore elevated levels of TAFIa are also expected leading to lowering in the efficiency of fibrinolysis in removing clots. This is thought to be another pathophysiological pathway by which AT deficiency causes VTE. In addition, this may be an additive factor in increasing hypercoagulability in cases with Prothrombin G20210A mutation in which there is an elevated level of plasma prothrombin. However, studies on association between TAFI level and VTE gave inconsistent results. At least three genetic variations in the TAFI gene were identified, but linkage with risk of developing VTE is not very evident. Focus is now on developing inhibitors of TAFI as a possible anticoagulant therapy (Mosnier & Bouma, 2006; Bunnage & Owen, 2008; Meltzer et al., 2010a & b; Miljić et al., 2010).

3.10 Activated Protein C Resistance (APC-R) and Factor V Leiden Mutation (FVL)

In 1993, Dahlbäck and his colleagues in Sweden were involved in studying patients with VTE. They added external APC to plasma of patients with VTE and recorded the effect of that on the Coagulation process. As explained earlier, APC inactivates co-factors V and VIII and therefore down-regulates the Coagulation process. Therefore, the addition of external APC should prolong the clotting time of the plasma under test. When they tried that on the plasma samples of VTE patients, they noticed that the expected prolongation effect did not happen in all cases (Figure 4). They discussed that there is a "resistance" to the action of APC, and therefore they called it "APC resistance or APC-R", a name which persisted until now. The team originally though that there must have been a yet unknown clotting co-factor that co-helps APC in inactivating factors V and VIII, and these patients showing APC-R should have had a deficiency in this yet-to-find co-factor. However, they could not find such a proposed co-factor. One year later, Bertina and his research team in the Netherlands could identify a missense point mutation in the factor V gene (guanine to adenine; G→A) at nucleotide number 1691 of exon 10 of the factor V gene, only eleven nucleotides upstream to intron 10. This new mutation was termed Factor V Leiden mutation (FVL) after the Dutch city where they made their discovery in. This nucleotide change causes a change in the translated factor V molecule at amino acid residue number 506 (arginine to glutamine; CGA→CAA). Arginine 506 is an important cleavage site for APC. In other words, APC has to recognise arginine at position 506 of the factor V molecule in order to be able to inactivate factor V. This change in amino acid residue at position 506 of the mutant FVL molecule makes the FVL molecule "resistant" to the action of APC, and therefore the mutant FVL remains active. Mutant FVL was found to retain its coagulation function, and therefore the Coagulation process is not down-regulated by APC in regards to factor V. This explains why FVL leads to hypercoagulability and henceforth VTE (figure 5). Since then, the terms APC-R and FVL were linked together and used interchangeably. Several studies quickly followed that discovery and proved a positive association between FVL and VTE, showing that heterozygous carriers of the mutation are at higher risk of developing VTE by 10-fold while homozygous carriers have a much higher risk ratio reaching 140-fold (Dahlbäck et al., 1993; Zöller et al., 1994; Bertina et al., 1994; Hoagland et al., 1996; Dahlbäck, 1997; Faioni et al., 1997; Alderborn et al., 1997; Bontempo et al., 1997). Moreover, most homozygous cases were found to get at least one VTE event in their life time, and at an earlier time of their life (Samama et al., 1996; Florell & Rodgers, 1997).

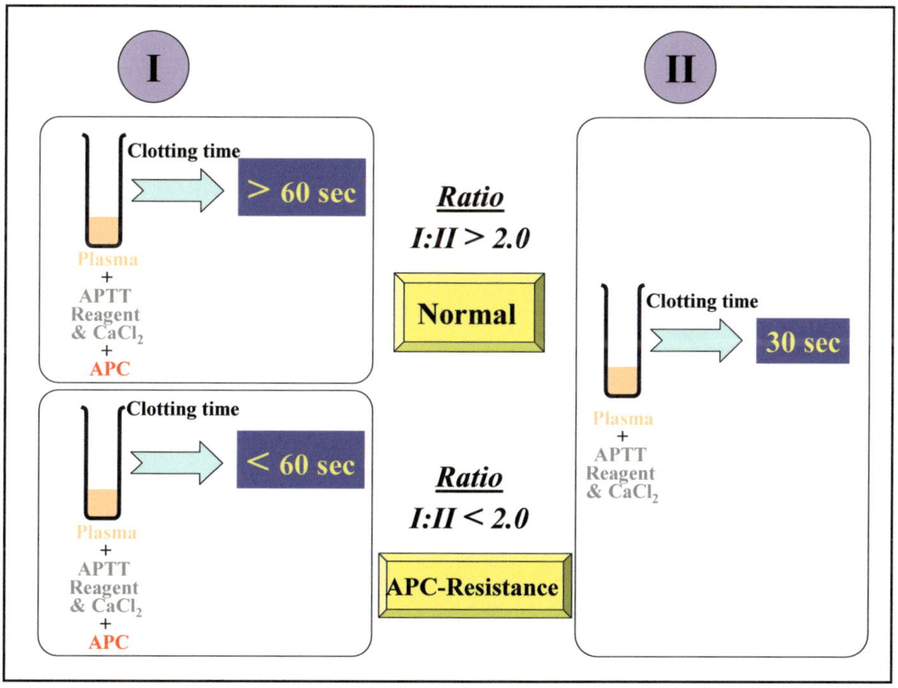

Fig. 4. APC-R test as developed originally by Dahlbäck et al., 1993 (prepared and drawn by the author).

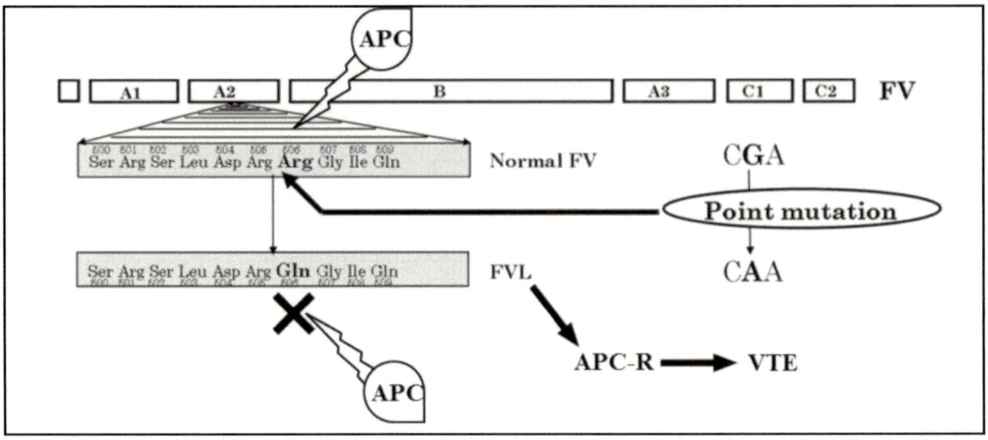

Fig. 5. Factor V molecule showing the site of amino acid 506 where FVL is present and how this leads to APC-R and VTE (prepared and drawn by the author).

The identification of APC-R/FVL and its high risk value have exploded a massive rush in researches to study this new disease, its prevalence and its relationship with VTE in almost every part of the world. First researches were conducted in Europe which concentrated on Caucasian populations. Results showed that FVL was present in a quite high percentage of patients with VTE (15-65%) and healthy subjects (1-15%). Other studies on Caucasians living in non-European countries, like the USA, Australia and Israel, revealed similar numbers (table 1). However, when studies started to appear in other ethnic groups and in other countries, FVL was astonishingly found to be very rare and in most occasions absent, like in Africans, South-East Asians, Chinese, Japanese, American Indians (native nations of America), Greenland Inuit (Eskimos) and native populations of Australia (table 2 and figure 6).

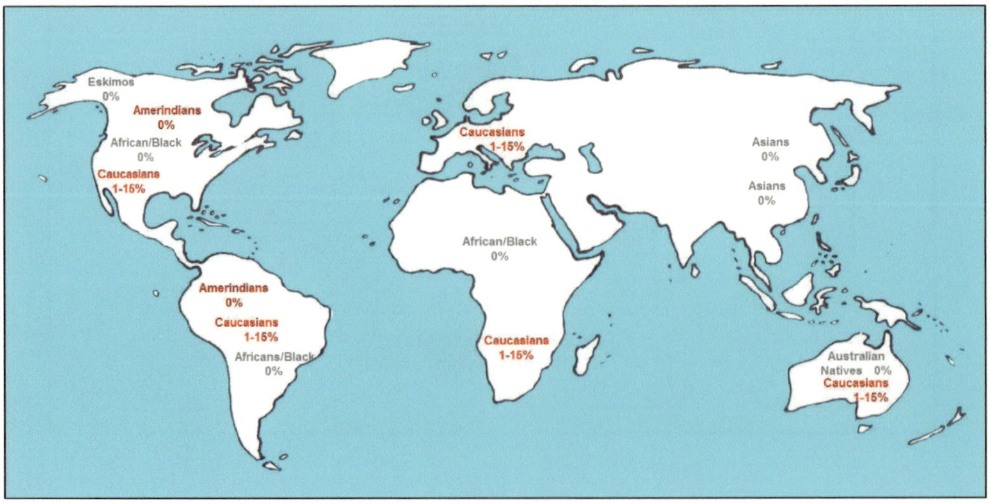

Fig. 6. Prevalence of FVL worldwide in different ethnic groups (prepared and drawn by the author).

	Country	VTE patients (%)	Normal Population (%)	References
European	UK	----	1.74-5.6	Beauchamp et al., 1994; Bengtsson et al., 1996
	Sweden	41.5-50	7.5-11.4	Zöller et al., 1994; Bengtsson et al., 1996; Alderborn et al., 1997
	Poland	----	5	Herrmann et al, 1997
	Netherlands	21	2	Bertina et al., 1994; Beauchamp et al., 1994
	Germany	30	7.1-12	Aschka et al, 1996; Schröder et al., 1996
	Belgium	22	3.3	Hainaut et al., 1997
	Slovakia	29.5-37.0	4	Hudecek et al., 2003; Simkova et al., 2004
	Austria	26	----	Melichart et al., 1996
	Hungary	44	6.9	Nagy et al., 1997; Stankovics et al., 1998
	Serbia	29.9	5.8	Djordjevic et al., 2004
	Azerbaijan	----	14	Gurgey & Mesci, 1997
	Spain	9.2-26.3	1.6-5.8	Olave et al., 1998; González Ordóñez et al., 1999; Vargas et al., 1999; Aznar et al., 2000; Ricart et al., 2006; García-Hernández et al., 2007
	France	9-18	3.5-5.0	Leroyer et al., 1997; Mansourati et al., 2000; Meyer et al., 2001; Mazoyer et al., 2009
	French/ Spanish Basques	----	0-0.7	Bauder et al., 1997; Zabalegui et al., 1998
	Italy	9.0-42.8	2-13.1	Faioni et al., 1997; Simioni et al., 1997; Martinelli et al., 2004; Sottilotta et al., 2009; Gessoni et al., 2010
	Yugoslavia	15.5	4.0	Mikovic et al., 2000
	Slovenia	12.9	6.3	Bedencic et al., 2008
	Croatia	21.0-28.2	2.4-4.0	Coen et al., 2001; Cikes et al., 2004; Jukic et al., 2009
	Albania/ Kosovo	----	3.4	Mekaj et al., 2009
	Greece	16.2-31.9	2.5-7.0	Rees et al., 1995; Lambropoulos et al., 1997; Antoniadi et al., 1999; Ioannou et al., 2000; Hatzaki et al., 2003
Non-European	USA	8.6	3.2-6.0	Ridker et al., 1997; Bontempo et al., 1997; Limdi et al., 2006
	Australia	----	4-10.2	Aboud & Ma, 1997; Bennett et al., 2001; Gibson et al., 2005;
	Israel	----	4.3	Rosen et al., 1999
	Brazil	20	2	Arruda et al., 1995

Table 1. Prevalence of FVL in Caucasian patients with VTE and healthy populations living in European and non-European countries.

	Country/ Ethnic groups	VTE patients (%)	Normal Population (%)	References
Asians	Japan	0	0	Fujimura et al., 1995; Zama et al., 1996; Kodaira et al., 1997; Ro et al., 1999
	Korea	0	----	Kim et al., 1998
	China	0	0	Pepe et al., 1997; Ho et al., 1999
	Indonesia	----	0	Pepe et al., 1997
	Malaysia	0.5	----	Lim et al., 1999
	Singapore	5	----	Lim et al., 1999; Lee, 2002
	India	3	1.3	Herrmann et al., 1997; Ghosh et al., 2001; Mishra & Bedi, 2010
	Pakistan	1.25	----	Nasiruddin et al., 2005
	USA	----	0	Gregg et al., 1997
Africans/ Black	Ethiopia	----	0	Pepe et al., 1997; Abdulkadir et al., 1997
	USA	1.4	0.9	Gregg et al., 1997; Limdi et al., 2006
	Sub-Sahara	----	0	Pepe et al., 1997
	Ecuador	----	0	Pepe et al., 1997
	Venezuela	----	4.4	Vizcaino et al., 2000
Amerindians	Ecuador	----	0	Pepe et al., 1997
	Venezuela	----	1.25	Vizcaino et al., 2000
	USA	----	0	Gregg et al., 1997
Eskimos	Greenland	----	0	De Maat et al., 1996
Indigenous Australians	Australia	----	0	Bennett et al., 2001; Erber et al., 2004

Table 2. Prevalence of FVL in non-Caucasian patients with VTE and healthy populations in different parts of the world.

Finding FVL to be mostly confined to Caucasian populations have brought speculations that FVL might have occurred as a single event in one European Caucasian ancestor, and the current carriers of the mutation descended from that ancestor. To prove a single origin of FVL, several molecular studies were conducted on different single nucleotides polymorphisms (SNPs) in the factor V gene trying to identify any association of FVL with such SNPs. At least 9 SNPs were found to be always associated with FVL. These studies included carriers and non-carriers of FVL, as well factor V gene in chimpanzees to elucidate when FVL might have first appeared (figure 7). These studies, combined with the distribution of FVL worldwide and the anthropological knowledge on movement of Mankind in the far past suggested that FVL should have occurred after the separation between Caucasoid (who settled in Europe) and Mongoloid (who moved to East Asia) populations, which is estimated to occur around 32,000 years ago (figure 8). This means that FVL is less than 32 thousand years old and this is why it is present in Caucasians only. The next question is: where in Europe has it happened? Since 1997 Castoldi et al suggested that FVL probably occurred outside Europe. It was observed that FVL was very rare in the

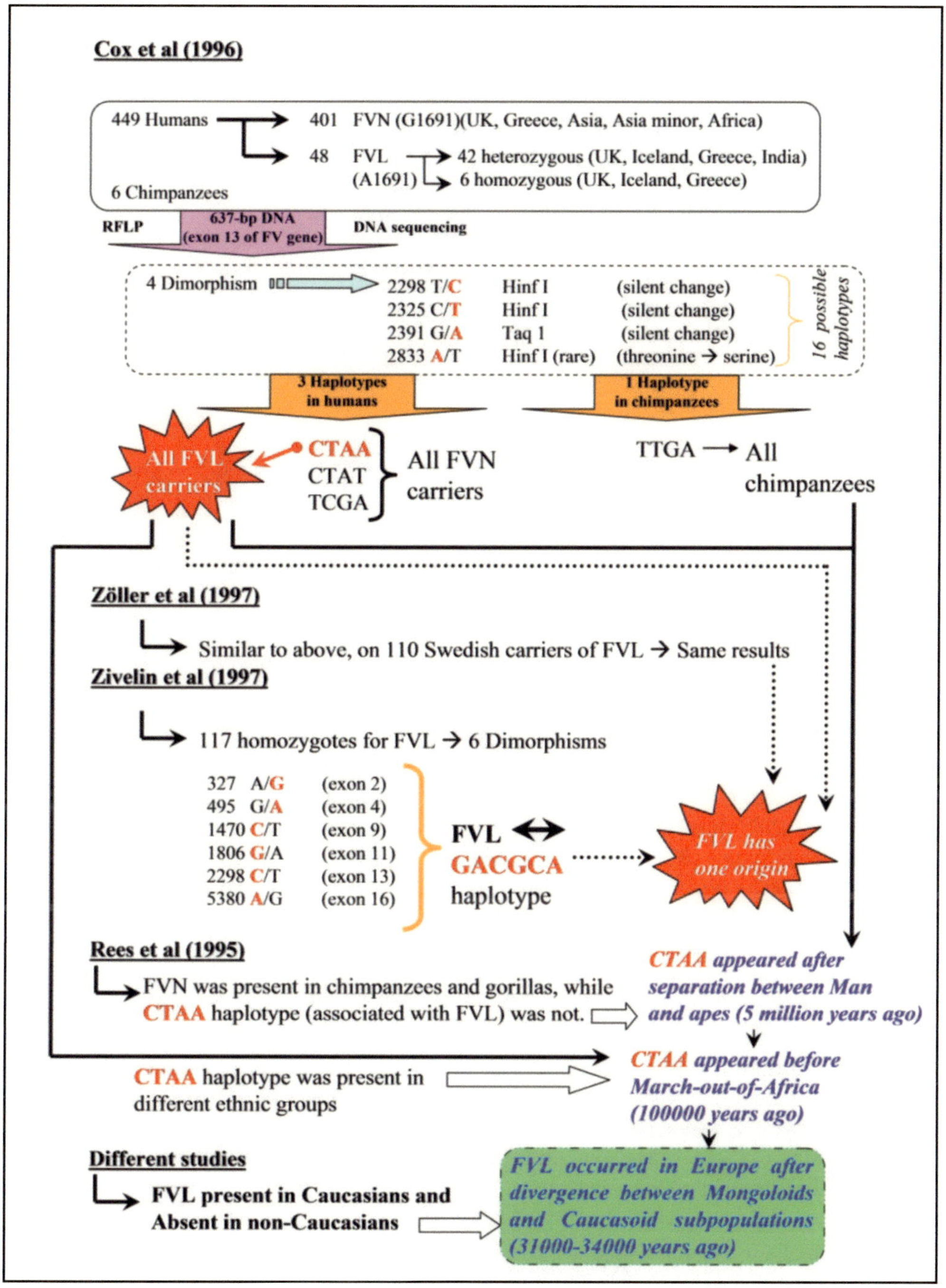

Fig. 7. Molecular studies exploring the origin of FVL (prepared and drawn by the author).

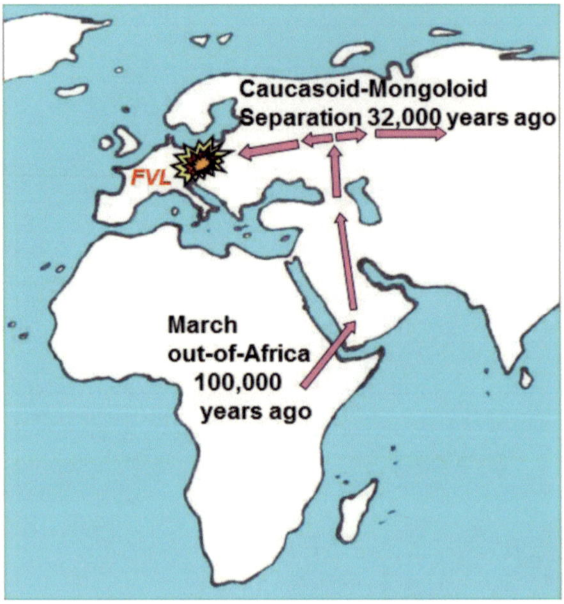

Fig. 8. Map showing movement of humans in the far past from Africa to the Middle East (March out-of-Africa), then to Europe and Asia. FVL event is thought to occur earlier than 32,000 years ago after the divergence of Caucasoid and Mongoloid populations (prepared and drawn by the author).

French and Spanish Basque populations, who are thought to be the oldest ethnic groups in Europe. This suggested FVL to occur outside Europe first (Bauder et al., 1997; Zabalegui et al., 1998). The prevalence of FVL in Eastern Mediterranean countries have shown the highest numbers in the world (table 3), bringing speculations that FVL might have occurred somewhere there and then spread to Europe (Castoldi et al., 1997; Bauder et al., 1997; Zabalegui et al., 1998; Irani-Hakime et al., 2000; Taher et al., 2001; Lucotte & Mercier et al., 2001, Dashti & Jadaon, 2011). Lucotte & Mercier (2001) proposed that FVL expanded in Europe during the Neolithic period, from a probable Anatolian center of origin in Turkey, which has occurred around 10,000 years ago. This may explain the highest prevalence of FVL in East Mediterranean countries, with noticeable gradual decrease in prevalence when radiating away from this region towards Europe and other parts of the world (Figure 9). Our research team in Kuwait has found that Arabs from Eastern Mediterranean countries who carry FVL also carried the same SNPs found to be associated with FVL in European carriers of the mutation (Jadaon et al., 2011). This gives another confirmation that FVL had most probably occurred as a single event in the past in the Eastern Mediterranean region.

The large number of cases having FVL in our days suggests that FVL should have an evolutionary survival advantage explaining its persistence until now. For example, Man had faced many challenges since long time in the past, like fighting wild animals, diseases or each other which should have caused a lot of injuries and fatal bleeding incidences. Increased clotting tendency due to FVL might have an advantageous effect in such occasions giving carriers of FVL some privilege. Women with FVL have higher clotting tendency which may be advantageous in preventing fatal blood loss during menstruation and childbirth. Less blood loss also improves the haemoglobin level in these women creating better life expectancy (Lindqvist et al., 2001; Lindqvist & Dahlbäck, 2008; Franchini & Lippi, 2011). This is also true in cases having both FVL and haemophilia, in which increased clotting due to FVL compensates for the bleeding tendency due to haemophilia, and hence better survival chances (Yan & Nelson, 2004; Franchini & Lippi, 2010). In addition, recent studies showed that FVL decreased risk of developing severe sepsis from infections to some extent, again another privilege to think of. That was also proved in animal models (Kerlin et al., 2003).

	Country/ Ethnic groups	VTE patients (%)	Normal Population (%)	References
East Mediterranean	Lebanon	9.9-70.6	13.6-18.7	Irani-Hakime et al., 2000; Irani-Hakime et al., 2001; Taher et al., 2001; Tamim et al., 2002; Finan et al., 2002; Almawi et al., 2005; Bouaziz-Borgi et al., 2006; Isma'eel et al., 2006a &b; Zahed et al., 2006
	Syria	----	13.6	Irani-Hakime et al., 2000; Dashti et al., 2010
	Palestine (inside & outside Israel)	----	11.7-27.2	Rosen et al., 1999; Dashti et al., 2010; Hussein et al., 2010
	Jordan	23.9-25.7	10.5-27.2	Awidi et al., 1999; Eid & Rihani, 2004; Eid & Shubeilat, 2005; Nusier et al., 2007; Obeidat et al., 2009; Al-Sweedan et al., 2009; Dashti et al., 2010
	Cyprus	----	13.4	Angelopoulou et al., 2000
	Turkey	21-30.8	4.6-9.8	Ozbek & Tangün, 1996; Gurgey & Mesci, 1997; Gurgey et al., 2001; Atasay et al., 2003; Irdem et al., 2005; Kalkanli et al., 2006; Kabukcu et al., 2007; Celiker et al., 2009; Oguzulgen et al., 2009; Diz-Kucukkaya et al., 2010

Table 3. Prevalence of FVL in patients with VTE and normal populations in different East Mediterranean countries.

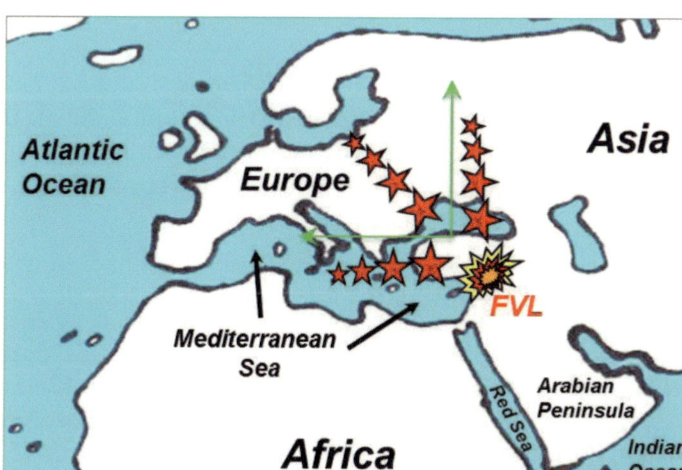

Fig. 9. Map of the Mediterranean area showing decrease in prevalence of FVL as moving from East Mediterranean to North and West Europe. This made many believe that the origin of FVL is somewhere in the Eastern Mediterranean region (prepared and drawn by the author).

Other mutations in the factor V gene were later identified, including Factor V Cambridge (Arg306Thr) (Williamson et al., 1998), Factor V Hong Kong (Arg306Gly) (Chan et al., 1998), Factor V Liverpool (Ile359Thr) (Mumford et al, 2003), and Factor V Kuwait (His1254Arg) (Jadaon et al., 2006). The number of cases reported to have these mutations were small and the relationship with VTE could not be well established like FVL, although many of these cases were reported in patients with VTE. Another mutation in the factor V gene called HR2 Haplotype (His1299Arg) was identified in 1996, which is discussed separately in the following section.

3.11 HR2 haplotype

In 1996, a new missense mutation in exon 13 of factor V gene (A4070G) was identified (Lunghi et al., 1996). This mutation leads to an amino acid change, replacing histidine with arginine at amino acid residue position 1299 (His1299Arg). The new mutation was first assigned the name R2 polymorphism because of the use of the restriction enzyme Rsa I in the test used to detect it. Later on, R2 polymorphism was found to be in tight association with at least 12 polymorphisms in the factor V gene. Therefore, these SNPs were collectively called HR2 (Haplotype R2) (Bernardi et al., 1997; Castoldi et al., 2000). Several studies in different parts of the world gave the prevalence of HR2 to be 9.5%-15.2% in VTE cases and 5.8%-10.4% in healthy controls, with an increased risk by at least 2.5-fold (Bernardi et al., 1997; Alhenc-Gelas et al., 1999; Castoldi et al., 2000; Pecheniuk et al., 2001; Margaglione et al., 2002; Castaman et al., 2003; Faioni et al., 2004; Jadaon & Dashti, 2005a). The exact mechanism by which HR2 haplotype increases the risk for development of VTE is still not that clear. However, Castoldi et al (2000) have studied the two isoforms of factor V, V1 and V2, in cases with or without HR2. V1 is 7-fold more thrombogenic than V2. They showed that V1 was present in cases with HR2 more than in cases without the haplotype. This may give a possible explanation for the hypercoagulation and increased risk of developing VTE in carriers of HR2. However, more studies may be needed before understanding the real mechanism involved in that.

4. Acquired risk factors for venous thrombosis

VTE due to genetic risk factors (familial or hereditary thrombophilia), discussed above, mostly occur at ages less than 40 years, and they often recurrent. However, there are several acquired risk factors that are usually associated with VTE at above 40 years of age (Florell & Rodgers, 1997).

4.1 Lupus Anticoagulants (LA)

LA is a member of a group of autoantibodies (immunoglobulins) against phospholipids, including anticardiolipin and anti-β_2-glycoprotein, which are produced in different autoimmune conditions. They often cause clinical manifestations like thrombosis, pregnancy loss and others, and the clinical condition is termed Antiphospholipid Syndrome (Hoffbrand et al., 2001; Laffan & Manning, 2002b; Ehsan & Plumbley, 2002). LA were given this name in 1972 because they were recognized initially in a patient with systemic lupus erythematosus (SLE) who had bleeding problems. However, later studies confirmed the association of LA with VTE, and not bleeding, but the name persisted (Greaves & Preston, 1991; Bengtsson et al, 1996; Ehsan & Plumbley, 2002). Although the mechanism of causing

VTE is still not clear, the involvement of phospholipids in the Coagulation process and its regulators may give a possible explanation. In fact, there are *in vitro* evidences that LA lead to inhibition of APC, AT and fibrinolysis, and increase in expression of TF. In addition, LA were shown to directly contribute to hypercoagulability in animal models (Roubey, 1994; Kinev & Roubey, 2008; Farmer-Boatwright & Roubey, 2009). The prevalence of LA was reported to be up to 20% of VTE cases, with up to 10-fold increased risk of developing VTE (Ghosh et al., 2001; Galli et al., 2002; Ehsan & Plumbley, 2002; Jadaon & Dashti, 2005b; Farmer-Boatwright & Roubey, 2009; Anderson & Weitz, 2010).

4.2 Pregnancy, childbirth and hormone therapy

Pregnancy and delivery (and post-delivery up to 6 weeks after childbirth) account for more than 6-fold increased risk of developing VTE. This may be due to changes in the Coagulation and Fibrinolysis processes happening during these events, which include increased levels of most clotting factors and their activators, with reduced fibrinolysis and PS level. Women taking oral contraceptives or receiving hormone replacement therapy were also found to have higher risk of developing VTE, which may again be attributed to increased clotting factors and decreased AT and tPA (Rosing et al., 1997; Hoffbrand et al., 2001; Ehsan & Plumbley, 2002; Chan, 2010; Anderson & Weitz, 2010).

4.3 Other acquired risk factors

VTE are common complications of major trauma like in surgery, fractures and blood transfusion, especially in elder and obese patients. VTE was also noticed to be secondary to other diseases like liver and kidney diseases, myeloproliferative disorders, disseminated intravascular coagulation (DIC), thrombotic thrombocytopenic purpura (TTP) and haemolytic uraemic syndrome (HUS) (Hoffbrand et al., 2001; Ehsan & Plumbley, 2002). Furthermore, patients with cancers of the gastrointestinal and urogenital tracts and the lungs were reported to have higher risk of VTE. This may be due to activation of clotting factors by the cancerous cells themselves or the chemotherapy these patients usually receive which affects the liver and vitamin K metabolism, or predisposes to DIC (Dahlbäck, 1995; Florell & Rodgers, 1997; Hoffbrand et al., 2001; Ehsan & Plumbley, 2002; Anderson & Weitz, 2010; Vossen et al., 2011). Therefore, such diseases affect the Coagulation and Fibrinolysis processes in favour of developing VTE. Also, VTE in such diseases, especially those involving chronic inflammation, maybe due to increased C4bBP which captures more PS and lowers the availability of the active free PS and therefore may cause hypercoagulation. VTE was also present in many cases challenged with prolonged immobilization like being confined to bed due to major illnesses or post-operation, or after long airplane journey. The latter attracted a lot of public attention and was referred to in the media as "traveller's thrombosis" or "economy-class syndrome" (Hoffbrand et al., 2001; O'Keeffe & Baglin, 2003; DeHart, 2003; Bhatia et al., 2009).

5. Combined genetic and acquired risk factors for VTE

All genetic and acquired risk factors discussed above are usually present as a "single" defect in a patient. However, many cases with VTE were reported to have more than one genetic/acquired risk factor at the same time, which may account for a higher risk of developing VTE (Jadaon & Dashti, 2005a & b). For example, several studies reported a number of individuals who had FVL in addition to other accompanying genetic defect(s) like hereditary AT, PC or PS deficiency. Both FV and AT genes are located on chromosome 1. As a result, a segregated inheritance pattern of APC-R and AT deficiency can persist in families for several generations (Ireland et al, 1995; Koeleman et al, 1997). In fact, van Boven et al (1996) found that the incidence of VTE in individuals having both FVL and AT deficiency was significantly higher than the incidence in individuals having only one of these two genetic defects. Similarly, coexistence of FVL and PC deficiency has 3 to 7-fold more risk of VTE than either of the two defects alone (Hallam et al, 1995; Zama et al, 1996; Koeleman et al, 1997, Jadaon & Dashti, 2005b). Moreover, more than half of patients with both APC-R and genetic PS deficiency were found to have thrombosis (Garcia de Frutos & Dahlbäck, 1995; Koeleman et al, 1997). It is interesting to mention here that a few isolated cases were reported to be double heterozygous for FVL and factor V deficiency, the mutations being present on opposite chromosomes. Plasma of such patients contain mutant FVL molecules only, similar to what is present in the plasma of people homozygous for the FVL mutation, resulting in what is called "Pseudohomozygous APC-R". Such cases have similar risk value to develop VTE as homozygous APC-R/FVL cases (Greengard et al, 1995; Simioni et al, 1996; Guasch et al, 1997).

Acquired risk factors, including trauma, surgery, immobilization, pregnancy, use of oral contraceptives and LA have been reported to greatly increase the risk of developing VTE in individuals who have FVL. This may explain why in women who have FVL mutation there is an increased incidence of VTE during pregnancy especially in the last trimester and during delivery (Samama et al, 1996; Florell & Rodgers, 1997; Perry & Pasi, 1997; Rotmensch et al, 1997; Hallak et al, 1997). Further, women who are heterozygous for the FVL and take oral contraceptives are at 34-fold increased risk for developing VTE (Melichart et al, 1996; Rosing et al., 1997). LA present in a patient's plasma may create a status similar to APC-R (acquired APC-R). FVL was found in more than half of the LA positive patients who had one thrombotic event, and in more than 90% of the LA positive patients who had recurrent thrombosis (Griffin et al, 1995; Bengtsson et al, 1996; Alarcon-Segovia et al, 1996).

Generally, there is a perception that familial thrombosis may be better considered as a complex genetic disorder caused by segregation of two (or more) genetic defects (known or yet unknown) in a family. Moreover, combination of these genetic defects with other acquired or circumstantial risk factors (like pregnancy, surgery, immobilization, etc.) or disorders (like LA) may greatly increase the risk for development of thrombosis in this group of patients. For example, it has been perceived that APC-R/FVL alone may be only a mild risk factor for developing VTE, especially when it is in heterozygous state. This may be partially explained by the fact that only FVL resists inactivation by APC, but the inactivation function of APC on FVIII is not affected by the FVL mutation. Thus, additional genetic or acquired factors may significantly enhance the risk of developing VTE in patients with FVL. The same may be said about the other genetic/acquired risk factors for VTE.

6. Conclusions

VTE are serious disorders with high morbidity and mortality rates. Several different genetic abnormalities were found to cause VTE, with different prevalence and risk ratios in different populations and ethnic groups. Also, several acquired risk factors were found to cause VTE by different methods. Combination of more than one risk factor (genetic or acquired) in the same patient is not uncommon and it leads to higher risk of developing VTE.

7. References

Abdulkadir, J.; Feleke, Y.; Berg, JP.; Falch, JA. & Odegaard, OR. (1997). Absence of the factor V Leiden mutation in Ethiopians. *Thrombosis Research,* Vol.86, No.5, (June 1997), pp. 431-432, ISSN 0049-3848

Aboud, MR. & Ma, DD. (1997). A comparrision between two activated protein C resistance methods as routine diagnostic tests for factor V Leiden mutation. *British Journal of Haematology,*Vol.97, No.4, (June 1997), pp. 798-803, ISSN 0007-1048

Acharya, SS. & Dimichele, DM. (2008). Rare inherited disorders of fibrinogen. *Haemophilia,* Vol.14, No.6, (November 2008), pp. 1151-1158, ISSN 1351-8216

Alarcon-Segovia, D.; Ruiz-Arguelles, GJ.; Garces-Eisele, J. & Ruiz-Arguelles, A. (1996). Inherited acitvated protein C resistance in a patient with familial primary antiphospholipid syndrome. *Journal of Rheumatology,* Vol.23, No.12, (December 1996), pp. 2162-2165, ISSN 1499-2752

Alderborn, A.; Siegbahn, A. & Wadelius, C. (1997). Venous thrombosis: factor V G1691A genetypeing related to APC resistance measured by 2 methods. *European Journal of Haematology,* Vol.58, No.4, (April 1997), pp. 229-232, ISSN 0902-4441

Alhenc-Gelas, M.; Le Cam-Duchez, V.; Emmerich, J.; Frebourg, T.; Fiessinger, JN.; Barg, JY. & Aiach, M. (1997). The A20210 allele of the prothrombin gene is not frequently associated with the factor V Arg506 to Gln mutation in thrombophilic families. *Blood,* Vo.96, No.4, (August 1997), pp. 1711, ISSN 0006-4971

Alhenc-Gelas, M.; Nicaud, V.; Gandrille, S.; van Dreden, P.; Amiral, J.; Aubry, ML.; Fiessinger, JN.; Emmerich, J. & Aiach, M. (1999). The factor V gene A4070G mutation and the risk of venous thrombosis. *Thrombosis and Haemostasis,*Vol.81, No.2, (February 1999), pp. 193–719, ISSN 0340-6245

Almawi, WY.; Keleshian, SH.; Borgi, L.; Fawaz, NA.; Abboud, N.; Mtiraoui, N. & Mahjoub, T. (2005). Varied prevalence of factor V G1691A (Leiden) and prothrombin G20210A single nucleotide polymorphisms among Arabs. *Journal of Thrombosis and Thrombolysis,* Vol. 20, Vol.3, (December 2005), pp. 163-168, ISSN 0929-5305

Al-Sweedan, SA.; Jaradat, S.; Iraqi, M. & Beshtawi, M. (2009). The prevalence of factor V Leiden (G1691A), prothrombin G20210A and methylenetetrahydrofolate reductase C677T mutations in Jordanian patients with beta-thalassemia major. *Blood Coagulation and Fibrinolysis,* Vol.20, No.8, (December 2009), pp. 675-678, ISSN 0957-5235

Anderson, JA. & Weitz, JI. (2010). Hypercoagulable states. *Clinics in Chest Medicine,*Vol.31, No.4, (December 2010), pp. 659-673, ISSN 0272-5231

Angelopoulou, K.; Nicolaides, A. & Constantinou Deltas, C. (2000). Prevalence of genetic mutations that predispose to thrombophilia in a Greek Cypriot population. *Clinical and Applied Thrombosis/Hemostasis,*Vol.6, No.2, (April 2000), pp. 104-107, ISSN 1076-0296

Antoniadi, T.; Hatzis, T.; Kroupis, C.; Economou-Petersen, E. & Petersen, MB. (1999). Prevalence of factor V Leiden, prothrombin G20210A, and MTHFR C677T mutations in a Greek population of blood donors. *American Journal of Hematology,* Vol.61, No.4, (August 1999), pp. 265-267, ISSN 1096-8652

Aoki, N.; Moroi, M.; Sakata, Y.; Yoshida, N. & Matsuda, M. (1978). Abnormal plasminogen. A hereditary molecular abnormality found in a patient with recurrent thrombosis.

Journal of Clinical Investigation, Vol.61, No.5, (May 1978), pp. 1186-1195, ISSN 0021-9738

Arruda, VR.; Annichino-Bizzacchi, JM.; Costa FF. & Reitsma, PH. (1995). Factor V Leiden (FVQ 506) is common in a Brazilian population. *American Journal of Hematology,*Vol.49, No.3, (July 1995), pp. 242-243, ISSN 1096-8652

Arya, R. (2005). Detection of prothrombin gene polymorphism at position 20209 (PT20209C/T): pilot study in a black population in the United Kingdom. *Thrombosis and Haemostasis,* Vol.93, No.1, (January 2005), pp. 179-180, ISSN 0340-6245

Aschka, I.; Aumann, V.; Bergmann, F.; Budde, U.; Ebert, W.; Eckhof-Donovan, S.; Krey, S.; Nowak-Gottl, U.; Schobess, R.; Sutor, AH.; Wendisch, J. & Schneppenheim, R. (1996). Prevalence of factor V Leiden in children with thrombo-embolism. *European Journal of Pediatrics,*Vol.155, No.12, (December 1996), pp. 1009-1014, ISSN 0340-6199

Atasay, B.; Arsan, S.; Günlemez, A.; Kemahli, S. & Akar, N. (2003). Factor V Leiden and prothrombin gene 20210A variant in neonatal thromboembolism and in healthy neonates and adults: a study in a single center. *Pediatric Hematology and Oncology,* Vol.20, No.8, (December 2003), pp. 627-634, ISSN 0888-0018

Awidi, A.; Shannak, M.; Bseiso, A.; Kailani, MAM.; Kailani, MA.; Omar, N.; Anshasi, B. & Sakarneh, N. (1999). High Prevalence of Factor V Leiden in Healthy Jordanian Arabs. *Thrombosis and Haemostasis,*Vol.41, No.4, (April 1999), pp. 582-584, ISSN 0340-6245

Aznar, J; Vayá, A.; Estellés, A.; Mira, Y.; Seguí, R.; Villa, P.; Ferrando, F.; Falcó, C.; Corella, D. & España, F. (2000). Risk of venous thrombosis in carriers of the prothrombin G20210A variant and factor V Leiden and their interaction with oral contraceptives. *Haematologica,*Vol.85, No.12, (December 2000), pp. 1271-1276, ISSN 0390-6078

Bauder, F.; Ducout, L.; Guerre, C. & Freyburger, G. (1997). Activated protein C (APC) resistance: does it exist in Basques? *British Journal of Haematology,*Vol.99, No.3, (December 1997), pp. 712-713, ISSN 0007-1048

Beauchamp, NJ.; Daly, ME.; Hampton, KK.; Cooper, PC.; Preston, FE. & Peake, IR. (1994). High prevalence of a mutation in the factor V gene within the U.K. population: relationship to activated protein C resistance and familial thrombosis. *British Journal of Haematology,* Vol.88, No.1, (September 1994), pp. 219-222, ISSN 0007-1048

Beauchamp, NJ.; Dykes, AC.; Parikh, N.; Campbell Tait, R. & Daly, ME. (2004). The prevalence of, and molecular defects underlying, inherited protein S deficiency in the general population. *British Journal of Haematology,* Vol.125, No.5, (June 2004), pp. 647–654, ISSN 0007-1048

Beck, EA.; Charache, P. & Jackson, DP. (1965). A new inherited coagulation disorder caused by abnormal fibrinogen (fibrinogen Baltimore). *Nature,* Vol.208, No.5006, (October 1965), pp. 143–145, ISSN 0028-0836

Bedencic, M.; Bozic, M.; Peternel, P. & Stegnar, M. (2008), Major and potential prothrombotic genotypes in patients with venous thrombosis and in healthy subjects from Slovenia. *Pathophysiology of Haemostasis and Thrombosis,* Vol.36, No.2, (January 2009), pp. 58-63, ISSN 1424-8840

Bengtsson, A.; Zöller, B.; de Frutos, PG.; Dahlbäck, B. & Sturfelt, G. (1996). Factor V:Q506 mutation and anticardiolipin antibodies in systemic lupus erythematosus. *Lupus,* Vol.5, No.6, (December 1996), pp. 598-601, ISSN 0961-2033

Bennett, JS. (1997). Both sides of the hypercoagulable state. *Hospital Practice,* Vol.32, No.11, (November 1997), pp. 105-108, ISSN 8750-2836

Bennett, JA.; Palmer, LJ.; Musk, AW. & Erber, WN. (2001). Prevalence of factor V Leiden and prothrombin 20210A mutations in indigenous Australians. *Thrombosis and Haemostasis,* Vol.86, No.6, (December 2001), pp. 1592-1593, ISSN 0340-6245

Bereczky, Z.; Kovács, KB. & Muszbek, L. (2010). Protein C and protein S deficiencies: similarities and differences between two brothers playing in the same game. *Clinical Chemistry and Laboratory Medicine,* Vol.48, No.Suppl 1, (December 2010), pp. S53-66, ISSN 1434-6621

Bernardi, F.; Faioni, EM.; Castoldi, E.; Lunghi, B.; Castaman, G.; Sacchi, E. & Mannucci, PM. (1997). A factor V genetic component differing from factor V R506Q contributes to the activated protein C resistance phenotype. *Blood,* Vol.90, No.4, (August 1997), pp. 1552–1557, ISSN 0006-4971

Bertina, RM.; Koeleman, BPC.; Koster, T.; Rosendaal, FR.; Dirven, RJ.; de Ronde, HD.; van der Velden, PA. & Reitsma, PH. (1994). Mutation in blood coagulation factor V associated with resistance to activated protein C. *Nature,* Vol.369, No.6475, (May 1994), pp. 64-67, ISSN 0028-0836

Bertina, RM. (1997). Factor V Leiden and other coagulation factor mutations affecting thrombotic risk. *Clinical Chemistry,* Vol.43, No.9, (September 1997), pp. 1678–1683, ISSN 0009-9147

Bertina, RM.; Poort, SR.; Vos, HL. & Rosendaal, FR. (2005). The 46C→T polymorphism in the factor XII gene (F12) and the risk of venous thrombosis. *Journal of Thrombosis and Haemostasis,* Vol.3, No.3, (Mars 2005), pp. 597-599, ISSN 1538-7933

Bhatia, V.; Arora, P.; Parida, AK.; Mittal, A.; Pandey, AK. & Kaul, U. (2009). Air travel and pulmonary embolism: "economy class syndrome". *Journal of Association of Physicians of India,*Vol.57, (May 2009), pp. 412-414

Bontempo, FA.; Hassett, AC.; Faruki, H.; Steed, DL.; Webster, MW. & Makaroun, MS. (1997). The factor V Leiden mutation: spectrum of thrombotic events and laboratory evaluation. *Journal of Vascular Surgery,* Vol.25, No.2, (February 1997), pp. 271-275, ISSN 0741-5214

Bouaziz-Borgi, L.; Almawi, WY.; Mtiraoui, N.; Nsiri, B.; Keleshian, SH.; Kreidy, R.; Louzir, B.; Hezard, N. & Mahjoub, T. (2006). Distinct association of factor V-Leiden and prothrombin G20210A mutations with deep venous thrombosis in Tunisia and Lebanon. *American Journal of Hematology,* Vol.81, No.8, (August 2006), pp. 641-643, ISSN 1096-8652

Brandt JT. (2002). Plasminogen and tissue-type plasminogen activator deficiency as risk factors for thromboembolic disease. *Archives of Pathology and Laboratory Medicine,* Vol.126, No.11, (November 2002), pp. 1376-1381, ISSN 0003-9985

Broze, GJ Jr. (1998). Tissue factor pathway inhibitor gene disruption. *Blood Coagulation and Fibrinolysis,* Vol.9, No.Suppl 1, (Mars 1998), pp. S89-92, ISSN 0957-5235

Bunnage, ME. & Owen, DR. (2008). TAFIa inhibitors in the treatment of thrombosis. *Current Opinion in Drug Discovery and Development,* Vol.11, No.4, (July 2008), pp. 480-486, ISSN 1367-6733

Carmeliet, P.; Stassen, JM.;, Schoonjans, L.; Ream, B.; van den Oord, JJ.; De Mol, M.; Mulligan, RC. & Collen, D. (1993). Plasminogen activator inhibitor-1 gene-deficient mice. II. Effects on hemostasis, thrombosis, and thrombolysis. *Journal of Clinical Investigation,* Vol.92, No.6, (December 1993), pp. 2756-2760, ISSN 0021-9738

Castaman, G.; Faioni, EM.; Tosetto, A. & Bernardi, F. (2003). The factor V HR2 haplotype and the risk of venous thrombosis: a meta-analysis. *Haematologica,* Vol.88, No.10, (October 2003), pp. 1182–1189, ISSN 0390-6078.

Castoldi, E.; Lunghi, B.; Mingozzi, F.; Ioannou, P.; Marchetti, G. & Bernardi, F. (1997). New coagulation factor V gene polymorphisms define a single and infrequent haplotype underlying the factor V Leiden mutation in Mediterranean populations and Indians. Thrombo*sis and Haemostasis,* Vol.78, No.3, (September 1997), pp. 1037-1041, ISSN 0340-6245

Castoldi, E.; Rosing, J.; Girelli, D.; Hoekema, L.; Lunghi, B.; Mingozzi, F.; Ferraresi, P.; Friso, S.; Corrocher, R.; Tans, G. & Bernardi F. (2000). Mutations in the R2 FV gene affect the ratio between the two FV isoforms in plasma. *Thrombosis and Haemostasis,* Vol.83, No.3, (Mars 2000), pp. 362–536, ISSN 0340-6245

Ceelie, H.; Spaargaren-van Riel, CC.; Bertina, RM. & Vos, HL. (2004). G20210A is a functional mutation in the prothrombin gene; effect on protein levels and 3'-end formation. *Journal of Thrombosis and Haemostasis,* 2, 1, (January 2004), pp. 119-127, ISSN 1538-7933

Celiker, G.; Can, U.; Verdi, H.; Yazici, AC.; Ozbek, N. & Atac, FB. (2009). Prevalence of thrombophilic mutations and ACE I/D polymorphism in Turkish ischemic stroke patients. *Clinical and Applied Thrombosis/Hemostasis,*Vol.15, No.4, (July-August 2009), 415-420, ISSN 1076-0296

Cella, G.; Cipriani, A.; Tommasini, A.; Rampin, E.; Sbarai, A.; Rocconi, R.; Mazzaro, G. & Luzzatto, G. (1997) Tissue factor pathway inhibitor (TFPI) antigen plasma level in patients with interstitial lung disease before and after heparin administration. *Seminars in Thrombosis and Hemostasis,* Vol.23, No.1, (February 1997), pp. 45-49, ISSN 0094-6176

Chan, JC. (2001). Gene targeting in hemostasis. Tissue factor pathway inhibitor. *Frontiers in Bioscience,* Vol.1, No.6, (February 2001), pp. D216-221, ISSN 1093-9946

Chan, WP.; Lee, CK.; Kwong, YL.; Lam, CK. & Liang, R. (1998). A novel mutation of Arg306 of factor V gene in Hong Kong Chinese. *Blood,*Vol.91, No.4, (February 1998), pp. 1135-1139, ISSN 0006-4971

Chan, WS. (2010). Venous thromboembolism in pregnancy. *Expert Review of Cardiovascular Therapy,* Vol.8, No.12, (December 2010), pp. 1731-1740, ISSN 1477-9072

Cikes, V.; Abaza, I.; Krzelj, V.; Terzić, IM.; Tafra, R.; Trlaja, A.; Marusić, E. & Terzić, J. (2004). Prevalence of factor V Leiden and G6PD 1311 silent mutations in Dalmatian population. *Archives of Medical Research,*Vol.35, No.6, (November-December 2004), pp. 546-548, ISSN 0188-4409

Coen, D.; Zadro, R.; Honović, L.; Banfić, L. & Stavljenić Rukavina, A. (2001). Prevalence and association of the factor V Leiden and prothrombin G20210A in healthy subjects and patients with venous thromboembolism. *Croatian Medical Journal,* Vol.42, No.4, (August 2001), pp. 488-492, ISSN 0353-9504

Comp, PC. & Esmon, CT. (1984). Recurrent venous thromboembolism in patients with a partial deficiency of protein S. *New England Journal of Medicine,* Vol.311, no.24, (December 1984), pp. 1525-1528, ISSN 0028-4793

Comp, PC.; Nixon, RR.; Cooper, MR. & Esmon, CT. (1984). Familial protein S deficiency is associated with recurrent thrombosis. *Journal of Clinical Investigation, Vol.*74, No.6, (December 1984), pp. 2082–2088, ISSN 0021-9738

Cox, MJ.; Rees, DC.; Martinson, JJ. & Clegg, JB. (1996). Evidence of a single origin of factor V Leiden. *British Journal of Haematology,* Vol.92, No.4, (Mars 1996), pp. 1022-1025, ISSN 0007-1048

D'Ursi, P.; Marino, F.; Caprera, A.; Milanesi, L.; Faioni, EM. & Rovida, E. (2007). ProCMD: a database and 3D web resource for protein C mutants. *BMC Bioinformatics*, Vol.8, No.Suppl 1, (December 2010), pp. S11, ISSN 1471-2105

Dahlbäck, B.; Carlsson, M. & Svensson, PJ. (1993). Familial thrombophilia due to a previously unrecognized mechanism characterized by poor anticoagulant response to ctivated protein C: Prediction of a cofactor to activated protein C. *Proceedings of the National Academiy of Sciences of the USA*, Vol.90, No.3, (February 1993), pp. 1004-1008, ISSN 1091-6490

Dahlbäck, B. (1995). Resistance to activated protein C, the Arg506 to Gln mutation in the factor V gene, and venous thrombosis. Functional tests and DNA-based assays. Pros and Cons. *Thrombosis and Haemostasis,* Vol.73, No.5, (May 1995), pp. 739-742, ISSN 0340-6245

Dahlbäck, B. (1997). Resistance to activated protein C caused by the factor V R506Q mutation is a common risk factor for venous thrombosis. *Thrombosis and Haemostasis,* Vol.78, pp. 483-488, ISSN 0340-6245

Dahlbäck, B. (2008). Advances in understanding pathogenic mechanisms of thrombophilic disorders. *Blood,* Vol.112, No.1, (July 2008), pp. 19-27, ISSN 0006-4971

Danckwardt, S.; Hartmann, K.; Katz, B.; Hentze, MW.; Levy, Y.; Eichele, R.; Deutsch, V.; Kulozik, AE. & Ben-Tal, O. (2006). The prothrombin 20209 C-->T mutation in Jewish-Moroccan Caucasians: molecular analysis of gain-of-function of 3' end processing. *Journal of Thrombosis and Haemostasis,* Vol.4, No.5, (May 2006), pp. 1078-1085, ISSN 1538-7933

Dashti, AA.; Jadaon, MM. & Lewis, HL. (2010). Factor V Leiden mutation in Arabs in Kuwait by real-time PCR: different values for different Arabs. *Journal of Human Genetics,*Vol.55, No.4, (April 2010), pp. 232-235, ISSN 1434-5161

Dashti, AA. & Jadaon, MM. (2011). Race differences in the prevalence of the factor V Leiden mutation in Kuwaiti nationals. *Molecular Biology Reports,* Vol.38, No.6, (August 2011), pp. 3623-3628, ISSN 0301-4851

Davie, EW. (1995). Biochemical and molecular aspects of the coagulation cascade. *Thrombosis and Haemostasis,* Vol.74, No.4, (July 1995), pp. 1-6, ISSN 0340-6245

De Maat, MPM.; Kluft, C.; Jespersen, J. & Gram, J. (1996). World distribution of factor V Leiden mutation. *Lancet,* Vol.347, No. 8993, (January 1996), pp. 58, ISSN 0140-6736

de Visser, MC.; Poort, SR.; Vos, HL.; Rosendaal, FR. & Bertina, RM. (2001). Factor X levels, polymorphisms in the promoter region of factor X, and the risk of venous thrombosis. *Thrombosis and Haemostasis,* Vol.85, No.6, (June 2001), pp. 1011-1017, ISSN 0340-6245

DeHart, RL. (2003). Health issues of air travel. *Annual Review of Public Health,*Vol.24, (January 2003), pp. 133-151

Dilley, A.; Austin, H.; Hooper, WC.; El-Jamil, M.; Whitsett, C.; Wenger, NK.; Benson, J. & Evatt, B. (1998). Prevalence of the prothrombin 20210 G-to-A variant in blacks:

infants, patients with venous thrombosis, patients with myocardial infarction, and control subjects. *Journal of Laboratory and Clinical Medicine,* Vo.132, No.6, (December 1998), pp. 452-455, ISSN 0022-2143

Diz-Kucukkaya, R.; Hancer, VS.; Artim-Esen, B.; Pekcelen, Y. & Inanc, M. (2010). The prevalence and clinical significance of inherited thrombophilic risk factors in patients with antiphospholipid syndrome. *Journal of Thrombosis and Thrombolysis,*Vol.29, No.3, (April 2010), pp. 303-309, ISSN 0929-5305

Djordjevic, V.; Rakicevic, LJ.; Mikovic, D.; Kovac, M.; Miljic, P.; Radojkovic, D. & Savic, A. (2004). Prevalence of factor V leiden, factor V cambridge, factor II G20210A and methylenetetrahydrofolate reductase C677T mutations in healthy and thrombophilic Serbian populations. *Acta Haematol,* Vol.112, No.4, (November 2004), pp. 227-229, ISSN 0001-5792

Dolan, G.; Greaves, M.; Cooper, P. & Preston, FE. (1988). Thrombovascular disease and familial plasminogen deficiency: a report of three kindreds. *British Journal of Haematology,* Vol.70, No.4, (December 1988), pp. 417-421, ISSN 00071048

Dykes, AC.; Walker, ID.; McMahon, AD.; Islam, SI. & Tait RC. (2001). A study of Protein S antigen levels in 3788 healthy volunteers: influence of age, sex and hormone use, and estimate for prevalence of deficiency state. *British Journal of Haematology,*Vol.113, No.3, (June 2001), pp. 636–641, ISSN 0007-1048

Egeberg, O. (1965). On the natural blood coagulation inhibitor system. Investigations of inhibitor factors based on antithrombin deficient blood. *Thrombosis et diathesis haemorrhagica,* Vol.14, No.3-4, (November 1965), pp. 473-489, ISSN 0340-5338

Ehsan, A. & Plumbley, JA. (2002). Introduction to Thrombosis and Anticoagulant Therapy, In: *Clinical Hematology and Fundamentals of Hemostasis* (4th Edition), Harmening DM., pp. 534-562, F. A. Davis Company, ISBN 0-8036-0783-0, Philadelphia, USA

Eid, SS. & Rihani, G. (2004). Prevalence of factor V Leiden, prothrombin G20210A, and MTHFR C677T mutations in 200 healthy Jordanians. *Clinical Laboratory Science,* 2004; Vol.17, No.4, (Fall 2004), pp. 200-202, ISSN 0894-959X

Eid, SS. & Shubeilat, T. (2005). Prevalence of Factor V Leiden, prothrombin G20210A, and MTHFR G677A among 594 thrombotic Jordanian patients. *Blood Coagulation and Fibrinolysis,* Vol.16, No.6, (September 2005), pp. 417-421, ISSN 0957-5235

El-Karaksy, H.; El-Koofy, N.; El-Hawary, M.; Mostafa, A.; Aziz, M.; El-Shabrawi, M.; Mohsen, NA.; Kotb, M.; El-Raziky, M.; El-Sonoon, MA. & A-Kader, H. (2004). Prevalence of factor V Leiden mutation and other hereditary thrombophilic factors in Egyptian children with portal vein thrombosis: results of a single-center case-control study. *Annals of Hematology,*Vol.83, No.11, (November 2004), pp. 712-715, ISSN 0939-5555

Esmon, CT.; Ding, W.; Yasuhiro, K.; Gu, JM.; Ferrell, G.; Regan, LM.; Stearns-Kurosawa, DJ.; Kurosawa, S.; Mather, T.; Laszik, Z. & Esmon, NL. (1997). The protein C pathway: new insights. *Thrombosis and Haemostasis,* Vol.78, No.1, (July 1997), pp. 70-74, ISSN 0340-6245

Erber, WN.; Buck, AM. & Threlfall, TJ. (2004). The haematology of indigenous Australians. *Hematology,* Vol.9, No.5-6, (October 2004), pp. 339-350

Escobar, CE.; Harmining, DM.; Joiner Maier, DM.; Simmons, VL.; Smith-Moore, KM. & Wyrick-Glatzel, J. (2002). Introduction to Hemostasis, In: *Clinical Hematology and*

Fundamentals of Hemostasis (4th Edition), Harmening, DM., pp. 441-470, F. A. Davis Company, ISBN 0-8036-0783-0, Philadelphia, USA

Faioni, EM.; Razzari, C.; Martinelli, I.; Panzeri, D.; Franchi, F. & Mannucci, PM. (1997). Resistance to activated protein C in unselected patients with arterial and venous thrombosis. *American Journal of Hematology*, Vol.55, No.2, (June 1997), pp. 59-64, ISSN 1096-8652

Faioni, EM.; Castaman, G.; Asti, D.; Lussana, F. & Rodeghiero, F. (2004). Association of factor V deficiency with factor V HR2. *Haematologica*,Vol.89, No.2, (February 2004), pp. 195–200, ISSN 0390-6078

Farmer-Boatwright, MK. & Roubey, RA.(2009). Venous thrombosis in the antiphospholipid syndrome. *Arteriosclerosis, Thrombosis, and Vascular Biology*, Vol.29, No.3, (Mars 2009), pp. 321-325, ISSN 1079-5642

Finan, RR.; Tamim, H.; Ameen, G.; Sharida, HE.; Rashid, M. & Almawi, WY. (2002). Prevalence of factor V G1691A (factor V-Leiden) and prothrombin G20210A gene mutations in a recurrent miscarriage population. *American Journal of Hematology*, Vol.71, No.4, (December 2002), pp. 300-305, ISSN 1096-8652

Finazzi, G.; Caccia, R. & Barbui, T. (1987). Different prevalence of thromboembolism in the subtypes of congenital antithrombin III deficiency: Review of 404 cases. *Thrombosis and Haemostasis*, Vol.58, No.4, (December 1987) 1094, ISSN 0340-6245

Florell, SR. & Rodgers, GM. (1997). Inherited thrombotic disorders: An update. *American Journal of Hematology*, Vol.54, No.1, (January 1997), pp. 53-60, ISSN 1096-8652

Franchini, M. & Lippi, G. (2010). Factor V Leiden and hemophilia. *Thrombosis Research*, Vol.125, No.2, (February 2010), pp. 119-123, ISSN 0049-3848

Franchini, M. & Lippi, G. (2011). Factor V Leiden in women: a thrombotic risk factor or an evolutionary advantage? *Seminars in Thrombosis and Hemostasis*, Vol.37, No.3, (April 2011), pp. 275-259, ISSN 0094-6176

Franco, RF.; Santos, SE.; Elion, J.; Tavella, MH. & Zago, MA. (1998). Prevalence of the G20210A polymorphism in the 3'-untranslated region of the prothrombin gene in different human populations. *Acta Haematologica*, Vol.100, No.1, (July 1998), pp. 9-12, ISSN 0001-5792

Fujimura, H.; Kambayashi, J.; Monden, M.; Kato, H. & Miyata, T. (1995). Coagulation factor V Leiden mutation may have a racial background. *Thrombosis and Haemostasis, Vol.*74, No.5, (November 1995), pp. 1381-1382, ISSN 0340-6245

Furie, B. & Furie, BC. (1988). The molecular basis of blood coagulation. *Cell*, Vol.53, No.4, (May 1988), pp. 505-518, ISSN 0092-8674

Galli, M.; Luciani, D.; Bertolini, G. & Barbui, T. (2002). Lupus anticoagulants are stronger risk factors for thrombosis than anticardiolipin antibodies in the antiphospholipid syndrome: a systematic review of the literature. *Blood*, Vol.101, No.5, (Mars 2002), pp. 1827-1832, ISSN 0006-4971

Garcia de Frutos, PG. & Dahlbäck, B. (1995). Resistance to activated protein C as an additional risk factor in hereditary deficiency of protein S. *Thrombosis and Haemostasis*, Vol.73, No.6, (June 1995), pp. 1360, ISSN 0340-6245.

García-Hernández, MC.; Romero Casanova, A. & Marco Vera, P. (2007). Clinical comments on genetic marker prevalence (factor V Leiden, prothrombin 20210A and homozygous methylenetetrahydrofolate reductase form [Ho-MTHFR]): based on a study conducted in Health Department No. 19 of the Valencian Community. *Revista Clininica Espanola,* Vol.207, No.1, (January 2007), pp. 26-28, ISSN 0014-2565

Gessoni, G.; Valverde, S.; Canistro, R. & Manoni, F. (2010). Factor V Leiden in Chioggia: a prevalence study in patients with venous thrombosis, their blood relatives and the general population. *Blood Transfusion,* Vol.8, No.3, (July 2010), pp. 193-195, ISSN 1723-2007

Ghosh, K.; Shetty, S.; Madkaikar, M.; Pawar, A.; Nair, S.; Khare, A.; Pathare, A.; Jijina, F. & Mohanty, D. (2001). Venous thromboembolism in young patients from western India: a study. *Clinical and Applied Thrombosis/Hemostasis,* Vol.7, No.2, (April 2001), pp. 158-165, ISSN 1076-0296

Gibson, CS.; MacLennan, AH.; Rudzki, Z.; Hague, WM.; Haan, EA.; Sharpe, P.; Priest, K.; Chan, A.; Dekker, GA. & South Australian Cerebral Palsy Research Group. (2005). The prevalence of inherited thrombophilias in a Caucasian Australian population. *Pathology,* Vol.37, No.2, (April 2005), pp. 160-163, ISSN 0031-3025

González Ordóñez, AJ.; Medina Rodriguez, JM.; Martín, L.; Alvarez, V. & Coto, E. (1999). The O blood group protects against venous thromboembolism in individuals with the factor V Leiden but not the prothrombin (factor II G20210A) mutation. *Blood Coagulation and Fibrinolysis,* Vol.10, No.5, (July 1999), pp. 303-307, ISSN 0957-5235

Greaves, M. & Preston, FE. (1991). Hypercoagulable state in clinical practice. *British Journal of Haematology,* Vol.79, No.2, (October 1991), pp. 148-151, ISSN 0007-1048

Greengard, JS.; Alhenc-Gelas, M.; Gandrille, S.; Emmerich, J.; Aiach, M. & Griffin, JH. (1995). Pseudo-homozygous activated protein C resistance due to coinheritance of heterozygous factor V-R506Q and type I factor V deficiency associated with thrombosis. *Thrombosis and Haemostasis,* Vol.73, No.6, (June 1995), pp. 1361, ISSN 0340-6245.

Gregg, JP.; Yamane, AJ. & Grody, WW. (1997). Prevalence of the factor V-Leiden mutation in four distinct American ethnic populations. *American Journal of Medical Genetics,* Vol.73, No.3, (December 1997), pp. 334-336, ISSN 1552-4733

Griffin, JH.; Evatt, B.; Zimmerman, TS.; Kleis, AJ. & Wideman, C. (1981). Deficiency of protein C in congenital thrombotic disease. *Journal of Clinical Investigation,* Vol.68, No.5, (November 1981), pp. 1370–1373, ISSN 0021-9738

Griffin, JH.; Heeb, MJ.; Kojima, Y.; Fernández, JA.; Kojima, K.; Hackeng, TM. & Greengard, JS. (1995). Activated protein C resistance: Molecular mechanisms. *Thrombosis and Haemostasis,* Vol.74, No.1, (January 1995), pp. 444-448, 1995, ISSN 0340-6245, ISSN 0340-6245

Guasch, JF.; Lensen, RPM. & Bertina, RM. (1997). Molecular characterization of a type I quantitative factor V deficiency in a thrombosis patient that is "pseudo homozygous" for activated protein C resistance. *Thrombosis and Haemostasis,* Vol.77, No.2, (February 1997), pp. 252-257, ISSN 0340-6245.

Gurgey, A. & Mesci, L. (1997). The prevalence of factor V Leiden (1691G → A) mutation in Turkey. *Turkish Journal of Pediatrics,* Vol.39, No.3, (July-September 1997), pp. 313-315, ISSN 0041-4301

Gurgey, A.; Haznedaroglu, IC.; Egesel, T.; Buyukasik, Y.; Ozcebe, OI.; Sayinalp, N.; Dundar, SV. & Bayraktar, Y. (2001). Two common genetic thrombotic risk factors: factor V Leiden and prothrombin G20210A in adult Turkish patients with thrombosis.

*American Journal of Hematology,*Vol.67, No.2, (June 2001), pp. 107-111, ISSN 1096-8652

Hainaut, P.; Azerad, MA.; Lehmann, E.; Schlit, AF.; Zech, F.; Heusterspreute, M.; Philippe, M.; Col, C.; Lavenne, E. & Mariau, M. (1997). Prevalence of activated protein C resistance and analysis of clinical profile in thromboembolic patients. A Belgian prospective study. *Journal of Internal Medicine,* Vol.241, No.5, (September -October 1997), pp. 427-433, ISSN 1365-2796

Hallak, M.; Senderowicz, J.; Cassel, A.; Shapira, C.; Aghai, E.; Auslender, R. & Abramovici, H. (1997). Activated protein C resistance (factor V Leiden) associated with thrombosis in pregnancy. *American Journal of Obstetrics & Gynecology,* Vol.176, No.4, (April 1997), pp. 889-893, ISSN 0002-9378

Hallam, PJ.; Millaer, DS.; Krawczak, M.; Kakkar, VV. & Cooper, DN. (1995). Population differences in the frequency of the factor V Leiden varient among people with clinically symptomatic protein C deficiency. *Journal of Medical Genetics,* Vol.32, No.7, (July 1995), pp. 543-545, ISSN 1468-6244

Hatzaki, A.; Anagnostopoulou, E.; Metaxa-Mariatou, V.; Melissinos, C.; Philalithis, P.; Iliadis, K.; Kontaxis, A.; Liberatos, K.; Pangratis, N. & Nasioulas, G. (2003). The impact of heterozygosity for the factor V Leiden and factor II G20210A mutations on the risk of thrombosis in Greek patients. *International Angiology,* Vol.22, No.1, (Mars 2003), pp. 79-82, ISSN 0392-9590

Heeb, MJ.; Espana, F. & Griffin, JH. (1989). Inhibition and complexation of activated Protein C by two major inhibitors in plasma. *Blood,* Vol.73, No.2, (February 1989), pp. 446-454, ISSN 0006-4971

Heijboer, H.; Brandjes, DP.; Büller, HR.; Sturk, A. & ten Cate, JW. (1990). Deficiencies of coagulation-inhibiting and fibrinolytic proteins in outpatients with deep-vein thrombosis. *New England Journal of Medicine,* Vol.323, No.22, (November 1990), pp. 1512-1516, ISSN 0028-4793

Herrmann, FH.; Koesling, M.; Schroder, W.; Altman, R.; Jimenez Bonilla, R.; Lopaciuk, S.; Perez-Requejo, JL. & Singh, JR. (1997), Prevalence of factor V Leiden mutation in various populations. *Genetic Epidemiology,* Vol.14, No.4, pp. 403-11, ISSN 1098-2272

Hillarp, A.; Zöller, B.; Svensson, PJ. & Dahlbäck, B. (1997). The 20210A allele of the prothrombine gene is a common risk factor among Swedish outpatients with verified deep venous thrombosis. *Thrombosis and Haemostasis,* Vol.78, No.3, (September 1997), pp. 990-992, ISSN 0340-6245

Ho, CH.; Chau, WK.; Hsu, HC.; Gau, JP. & Chih, CM. (1999). Prevalence of factor V Leiden in the Chinese population. *Zhonghua Yi Xue Za Zhi,* Vol.62, No.12, (December 1999), pp. 875-878, 1003-9406.

Hoagland, LE,; Triplett, DA.; Peng, F. & Barna L. (1996). APC-resistnace as measured by a Textarin time assay: comparison to the APTT-based method. *Thrombosis Research,* Vol.83, (September 1996), pp. 363-373, ISSN 0049-3848

Hoffbrand, AV.; Pettit, JE. & Moss, PAH. (2001). *Essential Haematology* (4th Edition), Blackwell Science Ltd, ISBN 0-63205-153-1, Oxford, UK

Huber, K. (2001). Plasminogen activator inhibitor type-1 (part one): basic mechanisms, regulation, and role for thromboembolic disease. *Journal of Thrombosis and Thrombolysis,*Vol.11, No.3, (May 2001), pp. 183-193, ISSN 0929-5305

Hudecek, J.; Dobrotová, M.; Hybenová, J.; Ivanková, J.; Melus, V.; Pullmann, R. & Kubisz, P. (2003). Factor V Leiden and the Slovak population. *Vnitr Lek,* Vol.49, No.11, (November 2003), pp. 845-850

Hussein, AS.; Darwish, H. & Shelbayeh, K. (2010). Association between factor V Leiden mutation and poor pregnancy outcomes among Palestinian women. *Thrombosis Research,* Vol.126, No.2, (August 2010), pp. e78-82, ISSN 0049-3848

Ioannou, HV.; Mitsis, M.; Eleftheriou, A.; Matsagas, M.; Nousias, V.; Rigopoulos, C.; Vartholomatos, G. & Kappas, AM. (2000). The prevalence of factor V Leiden as a risk factor for venous thromboembolism in the population of North-Western Greece. *International Angiology,* Vol.19, No.4, December 2000), pp. 314-318, ISSN 0392-9590

Irani-Hakime, N.; Tamim, H.; Elias, G.; Finan, RR.; Daccache, JL. & Almawi, WY. (2000). High prevalence of factor V mutation (Leiden) in the Eastern Mediterranean. *Clinical Chemistry,* Vol.46, No.1, (January 2000), pp. 134-136, ISSN 0009-9147

Irani-Hakime, N.; Tamim, H.; Elias, G.; Choueiry, S.; Kreidy, R.; Daccache, JL. & Almawi, WY. (2001). Factor V R506Q mutation-Leiden: an independent risk factor for venous thrombosis but not coronary artery disease. *Journal of Thrombosis and Thrombolysis,*Vol.11, No.2, (April 2001), pp. 111-1116, ISSN 0929-5305

Irdem, A.; Devecioglu, C.; Batun, S.; Soker, M. & Sucakli, IA. (2005). Prevalence of factor V Leiden and prothrombin G20210A gene mutation. *Saudi Medical Journal,*Vol.26, No.4, (April 2005), pp. 580-583, ISSN 0379-5284

Ireland, H.; Bayston, TA.; Chowdhury, V.; Thein, SL.; Conard, J.; Pabinger, I. & Lane, DA. (1995). Factor V Leiden as an independent risk factor for thrombosis in antithrombin deficiency type II: heparin binding site. *Thrombosis and Haemostasis,* No.73, No.6, (June 1995), pp. 1361, 1995, ISSN 0340-6245.

Isma'eel, H.; Arnaout, MS.; Shamseddeen, W.; Mahfouz, R.; Zeineh, N.; Jradi, O. & Taher, A. (2006a). Screening for inherited thrombophilia might be warranted among Eastern Mediterranean sickle-beta-0 thalassemia patients. *Journal of Thrombosis and Thrombolysis,* Vol.22, No.2, (October 2006), pp. 121-123, ISSN 0929-5305

Isma'eel, H.; El Accaoui, R.; Shamseddeen, W.; Taher, A.; Alam, S.; Mahfouz, R. & Arnaout, MS. (2006b). Genetic thrombophilia in patients with VTE in eastern Mediterranean located tertiary care center; is it time to change the algorithm for thrombophilia work up decision making? *Journal of Thrombosis and Thrombolysis,* Vol.21, No.3, (June 2006), pp. 267-270, ISSN 0929-5305

Isshiki, I.; Murata, M.; Watanabe, R.; Matsubara, Y.; Kawano, K.; Aoki, N.; Yoshino, H.; Ishikawa, K.; Watanabe, G. & Ikeda, Y. (1998). Frequencies of prothrombin 20210 G→A mutation may be different among races--studies on Japanese populations with various forms of thrombotic disorders and healthy subjects. *Blood Coagulation and Fibrinolysis,* Vol.9, No.1, (January 1998), pp. 105-106, ISSN 0957-5235

Jadaon, MM. & Dashti, AA. (2005a). HR2 haplotype in Arab population and patients with venous thrombosis in Kuwait. *Journal of Thrombosis and Haemostasis,*Vol.3, No.7, (July 2005), 1467-1471, ISSN 1538-7933

Jadaon, MM. & Dashti, AA. (2005b). The Risk of Venous Thrombosis Increases with Co-existence of Multiple Genetic Abnormalities: A Comprehensive Study in Kuwait. *Journal of Thrombosis and Haemostasis,* 2005; Vol.3, No.Supplement 1, (August 2005), abstract number P0077, ISSN 1538-7933

Jadaon, MM.; Dashti, AA. & Lewis, HL. (2006). Factor V Kuwait: a novel mutation in the coagulation factor V gene discovered in Kuwait. *Medical Principles and Practice,* Vol.15, No.2, (2006), pp. 102-105, ISSN 1011-7571

Jadaon, MM.; Dashti, AA. & Lewis HL. (2010). High prevalence of activated protein C resistance and factor V Leiden mutation in an Arab population and patients with venous thrombosis in Kuwait. *Diagnostic Molecular Pathology,* Vol.19, No.3, (September 2010), pp. 180-183, ISSN 1052-9551

Jadaon, MM.; Dashti, AA. & Lewis, HL. (2011). What is the origin of factor V Leiden mutation in Arabs? The first molecular proof. *Journal of Thrombosis and Haemostasis,* Vol.9, No.Supplement 2, (July 2011), abstract number P-MO-155, ISSN 1538-7933

Jankun, J. & Skrzypczak-Jankun, E. (2011). Val17Ile Single Nucleotide Polymorphisms Similarly as Ala15Thr Could be Related to the Lower Secretory Dynamics of PAI-1 Secretion - Theoretical Evidence. *Current Molecular Medicine,* Vol.11, No.6, (August 2011), pp.512-516, ISSN 1566-5240

Jukic, I.; Bingulac-Popovic, J.; Dogic, V.; Babic, I.; Culej, J.; Tomicic, M.; Vuk, T.; Sarlija, D. & Balija, M. (2009). ABO blood groups and genetic risk factors for thrombosis in Croatian population. *Croatian Medical Journal,* Vol.50, No.6, (December 2009), pp. 550-558, ISSN 0353-9504

Kabukcu, S.; Keskin, N.; Keskin, A. & Atalay, E. (2007). The frequency of factor V Leiden and concomitance of factor V Leiden with prothrombin G20210A mutation and methylene tetrahydrofolate reductase C677T gene mutation in healthy population of Denizli, Aegean region of Turkey. *Clinical and Applied Thrombosis/Hemostasis,* Vol.13, No.2, (April 2009), pp. 166-171, ISSN 1076-0296

Kalafatis, M.; Rand, MD. & Mann, KG. (1994). The mechanism of inactivation of human factor V and human factor Va by activated protein C. *The Journal of Biological Chemistry,* Vol.269, No.50, (December 1994), pp. 31869-31880, ISSN 0021-9258

Kalkanli, S.; Ayyildiz, O.; Tiftik, N.; Batun, S.; Isikdogan, A.; Ince, H.; Tekes, S. & Muftuoglu, E. (2006). Factor V Leiden mutation in venous thrombosis in southeast Turkey. *Angiology,*Vol.57, No.2, (Mars-April 2006), pp. 193-196, ISSN 0392-9590

Kamphuisen, PW.; Eikenboom, JC.; Rosendaal, FR.; Koster, T.; Blann, AD.; Vos, HL. & Bertina, RM. (2001). High factor VIII antigen levels increase the risk of venous thrombosis but are not associated with polymorphisms in the von Willebrand factor and factor VIII gene. *British Journal of Haematology,* Vol.115, No.1, (October 2001), pp. 156-158, ISSN 0007-1048

Kane, WH. & Davie, EW. (1988). Blood coagulation factor V and VIII: structural and functional similarities and their relationship to haemorrhegic and thrombotic disorders. *Blood,* Vol.71, No.3, pp. 539-555, ISSN 0006-4971

Kerlin, BA.; Yan, SB.; Isermann, BH.; Brandt, JT.; Sood, R.; Basson, BR.; Joyce, DE.; Weiler, H. & Dhainaut, JF. Survival advantage associated with heterozygous factor V Leiden mutation in patients with severe sepsis and in mouse endotoxemia. *Blood,* Vol.102, No.9, (November 2003), pp. 3085-3092, ISSN 0006-4971

Kim, TW.; Kim, WK.; Lee, JH.; Kim, SB.; Kim, SW.; Suh, C.; Lee, KH.; Lee, JS.; Seo, EJ.; Chi, HS. & Kim, SH. (1998). Low prevalence of activated protein C resistance and coagulation factor V Arg506 to Gln mutation among Korean patients with deep vein thrombosis. *Journal of Korean Medical Science,* Vol.13, No.6, (December 1998), pp. 587-590, ISSN 1011-8934

Kinev, AV. & Roubey, RA. (2008).Tissue factor in the antiphospholipid syndrome. *Lupus,* Vol.17, No.10, (October 2008), pp. 952-958, ISSN 0961-2033

Klammt, J.; Kobelt, L.; Aktas, D.; Durak, I.; Gokbuget, A.; Hughes, Q.; Irkec, M.; Kurtulus, I.; Lapi, E.; Mechoulam, H.; Mendoza-Londono, R.; Palumbo, JS.; Steitzer, H.; Tabbara, KF.; Ozbek, Z.; Pucci, N.; Sotomayor, T.; Sturm, M.; Drogies, T.; Ziegler, M. & Schuster, V. (2011). Identification of three novel plasminogen (PLG) gene mutations in a series of 23 patients with low PLG activity. *Thrombosis and Haemostasis,* Vol.105, No.3, (Mars 2011), pp. 454-460, ISSN 0340-6245

Kodaira, H.; Ishida, F.; Scimodaira, S.; Takamiya, O.; Furihata, K. & Kitano, K. (1997). Resistance to activated protein C and Arg506Gln factor V mutation are uncommon in eastern Asian populations. *Acta Haematologica,* Vol.98, No.1, pp. 22-25, ISSN 0001-5792

Koeleman, BPC.; Reitsma, PH. & Bertina, RM. (1997). Familial thrombophilia: a complex genetic disorder. *Seminars in Hematology,* Vol.34, No.3, (July 1997), pp. 256-264, ISSN 0037-1963

Koster, T.; Blann, AD.; Briët, E.; Vandenbroucke, JP. & Rosendaal, FR. (1995a). Role of clotting factor VIII in effect of von Willebrand factor on occurrence of deep-vein thrombosis. *Lancet,* Vol.345, No.8943, (January 1995), pp. 152-155, ISSN 0140-6736

Koster, T.; Rosendaal, FR.; Briet, E.; van der Meer, FJ.; Colly, LP.; Trienekens, PH.; Poort, SR.; Reitsma, PH. & Vandenbroucke, JP. (1995b). Protein C deficiency in a controlled series of unselected outpatients: an infrequent but clear risk factor for venous thrombosis. *Blood,* Vol.85, No.10, (May 1995), pp. 2756-2761, ISSN 0006-4971

Laffan, MA. & Manning, RA. (2002a). Investigation of Haemostasis, In: *Dacie and Lewis Practical Haematology* (9th Edition), Lewis, SM.; Bain, BJ. & Bates, I., pp. 339-390, Churchill Livingstone, ISBN 0-4430-6378-8,London, UK

Laffan, MA. & Manning, RA. (2002b). Investigation of Thrombotic Tendency, In: *Dacie and Lewis Practical Haematology* (9th Edition), Lewis, SM.; Bain, BJ. & Bates, I., pp. 391-413, Churchill Livingstone, 0-4430-6378-8,London, UK

Lambropoulos, AF.; Foka, Z.; Makris, M.; Daly, M.; Kotsis, A. & Makris, PE. (1997). Factor V Leiden in Greek thrombophilic patients: relationship with activated protein C resistance test and levels of thrombin-antithrombin complex and prothrombin fragment 1 + 2. *Blood Coagulation and Fibrinolysis,* Vol.8, No.8, (November 1997), pp. 485-489, ISSN 0957-5235

Lane, DA.; Mannucci, PM.; Bauer, KA.; Bertina, RM.; Bochkov, NP.; Boulyjenkov, V.; Chandy, M.; Dahlbäck, B.; Ginter, EK.; Miletich, JP.; Rosendaal, FR. & Seligsohn, U. (1996). Inherited thrombophilia: Part 1. *Thrombosis Haemostasis,* Vol.76, No.5, (November 1996), pp. 651-662, ISSN 0340-6245

Lee, LH. (2002). Clinical update on deep vein thrombosis in Singapore. *Annals of Academy of Medicine Singapore,* Vol.31, No.2, (Mars 2002), pp. 248-252

Leroyer, C.; Mercier, B.; Escoffre, M.; Ferec, C. & Mottier, D. (1997). Factor V Leiden prevalence in venous thromboembolism patients. *Chest,* Vol.111, No.6, (June 1997), pp. 1603-1606, ISSN 0012-3692

Lim, LC.; Tan, HH.; Lee, LH.; Tien, SL. & Abdul Ghafar, A.(1999). Activated protein C resistance: a study among 60 thromboembolic patients in the Singapore population. *Annals of Academy of Medicine Singapore,* Vol.28, No.2, (Mars 1999), pp. 252-255

Limdi, NA.; Beasley, TM.; Allison, DB.; Rivers, CA. & Acton, RT. (2006). Racial differences in the prevalence of Factor V Leiden mutation among patients on chronic warfarin therapy. *Blood Cells, Molecules, and Diseases,* Vol.37, No.2, (Septemebr-October 2006), pp. 100-106, ISSN 1079-9796

Lin, JS.; Shen, MC. & Tsay, W. (1998). The mutation at position 20210 in the 3'-untranslated region of the prothrombin gene is extremely rare in Taiwanese Chinese patients with venous thrombophilia. *Thrombosis and Haemostasis,* 80, 2, (August 1998), pp. 343, ISSN 0340-6245

Lindqvist, PG.; Zöller, B. & Dahlbäck, B. (2001). Improved hemoglobin status and reduced menstrual blood loss among female carriers of factor V Leiden--an evolutionary advantage? *Thrombosis and Haemostasis,* Vol.86, No.4, (October 2001), pp. 1122-123, ISSN 0340-6245

Lindqvist, PG. & Dahlbäck, B. (2008). Carriership of Factor V Leiden and evolutionary selection advantage. *Current Medical Chemistry,* Vol.15, No.15, 1541-1544, 0929-8673

Lisman, T.; de Groot, PG.; Meijers, JC. & Rosendaal, FR. (2005). Reduced plasma fibrinolytic potential is a risk factor for venous thrombosis. *Blood,* Vol.105, No.3, (February 2005), pp. 1102-1105, ISSN 0006-4971

Lucotte, G. & Mercier, G. (2001). Population genetics of factor V Leiden in Europe. *Blood Cells, Molecules, and Diseases,* (Mars-April 2001), Vol.27, No.2, pp. 362-367 , ISSN 1079-9796

Lunghi, B.; Lacoviello, L.; Gemmati, D.; Dilasio, MG.; Castoldi, E.; Pinotti, M.; Castaman, G.; Redaelli, R.; Mariani, G.; Marchetti, G. & Bernardi, F. (1996). Detection of new polymorphic markers in the factor V gene: association with factor V levels in plasma. *Thrombosis and Haemostasis,*Vol.75, No.1, (January 1996), pp. 45–48, ISSN 0340-6245

Machlus, KR.; Cardenas, JC.; Church, FC. & Wolberg, AS. (2011). Causal relationship between hyperfibrinogenemia, thrombosis, and resistance to thrombolysis in mice. *Blood,* Vol.117, No.18, (May 2011), pp. 4953-4963, ISSN 0006-4971

Mansourati, J.; Da Costa, A.; Munier, S.; Mercier, B.; Tardy, B.; Ferec, C.; Isaaz, K. & Blanc, JJ. (2000). Prevalence of factor V Leiden in patients with myocardial infarction and normal coronary angiography. *Thrombosis and Haemostasis,* Vol.83, No.6, (June 2000), pp. 822-825, ISSN 0340-6245

Manucci, PM. (2000). The molecular basis of inherited thrombophilia. *Vox Sanguinis,* Vol.78, No.Suppl 2, 39-45, ISSN 0042-9007

Margaglione, M.; Bossone, A.; Coalizzo, D.; D'Andrea, G.; Brancaccio, V.; Ciampa, A.; Grandone, E. & Di, MG. (2002). FV HR2 haplotype as additional inherited risk factor for deep vein thrombosis in individuals with a high-risk profile. *Thrombosis and Haemostasis,*Vol.87, No.1, (January 2002), pp. 32–36, ISSN 0340-6245

Maroney, SA. & Mast, AE. (2008). Expression of tissue factor pathway inhibitor by endothelial cells and platelets. *Transfusion and Apheresis Science,* Vol.38, No.1, (February 2008), pp. 9-14, ISSN 1473-0502

Martinelli, I.; Battaglioli, T.; Bucciarelli, P.; Passamonti, SM. & Mannucci, PM. (2004). Risk factors and recurrence rate of primary deep vein thrombosis of the upper extremities. *Circulation,* Vol.110, No.5, (August 2004), pp. 566-570, ISSN 0009-7322

Mazoyer, E.; Ripoll, L.; Gueguen, R.; Tiret, L.; Collet, JP.; dit Sollier, CB.; Roussi, J.; Drouet, L. & FITENAT Study Group. (2009). Prevalence of factor V Leiden and prothrombin G20210A mutation in a large French population selected for nonthrombotic history: geographical and age distribution. *Blood Coagulation and Fibrinolysis,* Vol.20, No.7, (October 2009), pp. 503-510, ISSN 0957-5235

Mehta, R. & Shapiro, AD. (2008). Plasminogen deficiency. *Haemophilia,* 14, 6, 1261-1268, ISSN 1351-8216

Meijers, JC.; Tekelenburg, WL.; Bouma, BN.; Bertina, RM. & Rosendaal, FR. (2000). High levels of coagulation factor XI as a risk factor for venous thrombosis. *New England Journal of Medicine,* ol.342, No.10, (Mars 2000), pp. 696-701, ISSN 0028-4793

Mekaj, Y.; Zhubi, B.; Hoxha, H.; Belegu, R.; Mekaj, A.; Miftari, E. & Belegu, M. (2009). Prevalence of resistence to activated protein C (APC-resistance) in blood donors in Kosovo. *Bosnian Journal of Basic Medical Science,* Vol.9, No.4, (November 2009), pp. 329-334, ISSN 1512-8601

Melichart, M.; Kyrle, PA.; Eichnger, S.; Rintelen, C.; Mannhalter, C. & Pabinger, I. (1996). Thrombotic tendency in 75 symptomatic, unrelated patients with APC resistance. *Wiener Klinische Wochenschrift,* Vol.108, No.19, pp. 607-610, ISSN 0043-5325

Meltzer ME, Lisman T, Doggen CJ, de Groot PG & Rosendaal FR. (2008). Synergistic effects of hypofibrinolysis and genetic and acquired risk factors on the risk of a first venous thrombosis. *PLoS Medicine,* Vol.5, No.5, (May 2008), pp. e97, ISSN 1549-1277

Meltzer, ME.; Lisman, T.; de Groot, PG.; Meijers, JC.; le Cessie, S.; Doggen, CJ. & Rosendaal, FR. (2010a). Venous thrombosis risk associated with plasma hypofibrinolysis is explained by elevated plasma levels of TAFI and PAI-1. *Blood,* Vol.116, No.1, (July 2010), pp. 113-121, ISSN 0006-4971

Meltzer, ME.; Bol, L.; Rosendaal, FR.; Lisman, T. & Cannegieter, SC. (2010b). Hypofibrinolysis as a risk factor for recurrent venous thrombosis; results of the LETS follow-up study. *Journal of Thrombosis and Haemostasis,* Vol.8, No.3, (Mars 2010), pp. 605-607, ISSN 1538-7933

Meyer, G.; Emmerich, J.; Helley, D.; Arnaud, E.; Nicaud, V.; Alhenc-Gelas, M.; Aiach, M.; Fischer, A.; Sors, H. & Fiessinger, JN. (2001). Factors V leiden and II 20210A in patients with symptomatic pulmonary embolism and deep vein thrombosis. *American Journal of Medicine,*Vol.110, No.1, (January 2001), pp. 12-15, ISSN 0002-9343

Miesbach, W.; Scharrer, I.; Henschen, A.; Neerman-Arbez, M.; Spitzer, S. & Galanakis, D. (2010). Inherited dysfibrinogenemia: clinical phenotypes associated with five different fibrinogen structure defects. *Blood Coagulation and Fibrinolysis,* Vol.21, No.1, (January 2010), pp. 35-40, ISSN 0957-5235

Mikovic, D.; Rakicevic, L.; Kovac, M. & Radojkovic, D. (2000). Prevalence of factor V Leiden mutation in Yugoslav thrombophilic patients and its relationship to the laboratory diagnosis of APC resistance. *Thrombosis and Haemostasis,* Vol.84, No.4, (October 2000), pp. 723-724, ISSN 0340-6245

Miletich, J.; Sherman, L. & Broze, G. (1987). Absence of thrombosis in subjects with heterozygous protein C deficiency. *New England Journal of Medicine,* Vol.317, No.16, (October 1987), pp. 991-996, ISSN 0028-4793

Miljić, P.; Heylen, E.; Willemse, J.; Djordjević, V.; Radojković, D.; Colović, M.; Elezović, I. & Hendriks, D. (2010). Thrombin activatable fibrinolysis inhibitor (TAFI): a molecular link between coagulation and fibrinolysis. *Srpski arhiv za celokupno lekarstvo,*Vol.138, No.Suppl 1, (January 2010), pp. 74-78, ISSN 0370-8179

Mishra, MN. & Bedi, VS. (2010). Prevalence of common thrombophilia markers and risk factors in Indian patients with primary venous thrombosis. *Sao Paulo Medical Journal,* Vol.128, No.5, (2010), pp. 263-267, ISSN 1516-3180

Mohanty, D.; al Hassan, H.; Neglen, P.; Eklof, BO. & Das, KC. (1995). Protein C Deficiency in Kuwait. *Journal of Laboratory and Clinical Medicine,* Vol.126, No.4, (October 1995), pp. 373-376, ISSN 0022-2143

Mosnier, LO. & Bouma, BN. (2006). Regulation of fibrinolysis by thrombin activatable fibrinolysis inhibitor, an unstable carboxypeptidase B that unites the pathways of coagulation and fibrinolysis. *Arteriosclerosis, Thrombosis, and Vascular Biology,* Vol.26, No.11, (November 2006), pp. 2445-2453, ISSN 1079-5642

Mumford, AD.; McVey, JH.; Morse, CV.; Gomez, K.; Steen, M.; Norstrom, EA.; Tuddenham, EG.; Dahlbäck, B. & Bolton-Maggs, PH. (2003). Factor V I359T: a novel mutation associated with thrombosis and resistance to activated protein C. *British Journal of Haematology,* Vol.123, No.3, (November 2003), pp. 496-501, ISSN 0007-1048

Nagy, A.; Melegh, B. & Losonczy, H. (1997). Study of the Leiden mutation (factor VQ506), the most frequent cause of thrombophilia, in 116 thrombosis patients. *Orvosi Hetilap,* Vol.138, No.44, (November 1997), pp. 2797-2800, ISSN 0030-6002

Nasiruddin; Rehman, Z.; Anwar, M.; Ahmed, S.; Ayyub, M. & Ali, W. (2005). Frequency of factor V leiden mutation. *Journal of College of Physicians and Surgeons Pakistan,* Vo.15, No.1, (January 2005), pp. 15-17, ISSN 1022-386X

Novotny, WF.; Girard, TJ.; Miletich, JP. & Broze, GJ. (1989). Purification and characterization of the lipoprotein-associated coagulation inhibitor from human plasma. *The Journal of Biological Chemistry,* Vol.264, No.31, (November 1989), pp. 18832-18837, ISSN 0021-9258

Novotny, WF. (1994) Tissue factor pathway inhibitor. *Seminars in Thrombosis and Hemostasis,* Vol.20, No.1, (January 1994), pp. 101-108, ISSN 0094-6176

Nusier, MK.; Radaideh, AM.; Ababneh, NA.; Qaqish, BM.; Alzoubi, R.; Khader, Y.; Mersa, JY.; Irshaid, NM. & El-Khateeb, M. (2007). Prevalence of factor V G1691A (Leiden) and prothrombin G20210A polymorphisms among apparently healthy Jordanians. *Neuroendocrinology Letters,* Vol.28, No.5, (October 2007), pp. 699-703, ISSN 0172-780X

Obeidat, NM.; Awidi, A.; Sulaiman, NA. & Abu-Khader, IB. (2009). Thrombophilia-related genetic variations in patients with pulmonary embolism in the main teaching hospital in Jordan. *Saudi Medical Journal,*Vol.30, No.7, (July 2009), pp. 921-925, ISSN 0379-5284

O'Donnell, J.; Tuddenham, EG.; Manning, R.; Kemball-Cook, G.; Johnson, D. & Laffan, M. (1997). High prevalence of elevated factor VIII levels in patients referred for thrombophilia screening: role of increased synthesis and relationship to the acute phase reaction. *Thrombosis and Haemostasis,* Vol.77, No.5, (May 1997), pp. 825-828, ISSN 0340-6245

Oguzulgen, IK.; Yilmaz, E.; Demirtas, S.; Erkekol, FO.; Ekim, N.; Demir, N.; Numanoglu, N.; Ozel, D.; Ulu, A. & Akar, N. (2009). The role of plasminogen activator inhibitor-1 polymorphism, factor-V-Leiden, and prothrombin-20210 mutations in pulmonary thromboembolism. *Clinical and Applied Thrombosis/Hemostasis,* Vol.15, No.1, (February 2009), pp. 73-77, ISSN 1076-0296

O'Keeffe, DJ. & Baglin, TP. (2003). Travellers' thrombosis and economy class syndrome: incidence, aetiology and prevention. *Clinical and Laboratory Haematology*, Vol.25, No.5, (October 2003), pp. 277-281, ISSN 0141-9854

Olave, T.; Cornudella, R.; Homs, C.; Azaceta, G.; Tirado, I. & Gutierrez, M. (1998). Incidence and clinical manifestations of activated protein C resistance and factor V Leiden in young patients with venous thromboembolic disease in Spain. *Haematologica*, Vol.83, No.4, (April 1998), pp. 378-80, ISSN 0390-6078

Ozbek, U. & Tangün, Y. (1996). Frequency of factor V Leiden in Turkey. *International Journal of Hematology*,Vol.64, No.2, (May 1996), pp. 291-292, ISSN 0925-5710

Patnaik, MM. & Moll, S. (2008). Inherited antithrombin deficiency: a review. *Haemophilia*, Vol.14, No.6, (November 2008), pp. 1229-1239, ISSN 1351-8216

Patrassi, GM.; Sartori, MT.; Viero, ML.; Boscaro, M.; Boeri, G. & Girolami, A. (1991). Venous thrombosis and tissue plasminogen activator release deficiency: a family study. *Blood Coagulation and Fibrinolysis*, Vol.2, No.2, April 1991), pp. 231-235, ISSN 0957-5235

Pecheniuk, NM.; Morris, CP.; Walsh, TP. & Marsh, NA. (2001). The factor V HR2 haplotype: prevalence and association of the A4070G and A6755G polymorphisms. *Blood Coagulation and Fibrinolysis*,Vol.12, No.3, (April 2001), pp. 201–206, ISSN 0957-5235

Pepe, G.; Rickards, O.; Vanegas, OC.; Brunelli, T.; Gori, AM.; Giusti, B.; Attanasio, M.; Prisco, D.; Gensini, GF. & Abbate, R. (1997). Prevalence of factor V Leiden mutation in non-European populations. *Thrombosis and Haemostasis*,Vol.77, No.2, (February 1997), pp. 329-331, ISSN 0340-6245

Perry, DJ. & Pasi, KJ. (1997). Resistance to activated protein C and factor V Leiden. *Quarterly Journal of Medicine*, Vol.90, No.6, (June 1997), pp. 379-385, ISSN 1460-2725

Poort, SR.; Rosendaal, FR.; Reitsma, PH. & Bertina, RM. (1996). A common genetic variation in the 3'-untranslated region of the prothrombin gene is associated with elevated plasma prothrombin levels and an increase in venous thrombosis. *Blood*, Vol.88, No.10, (November 1996), pp. 3698-3703, ISSN 0006-4971

Rees, DC.; Cox, M. & Clegg, JB. (1995). World distribution of factor V Leiden. *The Lancet*, Vol.346, No.8983, (October 1995), pp. 1133-1134, ISSN 0140-6736

Ricart, JM.; Vayá, A.; Todolí, J.; Calvo, J.; Villa, P.; Estellés, A.; España, F.; Santaolaria, M.; Corella, D. & Aznar, J. (2006). Thrombophilic risk factors and homocysteine levels in Behçet's disease in eastern Spain and their association with thrombotic events. *Thrombosis and Haemostasis*, Vol.95, No.4, (April 2006), pp. 618-624, ISSN 0340-6245

Ridker, PM.; Miletich, JP.; Hennekens, CH. & Buring JE. (1997). Ethnic distribution of Factor V Leiden in 4047 men and women. Implications for venous thromboembolism screening. *Journal of American Medical Association, Vol.*277, No.16, (April 1997), pp. 1305-1307, ISSN 0098-7484

Ro, A.; Hara, M. & Takada, A. (1999). The Factor V Leiden and the Prothrombin G20210A mutation was not found in Japanese patients with pulmonary thromboembolism. *Thrombosis and Haemostasis*, Vol.82, No.6, (December 1999), pp. 1769, ISSN 0340-6245

Rock, G. & Wells, P. (1997). New concepts in coagulation. *Critical Reviews in Clinical Laboratory Sciences*, Vol.34, No.5, (October 1997), pp. 475-501, ISSN 1040-8363

Rosen, E.; Renbaum, P.; Heyd, J. & Levy-Lahad, E. (1999). High frequency of factor V Leiden in a population of Israeli Arabs. *Thrombosis and Haemostasis,* Vol.82, No.6, (December 1999), pp. 1768, ISSN 0340-6245

Rosing, J. & Tans, G. (1997). Coagulation factor V: an old star shines again. *Thrombosis and Haemostasis,* Vol.78, No.1, pp. 427-433, (July 1997), ISSN 0340-6245

Rosing, J.; Tans, G.; Nicolaes, GA.; Thomassen, MC.; van Oerle, R.; van der Ploeg, PM.; Heijnen, P.; Hamulyak, K. & Hemker, HC. (1997). Oral contraceptives and venous thrombosis: different sensitivities to activated protein C in women using second and third-generation oral contraceptives. *British Journal of Haematology,* Vol.97, No.1, (April 1997), pp. 233-238, ISSN 0007-1048

Rotmensch, S.; Liberati, M.; Mittlemann, M. & Ben-Rafael, Z. (1997). Activated protein C resistance and adverse pregnancy outcome. *American Journal of Obstetrics & Gynecology,* Vol.177, No.1, (July 1997), pp. 170-173, ISSN ISSN 0002-9378

Roubey, RA. (1994). Autoantibodies to phospholipid-binding plasma proteins: a new view of lupus anticoagulants and other "antiphospholipid" autoantibodies. *Blood,* Vol.84, No.9, (November 1994), pp. 2854-2867, ISSN 0006-4971

Ruiz-Argüelles, GJ.; Garcés-Eisele, J.; Ruiz-Delgado, GJ. & Alarcón-Segovia, D. (1999). The G20210A polymorphism in the 3'-untranslated region of the prothrombin gene in Mexican mestizo patients with primary antiphospholipid syndrome. *Clinical and Applied Thrombosis/Hemostasis,* Vol.5, No. 3, (Ju;y 1999), 158-160, ISSN 1076-0296

Ruiz-Argüelles, GJ.; Garcés-Eisele, J.; Reyes-Núñez, V. & Ramírez-Cisneros, FJ. (2001). Primary thrombophilia in Mexico. II. Factor V G1691A (Leiden), prothrombin G20210A, and methylenetetrahydrofolate reductase C677T polymorphism in thrombophilic Mexican mestizos. *American Journal of Hematology,*Vol.66, No.1, (January 2001), pp. 28-31, ISSN 1096-8652

Samama, MM.; Simon, D.; Horellou, MH.; Trossaërt, M.; Elalamy, I. & Conard, J. (1996). Diagnosis and clinical characteristics of inherited activated protein C resistance. *Haemostasis,* Vol.26, No.Suppl 4, (October 1996), pp. 315-330, ISSN 0301-0147

Schröder, W.; Koesling, M.; Wulff, K.; Wehnert, M. & Herrmann, FH. (1996). Large-scale screening for factor V Leiden mutation in a north-eastern German population. *Haemostasis,* Vol.26, No.5, (September 1996), pp. 233-236, ISSN 0301-0147

Schuster, V.; Hügle, B. & Tefs, K. (2007). Plasminogen deficiency. *Journal of Thrombosis and Haemostasis,* Vol.5, No.12, (December 2007), pp.2315-2322, ISSN 1538-7933

Seligsohn, U. & Lubetsky, A. (2001). Genetic susceptibility to venous thrombosis. *New England Journal of Medicine,* Vol.344, No.16, (April 2001), pp. 1222–1231, ISSN 0028-4793

Simioni, P.; Scudeller, A.; Radossi, P.; Gavasso, S.; Girolami, B.; Tormene, D. & Girolami, A. (1996). "Pseudo Homozygous" activated protein C resistance due to double heterozygous factor V defects (factor V Leiden mutation and type I quantitave factor V defect) associated with thrombosis: Report of two cases belonging to two unrelated kinders. *Thrombosis and Haemostasis,* Vol.75, No.3, (Mars 1996), pp. 422-426, ISSN 0340-6245.

Simioni, P.; Prandoni, P.; Lensing, AW.; Scudeller, A.; Sardella, C.; Prims, MH.; Villatta, S.; Dazzi, F. & Girolami, A. (1997). The risk of recurrent venous thromboembolism in patients with an Arg506 → G mutation in the gene for factor V (factor V Leiden).

New England Journal of Medicine, Vol.336, No.6, (February 1997), pp. 399-403, ISSN 0028-4793

Simkova, M.; Batorova, A.; Dostalova, K.; Pozgayova, S.; Simko, F. & Kovacs, L. (2004). Factor V Leiden in patients with venous thrombosis in Slovak population. *General Physiology and Biophysics,* Vol.23, No. 4, (December 2004), pp. 435-442, ISSN 0231-5882

Simmonds, RE.; Ireland, H.; Lane, DA.; Zöller, B.; de Frutos, PG. & Dahlbäck, B. (1998). Clarification of the risk for venous thrombosis associated with hereditary protein S deficiency by investigation of a large kindred with a charaterized gene defect. *Annals of Internal Medicine,* Vol.128, No.1, (January 1998), pp. 8-14, ISSN 0003-4819

Song, KS.; Lee, SM. & Choi, JR. (2003). Detection of an Ala601Thr mutation of plasminogen gene in 3 out of 36 Korean patients with deep vein thrombosis. *Journal of Korean Medical Science,* Vol.18, No.2, (April 2003), pp. 167-170, ISSN 1011-8934

Sottilotta, G,l Mammì, C.; Furlò, G.; Oriana, V.; Latella, C. & Trapani Lombardo, V. (2009). High incidence of factor V Leiden and prothrombin G20210A in healthy southern Italians. *Clinical and Applied Thrombosis/Hemostasis,* Vol.15, No.3, (May-June 2009), pp. 356-359, ISSN 1076-0296

Stankovics, J.; Melegh, B.; Nagy, A.; Kis, A.; Molnar, J.; Losonczy, H.; Schuler, A. & Kosztolanyi, G. (1998). Incidence of factor V G1681A (Leiden) mutation in samplings from the Hungarian population. *Orvosi Hetilap,* Vol.139, No.19, (May 1998), pp. 1161-1163, ISSN 0030-6002

Svensson, PJ. & Dahlbäck, B. (1994). Resistance to activated protein C as a basis for venous thrombosis. *New England Journal of Medicine,* Vol.330, No.8, (February 1994), pp. 517-522, ISSN 0028-4793

Taher, A.; Khalil, I.; Shamseddine, A.; El-Ahdab, F. & Bazarbachi, A. (2001). High prevalence of Factor V Leiden mutation among healthy individuals and patients with deep venous thrombosis in Lebanon: is the eastern Mediterranean region the area of origin of this mutation? *Thrombosis and Haemostasis,* Vol.86, No.2, (August 2001), pp. 723-724, ISSN 0340-6245

Tait, RC.; Walker, ID.; Perry, DJ.; Carrell, RW.; Islam, SIA.; McCall, F.; Milchell, R. & Davidson, JF. (1991). Prevalence of antithrombin III deficiency subtypes in 4,000 healthy blood donors. *Thrombosis and Haemostasis,* Vol.65, No.6, (December 1991), pp. 839, ISSN 0340-6245

Tait, RC.; Walker, ID.; Reitsma, PH.; Islam, SI.; McCall, F.; Poort, SR.; Conkie, JA. & Bertina, RM. (1995). Prevalence of protein C deficiency in the healthy population. *Thrombosis and Haemostasis,*Vol.73, No.1, (January 1995), pp. 87-93, ISSN 0340-6245

Tamim, H.; Finan, RR. & Almawi, WY. (2002). Prevalence of two thrombophilia predisposing mutations: factor V G1691A (R506Q; Leiden) and prothrombin G20210A, among healthy Lebanese. *Thrombosis and Haemostasis,* Vol.88, No.4, (October 2002), pp. 691-692, ISSN 0340-6245

ten Kate, MK. & van der Meer, J. (2008). Protein S deficiency: a clinical perspective. *Haemophilia,* Vol.14, No.6, (November 2008), pp. 1222-1228, ISSN 1351-8216

Tollefsen, DM. & Blank, MK. (1981). Detection of a new heparin-dependent inhibitor of thrombin in human plasma. *Journal of Clinical Investigation,* Vol.68, No.3, (September 1981), pp. 589-596, ISSN 0021-9738

Tollefsen, DM.; Majerus, DW. & Blank, MK. (1982). Heparin cofactor II. Purification and properties of a heparin-dependent inhibitor of thrombin in human plasma. *Journal of Biological Chemistry,* Vol.257, No.5, (March 1982), pp. 2162-2169, ISSN 0021-9258

van Boven, HH.; Reitsma, PH.; Rosendaal, FR.; Bayston, TA.; Chowdhury, V.; Bauer, KA.; Scharrer, I.; Conard, J. & Lane DA. (1996). Factor V Leiden (FV R506Q) in families with inherited antithrombin deficiency. *Thrombosis and Haemostasis,* Vol.75, No.3, (Mars 1996), pp. 417-421 ISSN 0340-6245

Vargas, M.; Soto, I.; Pinto, CR.; Urgelles, MF.; Batalla, A.; Rodriguez-Reguero, J.; Cortina, A.; Alvarez, V. & Coto, E. (1999). The prothrombin 20210A allele and the factor V Leiden are associated with venous thrombosis but not with early coronary artery disease. *Blood Coagulation and Fibrinolysis,* Vol.10, No.1, (January 1999), pp. 39-41, ISSN 0957-5235

Vizcaino, G.; Torres, E.; Quintero, J.; Herrmann, F.; Grimm, R.; Diez-Ewald, M.; Arteaga-Vizcaino, M.; Perez-Requejo, JL. & Colina-Araujo, J. (2000), Prevalence of the activated protein C resistance in indigenous and Black populations of the western Venezuela. *Investigación Clínica,* Vol.41, No.1, (March 2000), pp. 29-36, ISSN 0535-5133

Vossen, CY.; Hoffmeister, M.; Chang-Claude, JC.; Rosendaal, FR. & Brenner, H. (2011). Clotting factor gene polymorphisms and colorectal cancer risk. *Journal of Clinical Oncology,* Vol.29, No.13, (May 2011), pp. 1722-1727, ISSN 0732-183X

Walker, FJ. & Fay, PJ. (1992). Regulation of blood coagulation by the protein C system. *The Journal of the Federation of American Societies for Experimental Biology,* Vol.6, No.8, (May 1992), 2561-2567, ISSN 0892-6638

Warshawsky, I.; Hren, C.; Sercia, L.; Shadrach, B.; Deitcher, SR.; Newton, E. & Kottke-Marchant, K. (2002). Detection of a novel point mutation of the prothrombin gene at position 20209. *Diagnostic Molecular Pathology,* Vol.11, No.3, (September 2002), pp. 152-156, ISSN 1052-9551

Williamson, D.; Brown, K.; Luddington, R.; Baglin, C. & Baglin, T. (1998). Factor V Cambridge: a new mutation (Arg306-->Thr) associated with resistance to activated protein C. *Blood,* Vol.91, No.4, (February 1998), pp 1140-1144, ISSN 0006-4971.

Wu, Q. & Zhao, Z. (2002). Inhibition of PAI-1: a new anti-thrombotic approach. *Current Drug Targets - Cardiovascular and Hematological Disorders,* Vol.2, No.1, (June 2002), pp. 1, 27-42, ISSN 1568-0061

Yan, SB. & Nelson, DR. (2004). Effect of factor V Leiden polymorphism in severe sepsis and on treatment with recombinant human activated protein C. *Critical Care Medicine,* Vol.32, No.5 Suppl, (May 2004), pp. S239-246, ISSN 0090-3493

Zabalegui, N.; Montes, R.; Orbe, J.; Ayape, ML.; Medarde, A.; Páramo, JA. & Rocha, E. (1998). Prevalence of FVR506Q and prothrombin 20210A mutations in the Navarrese population. *Thrombosis and Haemostasis,* Vol.80, No.3, (Septemebr 1998), pp. 522-523, ISSN 0340-6245

Zahed, LF.; Rayes, RF.; Mahfouz, RA.; Taher, AT.; Maarouf, HH. & Nassar, AH. (2006). Prevalence of factor V Leiden, prothrombin and methylene tetrahydrofolate reductase mutations in women with adverse pregnancy outcomes in Lebanon. *American Journal of Obstetrics & Gynecology,*Vol.195, No.4, (October 2006), pp. 1114-1118, ISSN 0002-9378

Zama, T.; Murata, M.; Ono, F.; Watanabe, K.; Watanabe, R.; Moriki, T.; Yokoyama, K.; Tokuhira M, & Ikeda, Y. (1996). Low prevalence of activated protein C resistance and coagulation factor V Arg506 to Gln mutation among Japanese patients with various forms of thrombosis, and normal individuals. *International Journal of Hematology,* Vol.65, No.1, (December 1996), pp. 71-78, ISSN 0925-5710

Zivelin, A.; Griffin, JH.; Xu, X.; Pabinger, I.; Samama, M.; Conard, J.; Brenner, B.; Eldor, A. & Seligsohn, U. (1997). A single genetic origin for a common Caucasian risk factor for venous thrombosis. *Blood,* Vol.89, No.2, (January 1997), pp. 397-402, ISSN 0006-4971

Zivelin, A.; Mor-Cohen, R.; Kovalsky, V.; Kornbrot, N.; Conard, J.; Peyvandi, F.; Kyrle, PA.; Bertina, R.; Peyvandi, F.; Emmerich, J. & Seligsohn, U. (2006). Prothrombin 20210G>A is an ancestral prothrombotic mutation that occurred in whites approximately 24,000 years ago. *Blood,* Vol.107, No.12, (June 2006), pp. 4666-4668, ISSN 0006-4971

Zöller, B.; Svensson, PJ.; He, X. & Dahlbäck, B. (1994). Identification of the same factor V gene mutation in 47 out of 50 thrombosis-prone families with inherited resistance to activated protein C. *Journal of Clinical Investigation,* Vol.94, No.6, (December 1994), pp. 2521-2524, ISSN 0021-9738

Zöller, B.; Hillarp, A. & Dahlbäck, B. (1997). Activated protein C resistance caused by a common factor V mutation has a single origin. *Thrombosis Research,* Vol.85, No.3, (February 1997), pp. 237-243, ISSN 0049-3848

2

Venous Thrombosis in Behcet's Disease

Selda Pelin Kartal Durmazlar
Department of Dermatology, Ministry of Health Ankara Diskapi Yildirim Beyazit Education and Research Hospital, Ankara, Turkey

1. Introduction

Behcet's Disease (BD) is manifested by a triad of relapsing hypopyon uveitis, aphthous stomatitis and genital ulcers. The disease initially described by a Turkish dermatologist Hulusi Behcet in 1937. The etiology and pathogenesis of Behçet's disease have not been fully clarified yet. However, it is now recognized as a multisystemic, immunoinflammatory disorder involving vessels of all sizes. The disease is most prevalent in the Mediterranean countries, Middle East, and Japan but has a worldwide distribution (Durmazlar et al., 2009; Kartal Durmazlar et al., 2008a).

2. History and diagnosis

The disease, currently known all over the world as "Behçet disease", "Behçet syndrome", "Behçet's triad", "Morbus Behçet" or "Tri-symptom Behçet" was first recognized by Dr. Hulusi Behçet (1889-1948) with a patient in 1924 (Tuzun, 2006; Ustun, 2002; Kartal Durmazlar & Kandi, 2011). This patient, who had been examined because of eye disturbances, recurrent oral and genital ulcers both in Istanbul and Vienna for 40 years, was given several diagnoses. Some doctors thought of tuberculosis or syphilis while some other doctors said a microorganism which was not present in Europe might have caused the disease. Hulusi Behçet, who continued to examine the patient after his loss of vision, thought that the causative agent was a virus. In the next several years he met two more patients with similar to that was seen in the previous patient. Hulusi Behçet thought the symptoms of these three patients were the symptoms of a new disease and reported his ideas on this topic firstly in 1936, in the Journal of Skin and Venereal Diseases (Tuzun, 2006; Ustun, 2002; Kartal Durmazlar & Kandi, 2011; Saylan, 1997). Later, in 1937 he wrote clear examples of symptomatic triad, which are still used as criterias worlwide for diagnosis of Behçet's disease, in Dermatologische Wochenschrift. In the same year at the meeting of the Society of Paris Dermatology he declared that several factors may cause the etiology of the disease, which still can be an acceptable statement. Later he diagnosed further patients and published in German as "Tri-Symptomenkomplex" in 1939, and in English as "Triple symptom complex" in 1940 (Tuzun, 2006; Ustun, 2002; Kartal Durmazlar & Kandi, 2011; Saylan, 1997; Evereklioglu, 2006). In subsequent years, this unique disorder drew the attention, and the term "Behçet syndrome" was first used by Jensen in 1941 (Jensen, 1941). The term "Behçet disease" was first used by Fiegenbaum and Kornblueth in 1946 (Kartal Durmazlar & Kandi, 2011; Figenbaum, 1946; Dilsen, 1996; Alpsoy, 2009). On 13 September

1947, international dermatologic societies came together in Zurich and named the disease as "Morbus Behçet", which honored the first describer of "triple symptom complex" after Zurich Medical Faculty Professor Mischner's proposal. In fact, several authors before Hulusi Behçet described one or several individual findings of this disorder. Among these physicians, for example, Hippocrates in the fifth century BC reported some individual symptoms attributed to an originally endemic and epidemic disease. But, due to sporadic appereance of the disease in the course of time, the disease became less significant and was forgotten. There were also other physicians who described one or several individual findings of this disorder, for example, Janin (1772), Reis (1906), Blüthe (1908), Gilbert (1920, 1921, 1923), Planner and Remenowsky (1922), Weve (1923), Shigeta (1924), Adamantiades (1930), Dascalopoulos (1932), Whitwell (1934), Nishimura (1936), Blobner (1937) reported several individual findings of this disorder. However, all these papers ascribed the findings either to another disease, such as tuberculosis, syphilis, sepsis or allergy, or to a coincidence and none of them indicated a new or a single syndrome with "classical triad" (Kartal Durmazlar & Kandi, 2011; Alpsoy 2009; Evereklioglu, 2006, 2007a, 2007b, 2007c; Freigenbaum, 1956). The disease is sometimes named as Adamantiades-Behcet's disease, however, Behcet's disease should be preferred as suggested by International Associations and Societies of "Behcet" (Mendes et al., 2009).

Several diagnostic criteria have been developed during the years, all have in common the 3 major features of oral ulceration, genital ulceration and eye lesion (16). Today, International Study Group criteria for the diagnosis of Behcet's disease is used worldwide (Table 1) (International Study Group diagnostic criteria, 1990.).

Recurrent oral ulceration	Minor aphthous, major aphthous, or herpetiform ulceration observed by physician or patient recurring at least three times in one 12-month period
	Plus any two of the following:
Recurrent genital ulceration	Aphthous ulceration or scarring, observed by physician or patient
Eye lesions	Anterior uveitis, posterior uveitis, cells in the vitreous on slit-lamp examination; or retinal vasculitis observed by ophthalmologist
Skin lesions	Erythema nodosum observed by the physician or patient, pseudofolliculitis, papulopustular lesions; or acneiform nodules observed by physician in post adolescent patients not on corticosteroids treatment
Pathergy	Read by physician at 24-48 hours (The test is performed by introducing a 20-gauge or smaller sterile needle 5 mm obliquely into the patient's flexor aspect of the avascular forearm skin without injection of saline under sterile conditions. The test is considered positive if there is an indurated erythematous small papule or pustule formation of more than 2 mm in diameter.

*Findings applicable only in the absence of other clinical explanations

Table 1. International Study Group diagnostic criteria, 1990.

As a systemic disease, Behcet's disease involves visceral organs also such as the gastrointestinal tract, pulmonary, musculoskeletal, and neurological systems (Table 2) (Evereklioglu, 2005).

Manifestations	Characteristics
Articular manifestations	Non-migratory monoarthritis or oligoarthritis, rarely polyarthritis, characterized by non-specific inflammatory-type synovitis. Favors large joints such as the knee (most commonly), ankle, wrist, and elbow as well as proximal interphalangeal and metacarpophalangeal joints. Spinal and sacroiliac involvements are uncommon. *Symptoms and signs:* arthralgia, tenderness, swelling, limitation of joint movement, warmth, morning stiffness, and redness at the articular site
Audio-vestibular features	Inner ear involvement cochlear and peripheral vestibular disturbances, tinnitus, deafness, dizziness, unilateral or bilateral sensorineural hearing, orthostatic disequilibrium
Thoracic involvement	Aorta and pulmonary artery aneurysms, infarct and hemorrhage, pleural effusion, pulmonary thromboembolism, tracheobronchial ulcerations, pneumonitis, mediastinitis, paranchymal fibrosis, arteriobronchial fistula, cor pulmonale, hilar and mediastinal lymphadenopathy, and lobular perfusion defects. *Symptoms:* hemoptysis, cough, dyspnea, and pleuritic chest pain
GIS involvement	Ulcerative lesions especially terminal ileum, cecum, occasionally in esophagus and stomach. *Symptoms:* anorexia, dysphagia, dyspepsia, vomiting, flatulence, vague abdominal discomfort, distention and pain, bloating, and diarrhea. Perforation can occur and malabsorbtion is common
Vascular involvement	Superficial and deep obliterative thrombophlebitis in lower extremity, varices, embolization, infarction, bleeding ulcers. Veins are affected more frequently than arteries. Large vessel thromboses in superior and inferior vena cava with a caput medusa, deep femoral and subclavian veins can occur. Occasionally, aorta, carotid, and popliteal aneurysms, radial artery occlusion, and thromboses of the hepatic (Budd-Chiari syndrome), mesenteric, pulmonary, iliac and renal veins with intracranial hypertension, mesenteric artery aneurysm
Cardiac involvement	Coronary artery disease, myocardial infarction, endocarditis, myocarditis, pericarditis, aortitis, valvular disease (aortic/mitral regurgitation), intracardiac thrombus, endomyocardial fibrosis, arrhythmia
Renal involvement	Microscopic hematuria and proteinuria (microalbuminuria) with normal renal functions, or rapidly progressive anti-neutrophylic antibody-associated vasculitis, cresentic or proliferative glomerulonephritis (focal segmental or sclerosing, diffuse or mesangial), IgA nephritis, renal vein thrombosis, amyloidosis, nephrotic syndrome, renal failure

Genitourinary involvement	Inflammation of the testis, typically epididymitis with painful swelling or uncommonly orchiepididymitis, urethritis, cystitis, voiding dysfunction
CNS involvement	5–10% of patients are affected. Focal or multifocal parenchymal , peripheral or CNS involvement with both motor and sensory manifestations, migraine-like headache (most frequent initial sign), hemiparesis, behavioral changes, stiff neck, pyramidal and extrapyramidal signs, cerebellar ataxia, cerebral vein thrombosis, isolated cerebral sinus thrombosis, cranial nerve palsies, peripheral neuropathy, seizures, benign intracranial hypertension, life-threatening brainstem and spinal cord lesions, aseptic meningitis, chronic meningoencephalitis, multiple sclerosis-like illness, organic confusional syndrome, acute myelitis, aneurysms, stroke, and pseudo-tumor cerebri.
Psychosomatic status	Character disorders, aggressiveness, anxiety, depression, dementia, cognitive deficits, memory disturbances, impairment in acquisition/information storage, personality change, attention deficit, bipolar disorder, and chorea

CNS _ central nervous system; GIS _ gastrointestinal system.

Table 2. Additional Systemic Features of Behcet Disease (From Evereklioglu, 2005).

3. Vascular involvement in Behcet's disease

Vasculo-Behcet Disease (VBD), which involves the arterial and venous system, is found in 15-38% of patients with BD. Three major manifestations of VBD have been identified: venous occlusion, arterial occlusion and aneurysm formation, with a clear preponderance of the venous lesions compared to arterial involvement. The coexistence of arterial and venous involvement is not frequent and is one of the major causes of morbidity and mortality. Venous involvement, including superficial thromboflebitis and deep venous thrombosis, is a characteristic manifestation. Thrombosis of superficial and deep vein is more frequent than arterial aneurism and thrombotic occlusions (Kartal Durmazlar et al., 2008a, 2009; Houman et al., 2001; Aksoy et al., 2010). Venous thrombosis appeared to be the major vascular involvement reported in 7 to 33% of cases with BD with a male predominance, and representing 85 to 93% of VBD (Houman et al., 2001). Deep vein thrombosis is seen in about one-fifth of Turkish patients with BD (Gul et al., 1999). Lower extremities is the most frequent site of thromboses but thromboses of other venous sites such as superior and inferior vena cava, coronary, portal, renal and pulmonary veins have been identified (Houman et al., 2001; La Regina et al., 2010). Leg ulcers in BD, which may be caused by vasculitis or deep vein thrombosis, have a chronic recurrent course and are refractory to treatment (Jung et al., 2008; Kartal Durmazlar et al, 2008b; Akgul & Kartal Durmazlar, 2008).

4. Pathogenesis of Behcet's disease and thrombosis

The main pathology in BD is an inflammatory process of small arteries and veins and thrombosis as a result of vasculitis of the vaso vasorum (Evereklioglu et al., 2002).

Histopathological studies revealed cellular infiltrations consisting of lymphocytes, plasmocytes, monocytes and PMN in varying degrees, depending on the stage of lesion in BD. Since cytokines are involved in the regulation of functions of lymphocytes and phagocytes, they are playing important role in the pathogenesis of the disease (Durmazlar et al, 2009). Chemotactic and phagocytic activity of neutrophils in patients with BD has been reported to be high (19). Increased spontaneous secretion of Tumor necrotizing factor (TNF-α), Interleukin-6 (IL-6) and Interleukin-8 (IL-8) in monocyte cultures obtained from BD patients have been reported (Mege et al., 1993). IL-8 secretion after incubation of human dermal microvascular endothelial cells with serum of BD patients indicates that chemotaxis is an initial process of inflammation. IL-8 upregulates neutrophil chemotaxis as mRNA expression have been reported to be more prominent in patients with active BD than in patients with inactive disease (Evereklioglu, 2005). IL-8, a major chemokine known as neutrofil activating factor, attract and activate leukocytes has been assumed to represent such a notable link between immune system activation and endothelial alterations in BD (Durmazlar et al., 2009; Evereklioglu, 2005; Tursen, 2009). It has been suggested that Th1 type cytokines and chemokines including IL-17, largely produced by activated $CD4^+$ and $CD8^+$ T cells, are involved in the recruitment of neutrophils to the site of inflammation. Activated neutrophils in BD patients produce significant quantities of IL-12 and IL-18 (Pay et al., 2007).

The pathogenesis of thrombotic events in BD is not fully understood. The primary abnormalities of the coagulation, anticoagulation, or fibrinolytic systems have not been confirmed yet in BD. The main factor responsible for the increased frequency of thrombosis in BD is thought to be endothelial dysfunction caused by vascular inflammation (Evereklioglu, 2005). There is accumulating evidence for inflammation markers as a result of thrombosis. Deep vein thrombosis significantly associates with the male gender and a positive pathergy test (Houman et al., 2001). A number of studies have explored the pathogenesis of thrombophilia in Behçet's disease. Neither deficiency in protein C, in protein S, in factor V Leiden and in antithrombin III nor resistance to activated protein C and anticardiolipin antibody levels seem to be correlated with vascular thrombosis in Behçet's disease (Houman et al., 2001; Espinosa et al., 2002; Hirohata & Kikuchi, 2003). In BD, there is an occlusive inflammatory thrombus formation, strictly adherent to inflamed vessel wall, which is typically not complicated with thromboembolism (Lakhanpal et al., 1985; Kobayashi et al., 2000; Matsumoto et al., 1991). There are increased thrombin generation, fibrinolysis, and thrombomodulin in Behçet's disease, but these abnormalities are not related to thrombosis (Espinosa et al., 2002). These results therefore suggest that thrombophilia in Behçet's disease may be related more to inflammation than to clotting disorder (Hirohata & Kikuchi, 2003). Studies have disclosed the occurrence of antiendothelial cell antibodies, increased E-selectin and myeloperoxydase expression in Behçet's disease (Houman et al., 2001; Espinosa et al., 2002; Hirohata & Kikuchi, 2003). As neutrophils from active Behçet's disease release increased amounts of myeloperoxydase, it is probable that neutrophil activation as well as the expression of antiendothelial cell antibodies may play an important role in the development of endothelial inflammatory damages, leading to thrombophilia (Houman et al., 2001; Espinosa et al., 2002; Hirohata & Kikuchi, 2003). Figure 1 summarizes the immunopathogenesis of Behcet's disease (Pay et al., 2007).

Homocysteine (Hcy) is an intermediary sulphydryl-containing aminoacid formed during the conversion of methionine to cysteine. Its sulphydryl group can cause direct endothelial cytotoxicity, inhibition of glutathione peroxidase and nitric oxide, interference with clotting

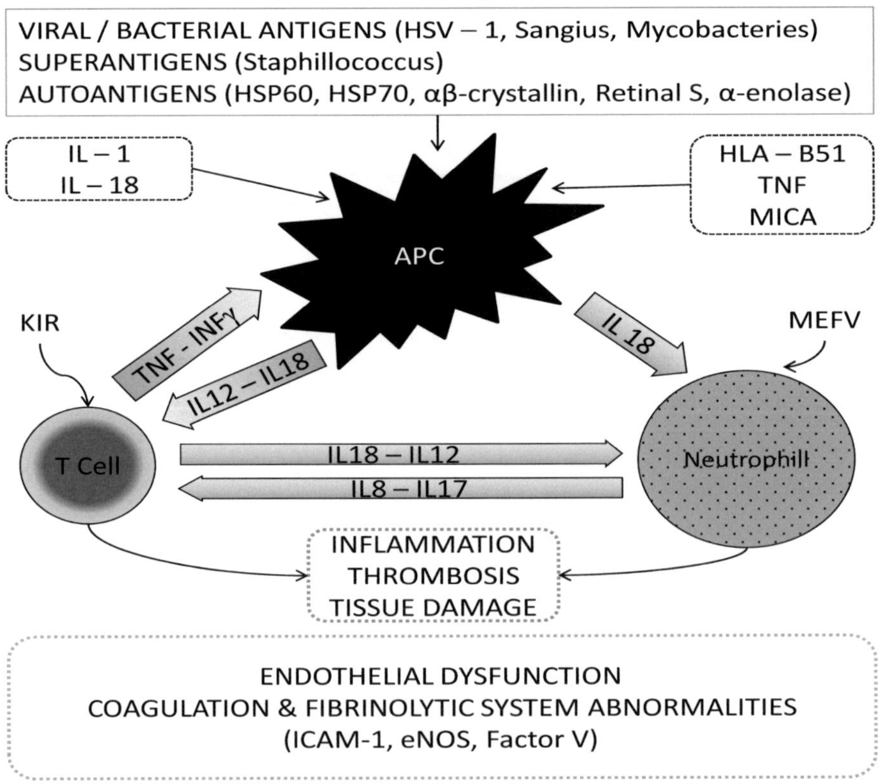

APC: Antigen presenting cell, MICA: MHC class I related gene, eNOS: Endothial NO synthetase, ICAM-1: intracellular adhesion molecule-1

Fig. 1. Immunopathogenesis of Behcet's disease (From Pay et al., 2007).

factor, and LDL oxidation (Kartal Durmazlar et al., 2008a, 2009). The association between Hcy levels and endothelial dysfunction and its correlation to the degree of endothelial damage have been shown in patients with BD. Hcy is thought to induce proinflammatory cytokines. Suggested mechanisms of Hcy in promoting such a clotting cascade are the inactivation of protein C, activation of coagulation factor V, and inhibition of thrombomodulin (Kartal Durmazlar et al., 2008a, 2009). The increase in Hcy concentration in patients at risk for vascular disease is expressed as odds ratio and for venous thrombosis, this odds ratio is approximately 1.6. In a study, a change of 1 μmol/l in Hcy concentration was found to correspond to a risk ratio of 1.01 (Willems et al., 2006). A study reported that 5 μmol/l increase of Hcy was associated with a 60% and 27% increased risk of venous thrombosis in retrospective and prospective studies, respectively (Omar et al., 2007). The association between Hcy levels and endothelial dysfunction and its correlation to the degree of endothelial damage has been shown in patients with BD (Ozdemir et al., 2004). Hcy generates superoxide and hydrogen peroxide, both of which have been linked to endothelial damage (Er et al., 2002). Hcy-induced vascular problems are thought to be multifactorial, including direct Hcy damage to the endothelium, enhanced lipid peroxidation and increased platelet aggregation by the effects on the coagulation system (Er et al., 2002; Sarican et al., 2007). Hcy has been shown in vivo and in vitro to promote inflammatory process such as the adhesion of neutrophils to endothelial cells as well as the release of the inflammatory cytokine IL-8 and monocyte chemoattractant protein-1 (MPC-1) (Koga et al., 2002). Hcy was shown to enhance the cytokine-stimulated expression of endothelial cell adhesion molecules and monocyte and T-cell adhesion to endothelial cells (Koga et al., 2002). Hcy was shown to promote TNF-*a* mediated induction of vascular cell adhesion molecule-1 (VCAM-1) in endothelial cells (Silverman et al., 2002). Some studies have shown hyperhomocysteinemia as a correctable risk factor for thrombosis in BD (Kartal Durmazlar et al., 2008a, 2009; Omar et al., 2007; Ozdemir et al., 2004; Er et al., 2002; Sarican et al., 2007). In a recent work, thrombogenesis in BD is discussed through the concept of Virchow's triad of venous thrombosis (La Regina et al., 2010). Based on this concept; abnormal blood flow, abnormal vessel wall, abnormal blood constituents are presented in Table 3.

Blood flow abnormalities	Enhanced erythrocyte aggregation, increased fibrinogen, high blood viscosity Impaired microcirculation Turbulent blood flow at sites of venous varices and arterial aneurysms Arterial and venous occlusion
Abnormal vessel wall	Perivasculitis Endothelial dysfunction Venous varices Aneurysms and pseudoaneurysms
Abnormal blood constituents	Endothelial factors such as vWF, t-PA, thrombomodulin, NO, VEGF, endothelin-1 Procoagulant factors such as factor V Leiden and prothrombin mutations, hyperhomocystenemia, factors VIII, IX, lipoprotein a Factors of fibrinolysis such as PAI-1, t-PA Anticoagulant factors (protein C, S, Z, antithrombin)

vWF: von Willebrand factor, t-PA: tissue plasminogen activator, NO: nitric oxide, VEGF: vascular endothelial growth factor, PAI-1: the type-1 inhibitor of plasminogen activators, t-PA: tissue plasminogen activator

Table 3. Thrombogenesis in Behcet's Disease according to Virchow's triad of venous thrombosis (From La Regina et al., 2010).

5. Medical management of Behcet's disease

The choice of treatment is generally based on the clinical presentation and the site affected. Although the treatment has become much more effective in recent years, BD still associates with severe morbidity and considerable mortality. Therefore, the main aim of the treatment should be the prevention of irreversible organ damage, especially, during the early, active phase of the disease. Male sex and a younger age of onset have been reported to be associated with severe disease, which in case may require aggressive treatment (Alpsoy & Akman, 2009).Recently, a group of experts developed recommendations for the management of BD by combining the current evidence from controlled trials (Hatemi et al., 2008). The European League against Rheumatism (EULAR) recommendations are summarized in Table 4.

Eye disease	• Affecting the posterior segment: Azathioprine and local and systemic corticosteroids • If refractory eye involvement (retinal vasculitis or macular involvement): Cyclosporine A or infliximab in combination with azathioprine and corticosteroids or IFN-a alone or with corticosteroids
Major vessel disease*	• Acute deep vein thrombosis: Corticosteroids, azathioprine, cyclophosphamide or cyclosporine A • Thrombosis of the vena cava and Budd–Chiari syndrome: Cyclophosphamide • Pulmonary and peripheral arterial aneurysms: Cyclophosphamide and corticosteroids; surgery • Anticoagulants, antiplatelet and antifibrinolytic agents are not recommended (there are no controlled data on, or evidence of benefit from uncontrolled experience with anticoagulants, antiplatelet or antifibrinolytic agents in the management of deep vein thrombosis pulmonary embolism is rare and there is the risk of major bleeding in case there are concomitant pulmonary aneurysms)
Gastrointestinal involvement**	Sulfasalazine, corticosteroids, azathioprine, TNF-a antagonists or thalidomide; surgery
Articular involvement	Colchicine; IFN-a, azathioprine, TNF-a antagonists in resistant cases
CNS involvement***	• Parenchymal disease: Corticosteroids, IFN-a, azathioprine, cyclophosphamide, methotrexate, TNF-a antagonists • Dural sinus thrombosis: Corticosteroids • Cyclosporine should be avoided in case of neurological involvement due to neurotoxicity, unless necessary for intraocular inflammation.
Mucocutaneous involvement (oral, genital and skin lesions)	• Isolated lesions: Topical measures such as corticosteroids preparations, lidocaine gel, chlorhexidine, sucralfate suspension • Acne-like lesions: Topical measures as used in acne vulgaris • Erythema nodosum: Colchicines • Resistant cases: Azathioprine, IFNa and TNFa antagonists may be considered in resistant cases.

CNS: Central nervous system; IFN: Interferon; TNF: Tumour necrosis factor.
* There is no firm evidence to guide the management of major vessel disease in BD
** There is no evidence-based treatment that can be recommended for the management of gastrointestinal involvement of BD
*** There are no controlled data to guide the management of CNS involvement in BD

Table 4. EULAR recommendations for treatment of Behcet's disease (Hatemi et al., 2008)

6. Conclusion

The pathogenesis of thrombotic events in BD is not fully understood. The primary abnormalities of the coagulation, anticoagulation, or fibrinolytic systems have not been confirmed yet in BD. In this review current knowledge of venous thrombosis in BD are summarized. There is no agreement on the treatment of thrombosis in BD. However, in general immunosuppressive agents such as corticosteroids, azathioprine, cyclophosphamide or cyclosporine are recommended for the treatment of venous thrombosis in BD. There is no enough evidence of benefit with anticoagulants or fibrinolytic agents in the management of thrombosis of BD (La Regina et al., 2010). Further studies are needed to clarify the safety and effectiveness of antithrombotic therapy in BD. However, owing to the complications of established thrombus, it would be reasonable to target different steps of the coagulation cascade for the prophylaxis and treatment of thrombosis in BD.

7. References

Akgul, A. & Kartal Durmazlar, SP. (2008). Medical treatment of venöz ulcers. *Turkiye Klinikleri Journal of Cardiovasc Surgery-Special Topics,* Vol.1, pp. 31-33

Aksoy, Y.; Ercan, A.; Dalmizrak, O.; Canpinar, H.; Kartal Durmazlar, SP. & Bayazit, M. (2010). The determination of matrix metalloproteinase 9 activity and gene expression levels in Behcet's disease patients with aneurismal complications. *Clinical Rheumatology,* DOI 10.1007/s10067-010-1559-1563

Alpsoy, E. & Akman, A., (2009). Behçet's disease: an algorithmic approach to its treatment. *Archives of Dermatological Research,* Vol.301, pp. 693-702

Alpsoy, E. (2009). Behcet's disease. *Turkderm,* Vol.43, Sup2, pp. 21-23

Dilsen, N. (1996). History and development of Behçet's disease. *Revue du Rhumatisme English Edition,* Vol.63, pp. 512-519

Durmazlar, SP.; Bahar Ulkar, G.; Eskioglu, F.; Tatlican, S.; Mert, A. & Akgul, A. (2009). Significance of serum interleukin-8 levels in patients with Behcet's disease: High levels may indicate vascular involvement. *International Journal of Dermatology,* Vol.48, No.3, pp. 259-264

Er, H.; Everekliogiu, C.; Cumurcu, T.; Türköz, Y.; Ozerol, E.; Sahin, K. & Doganay, S. (2002). Serum homocysteine level is increased and correlated with endothelin-1 and nitric oxide in Behçet's disease. *British Journal of Ophthalmology,* Vol.86, pp. 653–657

Espinosa, G.; Font, J.; Tassies, D.; Vidaller, A.; Deulofeu, R.; Lopez-Soto, A.; Cervera, R.; Ordinas, A.; Ingelmo, M. & Reverter, JC. (2002). Vascular involvement in Behcet's disease: relation with thrombophilic factors, coagulation activation, and thrombomodulin. *The American Journal of Medicine,* Vol.112, pp. 37-43

Everekliogiu, C.; Er, H.; Turkoz, Y. & Cekmen, M. (2002). Serum levels of TNF-alpha, sIL-2R, IL-6, and IL-8 are increased and associated with elevated lipid peroxidation in patients with Behcet's disease. *Mediators of Inflammation,* Vol.11, pp. 87-93

Everekliogiu, C. (2005). Current concepts in the etiology and treatment of Behcet Disease. *Survey of Ophthalmology,* Vol.50, pp. 297-350

Everekliogiu, C. (2006). Regarding neutrophil and lymphocyte responses to oral Streptococcus in Adamantiades-Behçet's disease. *FEMS Immunology and Medical Microbiology,* Vol.47, pp. 311-314

Everekliogiu, C. (2007a). The migration pattern, patient selection with diagnostic methodological flaw and confusing naming dilemma in Behçet disease. *European Journal of Echocardiography*, Vol.8, pp. 167-73

Everekliogiu, C. (2007b). Regarding the naming dilemma of Behçet disease in the 21st century. *Oral Diseases*, Vol.13, pp. 117-121

Everekliogiu, C. (2007c). The treatment schedule and historical naming process of Behçet disease. Journal of European Academy of Dermatology and Venereology, Vol.21, pp. 427-428

Everekliogiu, C. (2010). Behçet's disease or Adamantiades-Behçet disease? An evidence-based historical survey. *Medical Science Monitor*, Vol.16, pp.: RA136-142

Figenbaum, A. & Kornblueth, W. (1946). Behçet's disease as manifestation of a chronic septic condition connected with a constitutional disorder. With a report of 4 cases. *Acta Medical Orient*, Vol.5, pp. 139-151

Freigenbaum, A. (1956). Description of Behçet's syndrome in the Hippocratic third book of endemic diseases. *British Journal of Ophthalmology*, Vol.40, pp. 355-357

Gul, A.; Aslantas, AB.; Tekinay, T.; Konice, M. & Ozcelik, T. (1999). Procoagulant mutations and venous thrombosis in Behcet's disease. *Rheumatology*, Vol.38, pp. 1298-1299

Hatemi, G.; Silman, A.; Bang, D.; Bodaghi, B.; Chamberlain, AM.; Gul, A.et al; EULAR Expert Committee. (2008). EULAR recommendations for the management of Behçet disease. *Annals of the Rheumatic Diseases*, Vol.67, pp. 1656-1662.

Hirohata, S. & Kikuchi H. (2003). Behcet's disease. *Arthritis Research and Therapy*, Vol.5, pp. 139–146

Houman, MH.; Ben Ghorbel, I.; Khiari Ben Salah, I.; Lamloum, M.; Ben Ahmed, M. & Miled, M. (2001). Deep vein thrombosis in Behcet's disease. *Clinical and Experimental Rheumatology*, Vol.19, pp. 48-50

International study group for Behcet's disease. (1990). Criteria for diagnosis of Behcet's disease. *Lancet*, Vol,335, pp. 1078-1080

Jensen, T. (1941). Sur les ulcerations aphteuses de la muqueuse de la bouche et de la peau genitale combinees avec les symptomes oculaires (=Syndrome Behçet). *Acta Dermatology and Venereology*, Vol.22, pp. 64-79

Jung, JY.; Kim, DY. & Bang D. (2008). Leg ulcers in Behçet's disease. *British Journal of Dermatology*, Vol.158, pp. 172–203.

Kartal Durmazlar, SP.; Akgul, A.; Eskioglu, F. (2008a) Homocysteine may involve in the pathogenesis of Behcet's disease by inducing inflammation. *Mediators of Inflammmation* 2008: 407972, doi:10.1155/2008/407972

Kartal Durmazlar, SP.; Akgul, A. & Eskioglu, F. (2008b). Traditional wound care and wound dressings in venous ulcers. *Turkiye Klinikleri Journal of Cardiovasc Surgery-Special Topics*, Vol.1, pp. 59-64

Kartal Durmazlar, SP.; Akgul, A. & Eskioglu, F. (2009). B vitamin supplementation reduced serum homocysteine and interleukin-6 levels in patients with Behcet's disease with acute venous thrombosis: A prospective controlled study. *Turkiye Klinikleri Journal of Medical Science*, Vol.29, pp. 361-366

Kartal Durmazlar, SP. & Kandi, B. (2011). Naming dilemma of Behcet's disease. *Journal of Turkish Academy of Dermatolology*, Vol.5, No.1, jtad1151r1

Kobayashi, M.; Ito, M.; Nakagawa, A.; Matsushita, M.; Nishikimi, N.; Sakurai, T. & Nimura, Y. (2000). Neutrophil and endothelial cell activation in the vasa vasorum in vasculo-Behçet's disease. *Histopathology*, Vol.36, pp. 362–371

Koga, T.; Claycombe, K. & Meydani, M. (2002). Homocysteine increases monocyte and T-cell adhesion to human aortic endothelial cells. *Atherosclerosis*, Vol.161, pp. 365–374

Lakhanpal, S.; Tani, K.; Lie, JT.; Katoh, K.; Ishigatsubo, Y. & Ohokubo, T. (1985). Pathologic features of Behçet's syndrome: a review of Japanese autopsy registry data. *Human Pathology*, Vol.16, pp. 790-795

La Regina, M.; Gasparyan, AY.; Orlandini, F. & Prisco, D. (2010). Behcet's disease as a model of venous thrombosis. *Open Cardiovascular Medicine Journal*, Vol.4, pp. 71–77

Matsumoto, T.; Uekusa, T. & Fukuda, Y. (1991). Vasculo-Behçet's disease. A pathologic study of eight cases. *Human Pathology*, Vol.22, pp. 45–51.

Mege, JL.; Dilsen, N.; Sanguedolce, V. ; Gul, A.; Bongrand, P.; Roux, H.; Ocal, L.; Inanc, M. & Capo, C. (1993). Over production of monocyte derived tumor necrosis factor alpha, interleukin IL-6, IL-8 and increased neutrofil superoxide generation in Behcet's disease. A comporative study with familial mediterranean fever and healthy subjects. *Journal of Rheumatology*, Vol.20, pp. 1544-1549

Mendes, D.; Correia, M.; Barbedo, M.; Vaio, T.; Mota, M.; Gonçalves, O. & Valente, J. (2009). Behçet's disease--a contemporary review. *Journal of Autoimmunity*, Vol.32, pp. 178-188

Omar, S.; Ghorbel, IB.; Feki, H.; Souissi, M.; Feki, M.; Houman, H. & Kaabachi N. (2007). Hyperhomocysteinemia is associated with deep vein thrombosis of the lower extremities in Tunisian patients. *Clinical Biochemistry*, Vol.40, pp. 41-45.

Ozdemir, R.; Barutcu, I.; Sezgin, AT.; Acikgoz, N.; Ermis, N.; Esen, AM.; Topal, E.; Bariskaner, E. & Ozerol, I. (2004). Vascular endothelial function and plasma homocysteine levels in Behçet's disease. *American Journal of Cardiology*, Vol.94, pp. 522–525

Pay,S.; Simsek, I.; Erdem, H. & Dinc, A. (2007). Immunopathogenesis of Behcet's disease with special emphasize on the possible role of antigen presenting cells. *Rheumatology International*, Vol.27, pp. 417-424

Sarican, T.; Ayabakan, H.; Turkmen, S.; Kalaslioglu, V.; Baran, F. & Yenice N. (2007). Homocysteine: an activity marker in Behçet's disease? *Journal of Dermatological Science*, Vol.45, pp. 121–126

Saylan, T. (1997). Life story of the Dr. Hulusi Behçet. *Yonsei Medical Journal*, Vol.38, pp. 327-332

Silverman, MD.; Tumuluri, RJ.; Davis, M.; Lopez, G.; Rosenbaum, JT. & Lelkes, PI. (2002). Homocysteine upregulates vascular cell adhesion molecule-1 expression in cultured human aortic endothelial cells and enhances monocyte adhesion. *Arteriosclerosis Thrombosis and Vascular Biology*, Vol.22, pp. 587–592

Tursen, U. (2009). Activation markers in Behcet's disease. *Turkderm*, Suppl 2, pp. 74-86

Tuzun, Y. (2006). Hulusi Behçet, MD February 20, 1889 to March 8, 1948. *Clinical Dermatology*, Vol.24, pp. 548-550

Ustün, C. (2002). A famous Turkish dermatologist, Dr. Hulusi Behçet. *European Journal of Dermatology*, Vol.12, pp. 469-470

Willems, HP.; den Heijer, M.; Gerrits, WB.; Schurgers, LJ.; Havekes, M.; Blom, HJ. & Bos, GM. (2006). Oral anticoagulant treatment with coumarin derivatives does not influence plasma homocysteine concentration. *European Journal of Internal Medicine*, Vol.17, pp. 120-124.

3

Antiphospholipid Syndrome and Venous Thrombosis

Ertugrul Okuyan
Bagcilar Education and Research Hospital Istanbul
Turkey

1. Introduction

Antiphospholipid syndrome(APLS) is a prothrombotic state characterized by recurrent venous thrombotic events including deep venous thrombosis, as well as pulmonary embolism, arterial thrombosis, recurrent fatal loss due to placental thrombosis and the presence of circulating antiphospholipid antibodies(APA) (Roubey RAS, 2001). As both thrombosis and pregnancy morbidity have a large number of other origins, the diagnosis of APLS relies on the quality and reliability of the laboratory investigations, on the persistent positivity of the APA assays, and sometimes on the lack of any other cause. Although a broad spectrum of APA exists, the universally accepted diagnostic APA tests are lupus anticoagulant(LA) functional coagulation assay; anticardiolipin antibody(ACA) enzyme-linked immunosorbent assay(ELISA); and anti-β_2-glycoprotein I antibody(aβ_2GPI) ELISA.
Antiphospholipid antibodies were first described in 1906 in patients with syphilis. These complement-fixing antibodies reacting with extracts from bovine hearts(mitochondrial phospholipid cardiolipin) formed the basis for the serologic syphilis test(Venereal Disease Research Laboratory-VDRL assay). Mass population screening for syphilis demonstrated that patients with systemic lupus erythematosus(SLE) without clinical syphilis had persistently false-positive VDRL tests(Haserick J,et al 1952, Baker WF, et al 2008). As false-positive VDRL tests in patients with SLE were also found to be associated with prolonged in vitro coagulation, the term 'lupus anticoagulant' was introduced.
The lupus anticoagulant is an antibody that prolongs phospholipid dependent coagulation tests in vitro. It was given this name in 1972 because clear proof of its site of action was lacking, and because the anticoagulant had been recognized in patients with systemic lupus erythematosus(Donald I Feinstein 2009). It is a misnomer because the lupus anticoagulant is more frequently encountered in patients without lupus and is associated with thrombosis rather than with bleeding. Immunoglobulins reacting with other hemostatic factors, such as von Willebrand factor (VWF), factor VIII, factor IX, and factor XI, inhibitors of thrombin and fibrin polymerization, and factor XIII have also been described in patients with SLE(Donald I Feinstein 2009), but they are rare compared with the lupus anticoagulant.
Patients with the lupus anticoagulant who do not have established SLE fall into several different categories: (1) patients with "lupus-like"chronic autoimmune disorders but without findings that fit the criteria for the diagnosis of SLE; (2) patients with other chronic systemic autoimmune disorders; (3) patients presenting with a venous or arterial thrombotic

event for which no underlying cause may be apparent; (4) patients receiving certain drugs, including procainamide and phenothiazines(a high prevalence of the lupus anticoagulant and a positive antinuclear antibody test are observed in psychotic patients receiving long-term chlorpromazine therapy); other drugs or biologics that can induce the lupus anticoagulant include hydralazine, quinidine, and possibly α-interferon; (5) patients with a recent acute viral infection, in whom the antibody is usually transient; (6) patients with human immunodeficiency virus infection; (7) women with recurrent fetal wastage;(8) occasionally in older patients with malignancies and (9) patients seeking medical attention for a variety of disorders in whom the lupus anticoagulant is discovered as an incidental finding, usually discovered because of a prolonged partial thromboplastin time (PTT) performed as a routine preoperative evaluation.

2. Epidemiology

APA can be detected in the absence of thrombosis or pregnancy morbidity or other systemic autoimmune diseases. During ongoing infectious disease, during treatments with a variety of drugs and even in healthy individuals, APA positivity may occur. The prevalence of APA ranges from 1% to 10% in the general population, 16% in patients with rheumatoid arthritis, and 30% to 40% in patients with SLE(Petri M 2000, Lim W et al 2006). The prevalence of positive tests for lupus anticoagulant and anticardiolipin antibody in a normal population has been reported in several studies. Because of the non-Gaussian distribution of anticardiolipin antibody levels in normal subjects, the cut-off points between normal and abnormal results is difficult to determine. One study reported IgG and IgM anticardiolipin antibodies in approximately 5% of normal individuals, although only 2% had persistently elevated levels on repeat testing. Shi and colleagues detected anticardiolipin antibodies in 6% of normal blood donors, respectively, and detected lupus anticoagulant activity by kaolin clotting time in 4%Shi W 1993). The prevalence of anticardiolipin antibody appears to increase with age.

The prevalences of elevated levels of IgG and IgM anticardiolipin antibody in healthy pregnant women were 2% to 3% and 4%, respectively(Harris EN 1991, Aoki K 1994, Lockshin MD 1997). Most of these were low titer; only 0.2% were high titer. In other studies, the incidence of anticardiolipin antibodies in pregnant individuals ranged from 1% to 2% and lupus anticoagulant 1% to 4%(Petri M 2000).

When the patient does not exhibit any other symptom that would allow the diagnosis of another associated autoimmune disease, the antiphospholipid syndrome is considered primary, or isolated. The term 'secondary' APLS is sometimes used for patients suffering from another autoimmune or inflammatory disease.

3. Etiopathogenesis

Lupus anticoagulants and anticardiolipin antibodies are immunoglobulins that were originally thought to react only with phospholipid. However, it is now well established that these antibodies react directly with epitopes on β2-GPI(McNeil HP 1990, Galli M 1990) or prothrombin(Rao LVM 1996, Bevers EM 1991), that subsequently bind to anionic phospholipid. Anticardiolipin antibodies are low-affinity monovalent antibodies to β2-GPI when in solution, and the monovalent complexes bind weakly to anionic phospholipids. However, when the antigen density is high, bivalent complexes are formed that have a high affinity for phospholipid surfaces. The fact that β2-GPI antibodies are polyclonal reacting with different epitopes on the β2-GPI molecule and the increased affinity of the divalent antigen-antibody complexes for phospholipid surfaces explains why some anticardiolipin antibodies have anticoagulant activity and some do not(Arnout J 2003). This anticoagulant activity correlates best with the incidence of thrombosis(Galli M 2003), and a subset of lupus anticoagulants caused by anti–β2-GPI antibodies with specificity for an epitope on domain I. In some patients the anticardiolipin antibody will react with immobilized cardiolipin in vitro but not prolong phospholipid-dependent coagulation tests. Similarly, some of the antiprothrombin antibodies can prolong coagulation tests and some will not.

As with most autoimmune conditions, the etiology of APLS is not understood. It has been demonstrated that normal healthy individuals without APS have memory B cells that produce aPL antibodies; in a study of patients with infectious mononucleosis, 10 to 60 percent of immunoglobulin M aCL-producing cells expressed CD 27, the marker of memory B cells(Lieby P 2003).

Although antibodies against anionic phospholipid moieties arise during the course of infections such as syphilis and lyme disease, those are distinct from antibodies generated by patients with the syndrome because they generally recognize phospholipid epitopes directly and are not associated with the clinical manifestations of the syndrome.

Reports of familial clustering of raised aPL antibody levels indicate that genetic susceptibility can play a role in their development(Donald I. Feinstein 2007). In one study of 84 APLS patients, more than 35% had at least one relative, and more than 20% had two or more relatives, with evidence of at least one clinical feature of APS, such as thrombosis or recurrent fetal loss(Weber M 2000).

Many different mechanisms have been described for thrombosis during APLS, mainly after in-vitro experiments: (1) activation of endothelial cells by complexes of β2 GPI and anti-β2 GPI, these complexes could bind to annexin 2 or even Toll-like receptors on the surface of endothelial cells(Zhang J 2005, Fischetti F 2005); (2) platelet activation after direct binding of the β2 GPI, which targets the autoantibodies on the surface of these cells, the β2 GPI is selectively bound by the activator receptor apo ER 2(Lutters BC 2003); (3) functional dysregulation of hemostasis by the presence of autoantibodies against natural anticoagulant proteins like annexin 5 and activated protein C; (4) abnormal fibrinolysis directly linked to the presence of APL(Cesarman-Maus G 2006).

APL can stimulate platelet aggregation(Lin YL 1992), an effect that might be promoted via signalling through apolipoprotein E receptor 2(apoER2) receptors; the beta2GPI binding site for apo ER2 on platelets was localized to its domain V. Beta2GPI also has a dampening effect on platelet adhesion by interfering with the platelet-von Willebrand factor interaction, and consequently aPL antibodies, by interfering with this dampening, can increase platelet adhesion in flow systems(Hullstein JJ 2007).

Normal endothelial function includes control over thrombosis and thrombolysis, platelets and leukocyte interaction with the vessel wall, and regulation of vascular tone and smooth muscle proliferation. Several in vitro studies and studies on animal models have shown that incubation of endothelial cells with aPL from APLS patients generates different effects on endothelial function via β2 GPI. As a whole this might cooperate in sustaining endothelial perturbation that has been suggested to have a pivotal pathogenetic role in APS associated thrombosis(Stalc M 2006).

Because high-level aPLs may persist for years in asymptomatic persons, it is likely that vascular injury, endothelial cell activation, or both immediately precede the occurrence of thrombosis in those bearing the antibody (second-hit hypothesis). Of note, at least 50% of

APLS patients with vascular factors possess other acquired thrombosis risk factors at the time of their events(Kaul M 2006, Erkan D 2002).
Both persons congenitally lacking ß2GPI39 and ß2GPI knockout mice appear normal(Sheng Y 2001). ß2GPI polymorphisms influence the generation of aPLs in individuals, but they have only a weak relationship to the occurrence of APLS. A cluster of 50 upregulated genes may have an effect on the occurrence of thrombosis in aPL-positive individuals(Potti A 2006).

4. Diagnostic criteria of the antiphospholipid syndrome

The international preliminary classification criteria for APLS was published in 1999 after a workshop in Sapporo, Japan(Wilson WA 1999)-the so-called Sapporo criteria-. It was updated in 2006 after another workshop in Sydney, Australia(Miyakis S 2006). (table 1).

Clinical criteria 1. Vascular thrombosis One or more clinical episodes of arterial,venous or small vessel thrombosis, in any tissue or organ. 2. Pregnancy morbidity a. One or more unexplained deaths of a morphologically normal fetus at or beyond the 10th week of gestation, or b. One or more premature births of a morphologically normal neonate before the 34th week of gestation because of eclampsia, severe preeclampsia, or recognized features of placental insufficiency, or c. Three or more unexplained consecutive spontaneous abortions before the 10th week of gestation, with maternal anatomic or hormonal abnormalities and paternal and maternal chromosomal causes excluded.
Laboratory criteria 1. Lupus anticoagulant present in plasma, on 2 or more occasions at least 12 weeks apart, detected according to the guidelines of the International Society on Thrombosis and Hemostasis 2. Anticardiolipin antibody of IgG and/or IgM isotype in serum or plasma, present in medium or high titer(ie, >40 GPL or MPL, or greater than the 99th percentile),on 2 or more occasions at least 12 week apart, measured by a standardized ELISA. 3. Anti-β_2-glycoprotein I antibody of IgG and/or IgM isotype in serum or plasma(in titer greater than the 99th percentile) present one or more occasions, at least 12 week apart, measured by a standardized ELISA.

***Definite APLS is present if at least one of the clinical criteria and one of the laboratory criteria are met. Classification of APLS should be avoided if less than 12 weeks or more than 5 years seperate the positive APL test and the clinical manifestation.

Table 1. Updated Sapporo classification criteria for the antiphospholipid syndrome

The first clinical aspect of the APLS is thrombosis, which can affect arterial or venous vessels, as well as small vessels, and must be confirmed by means of imaging studies and/or histopathology. Arterial thrombosis mainly occurs in the central nervous system. But all arteries can be effected and myocardial infarction, peripheral gangrene, aseptic osteonecrosis and adrenal insufficency can develop with respect to effected arterial site. The venous thrombosis commonly localizes to the deep veins of the limbs and can be complicated by pulmonary embolism. As in arterial thrombosis, any segment of the venous vasculature can be effected, which will induce different manifestations.

A definitive diagnosis of APLS is based on fulfilling at least one of the Updated Sapporo Clinical criteria(vascular thrombotic event or pregnancy morbidity) and at least one of the laboratory criteria(Table 1). In general, medium titer aCL is considered 40 U or more and high titer, more than 80 U; titers between 20 and 40 U should be evaluated cautiously. Transient APL positivity is common during infections; thus documentation of the persistence(at least 12 weeks apart) of autoimmune APL is crucial for both diagnostic and therapeutic purposes.

The choice of initial APL tests remains a subject of debate. In general, the LA test is more specific for APL-related clinical events. The specificity of aCL for APL-related clinical events increases with higher titers. The IgG isotype is more strongly associated with APL-related clinical events than the IgM isotype. In a patient with suspected APS, testing for LA and IgG/IgM aCL should be ordered initially. If these tests are negative or low-titer and there is still a high level of suspicion for APS, then testing for antiβ_2GPI antibodies and IgA aCL/antiβ_2GPI can be pursued(George D 2009). Antiphospholipid antibody tests developed based on other phospholipids such as phosphatidylserine, phosphatidylinositol, or phosphatidylethanolamine or phospholipid-binding plasma proteins(such as prothrombin) are not yet well standardized and accepted.

5. Clinical features

Although any vasculature can be affected by thrombosis, stroke and transient ischemic attack are the most common presentations of arterial thrombosis, whereas deep vein thrombosis with or without pulmonary embolism is the most common presentation of venous thrombosis in APLS(George D 2009). Antiphospholipid antibodies can cause both arterial and venous thrombosis in the same patient. Reccurent thromboses tend to occur in the same vascular distribution(venous followed by venous and arterial followed by arterial). in some studies the incidence of venous thrombosis (70%) is greater than the incidence of arterial thrombosis.(Galli M 1997, Triplett DA 1995).

Superficial thrombophlebitis, superior vena cava syndrome, renal vein thrombosis, Budd Chiari syndrome, central retinal vein occlusion, pulmonary hypertension due to recurrent pulmonary embolism, and diffuse pulmonary hemorrhage due to microthrombosis are some of the thrombotic manifestations of APLS.

Of unselected patients with antiphospholipid antibody, 1% to 2.5% per year will develop thromboembolism(Galli M 2003, Finazzi G 1996),and 10% to 25% of patients with deep venous thrombosis will be found to have antiphospholipid antibodies(Ginsburg KS 1992).However, in a prospective population based study of 66140 individuals in Norway(Naess IA 2005), elevated anticardiolipin antibody levels were not a risk factor for

predicting an initial venous thrombosis. Thrombosis is more frequent as the level of anticardiolipin antibody increases, and medium and high titers (>40 GPL and/or MPL units) are more frequently associated with thrombotic events. Although some investigators believe that elevated levels of IgG or IgA isotypes are more common than IgM in patients with thrombotic complications, this has not been clearly established. The lupus anticoagulant or increased levels of anticardiolipin antibody must be persistently present on more than one occasion at least 12 weeks apart because the incidence of thrombotic complications is almost the same in patients with transiently positive tests as in patients with negative tests at two different time intervals. The persistent presence of elevated levels of anticardiolipin antibody has been shown to be associated with indices of in-vivo coagulation activation. In a study of patients with SLE(Ginsberg JS 1993) who were persistently anticardiolipin antibody- positive versus patients who were transiently positive or persistently negative, anticardiolipin antibody-positive patients had a higher mean level of F1+2 and fibrinopeptide A than patients who were transiently positive, persistently negative, or on warfarin therapy. The differences remained significant even if patients with prior thromboembolism were excluded from the analysis. These results suggest that the presence of persistently elevated levels of anticardiolipin antibody in SLE patients is associated with an ongoing prothrombotic state.
Patients who are persistently positive for the lupus anticoagulant or who have persistently elevated levels of anticardiolipin antibody and suffer a thromboembolic event have a recurrence rate of approximately 50% within 2 years(Rosove MH 1992, Khamashta MA 1995). Recurrences tend to occur in most of the patients on the same side of the circulation as the initial event—venous recurrences after an initial venous event and arterial recurrences after an initial arterial event.

6. Treatment of venous thrombosis in APLS

6.1 General treatment

The standard of care for venous thromboembolism is continous infusion of intravenously delivered unfractionated heparin(UFH) and, more recently, subcutaneous low-molecular weight heparins(LMWH). DVT is associated with several possible complications, including recurrent nonfatal venous thromboembolism, postthrombotic chronic venous insufficiency, and nonfatal/fatal pulmonary embolism. The goals of therapy for DVT include the prevention of thrombus propagation, embolization, and early and late thrombus recurrence. Proper anticoagulation is the first critical step in the effective treatment of DVT. Complications can develop soon after thrombus detection, presenting a narrow window of opportunity for a safe and effective intervention. The secondary stage of treatment involves the maintenance of adequate anticoagulation to prevent the development of recurrent thromboembolism.
LMWH or fondaparinux is preferred for the initial anticoagulation of patients with deep vein thrombosis(Table 2). LMWH and fondaparinux are as safe and as effective as continuous unfractionated heparin (UFH). Suitable patients can be safely treated with LMWH and fondaparinux in the outpatient setting. Heparin/fondaparinux should be continued for at least five days after the initiation of warfarin therapy and until International Normalized Ratio (INR) is > 2.0 for two consecutive days. Warfarin should be initiated 5 mg on day 1.

Treatment for venous thromboembolism with LMWH provides reliable anticoagulation levels when given subcutaneously on a weight-based dosing schedule. No laboratory monitoring of the intensity of anticoagulation is required for LMWH, except in special circumstances. Recent randomized controlled trials of the treatment of pulmonary embolism (PE) have shown LMWH to be as effective and safe as UFH. One randomized controlled trial of the treatment of venous thromboembolism (VTE) in 1,021 patients included 271 patients presenting with PE. In this study, there were no significant differences in outcomes following treatment with UFH versus LMWH. These studies used reviparin and tinzaparin. Two reviews agreed that LMWH may be efficacious in the treatment of PE, but cautioned that the LMWH products may not be equivalent to each other (Raskob 1999 ; Charland, 1998; Columbus Investigators, 1997; Simonneau, 1997).
LMWH may not be appropriate for patients with renal insufficiency (creatinine clearance less than 30 mL/min). Studies have shown modestly delayed clearance in patients with chronic renal failure. The clinician should weigh this evidence when considering outpatient therapy.
A high-loading dose of warfarin (greater than 10 mg) is of no clinical use and should be discouraged. A 10 mg initial dose of warfarin has been associated with early over-anticoagulation and, when compared to a 5 mg initial dose, was no more effective in achieving a therapeutic international normalized ratio (INR) by day four or five of therapy. A therapeutic range of anticoagulation to keep the INR at 2.5 (range 2.0-3.0) is recommended for patients with venous thromboembolism. Heparin and warfarin may be started at the same time. The anticoagulant effect of warfarin is delayed until clotting factors already circulating are cleared. Although Factor VII has a shorter half-life in the blood (six to seven hours), peak anticoagulant activity is delayed for up to 96 hours until factors with longer plasma half-lives (II, IX and X) have cleared . Heparin (UFH or LMWH) and warfarin may be started at the same time. Heparin (UFH or LMWH) and/or fondaparinux should be given for a minimum of five days. Patient should continue heparin until INR >=2.0 for two consecutive days. In patients with suspected hypercoagulable state (Protein C or Protein S deficiency), the patient should be adequately anticoagulated with heparin (UFH or LMWH) and/or fondaparinux before warfarin is started at a low dose (2-5 mg). This is to avoid warfarin-induced skin necrosis or other transient hypercoagulable complications.
Recommendations for the management of thrombosis in the APLS have been based largely on retrospective case series. Recently, several clinical trials have been published on the management of thrombosis in APLS.These new clinical trials have challenged the previous dogma of a target INR of 3 to 4(high-intensity warfarin).

6.2 Primary prophylaxis of thrombosis in patients with APL antibodies

The therapeutic approach in asymptomatic carriers of APL without prior thrombotic events is still controversial. Present evidence-based knowledge does not support the widespread use of aspirin in all these aPL-positive patients. Annual thrombosis risk in asymptomatic APL-positive patients range from 0% to 3.8%(Finazzi G 1996, Shah NM 1998), being equivalent to that of major bleeding associated with the use of aspirin. The only randomized clinical trial (APLASA study) in which 98 asymptomatic persistently APL-positive individuals were randomized to recieve a daily dose of 81 mg of aspirin or placebo showed that these patients have a low overall annual incidence rate of acute

thrombosis, and develop vascular events when additional risk factors are present(Erkan D 2007). Therefore, according to the results of this trial, asymptomatic, persistently APL-positive individuals seem not to benefit from low-dose aspirin for primary thromboprophylaxis.
However, a more realistic approach with a lower degree of evidence would be to stratify these individuals according to some clinical features such as the presence of traditional congenital or acquired procoagulant risk factors, the APL profile(persistently positive aCL and or anti-β_2GPI antibodies at moderate/high titers), and the coexistence of an underlying autoimmune disease, to consider primary prophylactic therapy with low-dose 75-100 mg aspirin daily. It is known that SLE represents a prothrombotic condition and acts as strong thrombophilic risk factor, primarily related to the chronic systemic inflammation and renal involvement. Furthermore, one study has shown that prophylactic aspirin should be given to all patients with SLE to prevent both arterial and venous thrombotic manifestations, especially in patients with APL(Wahl DG 2000). In the same study, the authors suggested that in selected patients with LA and a low bleeding risk, prophylactic oral anticoagulant therapy may provide higher utility. Therefore, there is currently consensus for primary thromboprophylaxis in these patients, mainly with low-dose aspirin.
An alternative to aspirin in SLE patients may be hydroxychloroquine. There are many evidences for the protective role of this old drug against the development of both venous and arterial thrombosis(Ruiz-Irastorza G 2006, Erkan D 2002).
All nonthrombotic APL-positive subjects should be encouraged to stop smoking. Cessation of oestrogen –містаing oral contraceptive use and treatment of other vascular risk factors if present are additional recommended therapeutic measures.
At least half of patients with APLS with vascular events also have another reversible risk factors which are not related to APLS at time of thrombosis(Erkan D 2002). Therefore, identification and elimination of these risk factors and agressive prophylaxis during high-risk periods, are crucial for the primary thrombosis prevention in asymptomatic persistently APL-positive individuals. Serious perioperative complications including catastrophic antiphospholipid syndrome(CAPS) may occur despite prophylaxis in APL-positive individuals as they are at additional risk for thrombosis when undergoing surgical procedures. Therefore, perioperative strategies should be clearly identified before any surgical procedure, pharmacological, and physical antithrombosis interventions should be vigorously used; periods without anticoagulation should be kept to an absolute minimum(George D 2009).

6.3 Therapy for acute thrombosis and secondary propylaxis of thrombosis in patients with antiphospholipid syndrome

Therapy for thrombosis associated with the APLS should be guided by the knowledge that recurrence is common. In one study, patients who had discontinued oral anticoagulation had a 50% probability of recurrence in 2 years and a 78% recurrence in 8 years(Derksen RHWM 1993). Similar results have been published by others with a recurrence rate of 10% to 30% per year(Galli M 2003, Rosove MH 1992, Khamashta MA 1995). Three prospective studies reported that there was an increased risk of recurrence that varied from 10% to 67% per year(Lim W 2006, Schulman S 1998, Kearon C 1999, Kearon C 2003, Ortel TL

2005). In most reports the incidence of recurrence is highest in the first 6 months after discontinuing anticoagulant therapy. Although it was initially thought that prevention of venous recurrence required high-intensity warfarin with a target INR of 3.5, evidence has been accumulating from recent studies that standard intensity warfarin (INR 2 to 3) can almost completely abrogate recurrence of venous thromboembolic disease(Crowther MA 2003, Finazzi G 2005). The pooled data from these two studies revealed no difference in recurrent thrombosis between moderate-intensity warfarin (INR 2 to 3) and high-intensity (INR 3 to 4), nor was there a greater bleeding risk. As the data from several studies have demonstrated that patients with antiphospholipid syndrome have a high risk for recurrent venous thromboembolic disease after anticoagulation is discontinued, many feel that anticoagulation should be continued indefinitely. The American College of Chest Physicians recommends treatment for 12 months and consideration of indefinite therapy after an initial event(Ortel TL 2005, Buller HR 2004). Because of the efficacy of warfarin therapy in preventing recurrences, the use of corticosteroids and other immunosuppressive agents to suppress antibody production in the absence of autoimmune disease is not recommended.

-	Objectively confirm DVT; provide short-term treatment with SC LMWH or IV UFH or SC UFH(1A)
-	High clinical suspicion for DVT: treat until diagnosis is confirmed(1C)
-	Initial treatment LMWH or UFH for ≥5 days
-	Warfarin should be started on the first day of treatment
-	IV UFH by weight based or standard dosing to achieve and maintain an aPTT prolongation that corresponds to plasma heparin levels of 0.3 to 0.7 IU/mL anti-Xa activity(1C)
-	UFH with large doses:measure anti-Xa to adjust dose(1B)
-	SC UFH at a dose of 17500 U,SC, Q 12 hours or 250 U/kg, sc, Q 12 hours with adjustment to achieve a therapeutic aPTT(1C).
-	SC fixed dose UFH at a dose of 333 U/kg, sc, Q 12 hours without monitoring for adjustment of dose(1C).
-	SC LMWH once or twice daily over UFH as an outpatient if possible(1C) or as an inpatient(1A).
-	Reccomend against monitoring with anti-Xa levels(1A).
-	Severe renal failure: suggest IV UFH over LMWH(2C).

Table 2. Venous thromboembolism(VTE) treatment guidelines adapted from the American College of Chest Physicians Evidence -based clinical practice guidelines-8th edition

Monitoring anticoagulant therapy may be difficult in patients with lupus anticoagulants and a prolonged PTT. It is mandatory when using unfractionated heparin to monitor therapy using a specific heparin assay, such as the one dependent on factor Xa inhibition (therapeutic range, 0.3 to 0.7). In most instances, it is preferable to use low-molecular-weight heparin in therapeutic doses, which usually eliminates the need for monitoring. When using warfarin, the optimal INR for patients with lupus anticoagulants is controversial, because patients with lupus anticoagulants may have a variably prolonged prothrombin time,and various thromboplastins have a different sensitivity in the presence of a lupus anticoagulant.Therefore, it is possible that in various studies of therapy in patients with lupus anticoagulants that the degree of anticoagulation is overestimated, and the target INR of 3.0 noted earlier might be an overestimate because of the presence of the lupus anticoagulant(Donald I. Feinstein 2007). Rarely, patients may continue to have recurrent venous thromboembolic events despite INR values in the therapeutic range. Recurrent thrombotic events despite therapeutic anticoagulation require evaluation and modification of all non-APL thrombosis risk factors. Warfarin therapy is generally increased to high-intensity(INR, 3.0-4.0). Other options include adding low-dose aspirin, hydroxychloroquine, and/or statins to warfarin or switching to low-molecular weight heparin. There are no randomized controlled studies investigating the effectiveness of any of these approaches.

Based on many cohort studies ,subgroup analysis and two randomized controlled studies, a recent review(Ruiz-Irastorza G 2007) suggests that patients with definite APLS with a first venous thrombosis should be treated with prolonged oral anticoagulation at a target INR of 2.0-3.0 and those with an arterial event at an 3.0-4.0.

So, the best secondary thromboprophylaxis in patients with definite APLS is long-term anticoagulation at a target INR of 2.0-3.0. Patients with recurrent venous thrombotic events despite optimal anticoagulation should be treated with warfarin at an INR of 3.0-4.0.

7. References

Roubey RAS. Antiphospholipid antibody syndrome. In:Koopman WJ, editor. Arthritis and allied conditions, 14th edition, vol2;2001.p.1446-61.

Haserick J, Long R: Systemic lupus erythematosus preceded by false positive serologic tests for syphillis, presentation of five cases. Ann Intern Med 37:559-565, 1952.

Baker WF, Bick RL, Fareed J: Controversies and unresolved issues in antiphospholipid syndrome pathogenesis and management. Hematology/Oncology Clinics of North America 22:155-174, 2008.

Donald I. Feinstein: Inhibitors of blood coagulation. Hematology Basic Principles Chapter 131-4th edition 2009.

Petri M. Epidemiology of the antiphospholipid antibody syndrome. J Autoimmun 15:145-151, 2000.

Lim W, Crowther MA, Eikelboom JW: Manegement of antiphospholipid antibody syndrome- a systematic review.JAMA 295:1050-1057,2006.

Shi, W., Chong, B. H., Hogg, P. J. & Chesterman, C. N. (1993) Thromb. Haemostasis 70, 342-345.

Harris EN, Spinnato JA: Should anticardiolipin tests be performed in otherwise healthy pregnant women?. Am J Obstet Gynecol 1991; 165:1272.

Aoki K, Matsuura E, Sasa H, et al: Beta2-glycoprotein I-dependent and independent anticardiolipin antibodies in healthy pregnant women. Hum Reprod 1994; 9:1849.

Lockshin MD: Antiphospholipid antibody: Babies, blood clots, biology. JAMA 1997; 277:1549.

McNeil HP, Simpson RJ, Chesterman CN, Krilis SA: Antiphospholipid antibodies are directed against a complex antigen that includes a lipid-binding inhibitor of

coagulation: b2-glycoprotein I (apolipoprotein H). Proc Natl Acad Sci U S A 1990; 87:4120.
Galli M, Comfurius P, Maasen C, et al: Anticardiolipin antibodies (ACA) directed not to cardiolipin but to a plasma protein cofactor. Lancet 1990; 335:1544.
Rao LVM, Hoang AD, Rapaport SI: Mechanism and effects of lupus anticoagulant IgG and prothrombin to surface phospholipid. Blood 1996; 11:4173.
Bevers EM, Galli M, Barbui T, et al: Lupus anticoagulant IgG's (LA) are not directed to phospholipid only, but to a complex of lipid-bound human prothrombin. Thromb Haemost 1991; 66:629.
Arnout J, Vermylen J: Current status and implications of autoimmune antiphospholipid antibodies in relation to thrombotic disease. Thromb Haemost 2003; 1:931.
Galli M, Luciani D, Bertolini G, et al: Lupus anticoagulants are stronger risk factors for thrombosis than anticardiolipin antibodies in the antiphospholipid syndrome: A systematic review of the literature. Blood 2003; 101(5):1827.
Lieby P, Soley A, Knapp AM, et al: Memory B cells producing somatically mutated antiphospholipid antibodies are present in healthy individuals. Blood 102;2459:2003.
Donald I. Feinstein. Lupus anticoagulant and acquired inhibitors of blood coagulation. Book chapter 131. Williams Hematology 2007, 5th edition.
Weber M, Hayem G, DeBandt M, et al: The family history of patients with primary or secondary antiphospholipid syndrome(APS). Lupus 9:258, 2000.
Zhang J, McCrae KR. Annexin A2 mediates endothelial cell activation by antiphospholipid/anti-beta2 glycoprotein I antibodies. Blood 2005;105:1964-1969.
Fischetti F, Durigutto P, Pellis V et al. Thrombus formation induced by antibodies to beta 2-glycoprotein I is complement dependent and requires a priming factor. Blood 2005;106:2340-2346.
Lutters BC, Derksen RH, Tekelenburg WL et al. Dimers of beta 2-glycoprotein I increase platelet deposition to collagen via interaction with phospholipids and the apolipoprotein E receptor 2. The journal of Biological Chemistry 2003;278:33831-33838.
Cesarman-Maus G, Rios-Luna N, Deora AB et al. Autoantibodies against the fibrinolytic receptor, annexin 2, in antiphospholipid syndrome. Blood 2006;107.4375-4382.
Lin YL, Wang CT: Activation of human platelets by the rabbit anticardiolipin antibodies. Blood 80:3135, 1992.
Hulstein JJ, Lenting PJ, de LB, et al: Beta2-glycoprotein I inhibits von Willebrand factor dependent platelet adhesion and aggregation. Blood 110:1483, 2007.
Stalc M, Poredos P, Peternel P, et al. Endothelial function is impaired in patients with primary antiphospholipid syndrome. Thrombosis Research 2006;118, 455-461.
Kaul M, Erkan D, Sammaritano L, et al: Assessment of the 2006 revised antiphospholipid syndrome (APS) classification criteria [abstract]. Arthritis Rheum 54:S796, 2006.

Erkan D, Yazici Y, Peterson MG, et al: A cross-sectional study of clinical thrombotic risk factors and preventive treatments in antiphospholipid syndrome. Rheumatology (Oxford) 41:924-929, 2002.

Sheng Y, Reddel SW, Herzog H, et al: Impaired thrombin generation in beta 2-glycoprotein I null mice. J Biol Chem 276:13817-13821, 2001.

Potti A, Bild A, Dressman HK, et al: Gene-expression patterns predict phenotypes of immune-mediated thrombosis. 107:1391-1396, 2006.

Wilson WA, Gharavi AE, Koike T, et al. International consensus statement on preliminary classification criteria for definite antiphospholipid syndrome: report of an international workshop. Arthritis Rheum 42:1309-1311,1999.

Miyakis S, Lockshin MD, Atsumi T, et al: International consensus statement on an update of the classification criteria for definite antiphospholipid syndrome. J Thromb Haemost 4:295-306, 2006.

George D, Erkan D. Antiphospholipid syndrome. Progress in Cardiovascular Diseases 52(2009):115-125.

Galli M, Finazzi G, Barbui T: Antiphospholipid antibodies: Predictive value of laboratory tests. Thromb Haemost 1997; 78:75.

Triplett DA: Protean clinical presentation of antiphospholipid-protein antibodies (APA). Thromb Haemost 1995; 74:329.

Galli M, Barbui T: Antiphospholipid antibodies and thrombosis: Strength of association. Hematol J 2003; 4:180.

Finazzi G, Brancaccio V, Moia M, et al: Natural history and risk factors for thrombosis in 360 patients with antiphospholipid antibodies: A four-year prospective study from the Italian Registry. Am J Med 1996; 100:530.

Ginsburg KS, Liang MH, Newcomer L, et al: Anticardiolipin antibodies and the risk for ischemic stroke and venous thrombosis. Ann Intern Med 1992; 117:997.

Naess IA, Christiansen SC, Cannegieter SC, et al: A prospective study of anticardiolipin antibodies as a risk factor for venous thrombosis in a general population (the HUNT study). Thromb Haemost 2005; 4:44-49.

Ginsberg JS, Demeers C, Brill-Edwards P, et al: Increased thrombin generation and activity in patients with systemic lupus erythematosus and anticardiolipin antibodies: Evidence for a prothrombotic state. Blood 1993; 81:2958.

Rosove MH, Brewer PM: Antiphospholipid thrombosis: Clinical course after the first thrombotic event in 70 patients. Ann Intern Med 1992; 117:303.

Khamashta MA, Cuadrado MJ, Mujic F, et al: The management of thrombosis in antiphospholipid-antibody syndrome. N Engl J Med 1995; 332:993.

Raskob GE. Heparin and low molecular weight heparin for treatment of acute pulmonary embolism. Curr Opin Pulm Med. 1999 Jul;5(4):216-21. Review.

Charland SL, Klinter DE. Low-molecular-weight heparins in the treatment of pulmonary embolism. Ann Pharmacother. 1998 Feb;32(2):258-64. Review.

The Columbus Investigators. Low-molecular-weight heparin in the treatment of patients with venous thromboembolism. N Engl J Med. 1997 Sep 4;337(10):657-62.

Simonneau G, Sors H, Charbonnier B, Page Y, Laaban JP, Azarian R, Laurent M, Hirsch JL, Ferrari E, Bosson JL, Mottier D, Beau B. A comparison of low-molecular-weight heparin with unfractionated heparin for acute pulmonary embolism. The THESEE Study Group. Tinzaparine ou Heparine Standard: Evaluations dans l'Embolie Pulmonaire. N Engl J Med. 1997 Sep 4;337(10):663-9.

Shah NM, Khamashta MA, Atsumi T et al. Outcome of patients with anticardiolipin antibodies: a 10 year follow-up of 52 patients. Lupus 1998 7:3-6

Erkan D, Harrison MJ, Levy R et al. Aspirin for primary thrombosis prevention in the antiphospholipid syndrome: a randomized, double-blind, placebo-controlled trial in asymptomatic antiphospholipid antibody-positive individuals. Arthritis Rheum 2007;56:2382-2391.

Wahl DG, Bounameaux H, de Moerloose P et al. Prophylactic antithrombotic therapy for patients with systemic lupus erythematosus with or without antiphospholipid antibodies: do the benefits outweigh the risks? A decision analysis. Arch Intern Med 2000;160:2042-2048.

Ruiz-Irastorza G, Egurbide MV, Pijoan JI et al(2006) Effect of antimalarials on thrombosis and survival in patients with systemic lupus erythematosus. Lupus 2006;15:577-583.

Derksen RHWM, DeGroot PG, Kateer L, Nieuweahuis HK: Patients with antiphospholipid antibodies and venous thrombosis should receive long-term anticoagulant treatment. Ann Rheum Dis 1993; 52:689.

Khamashta MA, Cuadrado MJ, Mujic F, et al: The management of thrombosis in antiphospholipid-antibody syndrome. N Engl J Med 1995; 332:993.

Lim W, Crowther MA, Eikelboom JW: Management of antiphospholipid antibody syndrome. JAMA 2006; 295(9):1050.

Schulman S, Svenungsson E, Granqvist S: Duration of anticoagulation study group. Anticardiolipin antibodies predict early recurrence of thromboembolism and death among patients with venous thromboembolism following anticoagulant therapy. Am J Med 1998; 104:332.

Kearon C, Gent M, Hirsh J, et al: A comparison of three months of anticoagulation with extended anticoagulation for a first episode of idiopathic venous thromboembolism. N Engl J Med 1999; 340:901.

Kearon C, Ginsberg JS, Kovacs MJ, et al: Comparison of low-intensity warfarin therapy with conventional-intensity warfarin therapy for long-term prevention of recurrent venous thromboembolism. N Engl J Med 2003; 349:631.

Ortel TL: Thrombosis and the antiphospholipid syndrome. Hematology Am Soc Hematol Educ Program 2005; 462:

Crowther MA, Ginsberg JS, Julian J, et al: A comparison of two intensities of warfarin for the prevention of recurrent thrombosis in patients with the antiphospholipid antibody syndrome. N Engl J Med 2003; 349:1133.

Finazzi G, Marchioli R, Brancaccio V, et al: A randomized clinical trial of high-tensity warfarin vs. conventional antithrombotic therapy for the prevention of recurrent thrombosis in patients with the antiphospholipid syndrome (WAPS). Thromb Haemost 2005; 3:848.

Buller HR, Agnelli G, Hull RD, et al: Antithrombotic therapy for venous thromboembolic disease. The seventh ACCP conference on antithrombotic and thrombolytic therapy. Chest 2004; 126(Suppl):401S.

Ruiz-Irastorza G, Hunt BJ, Khamashta MA. A systematic review of secondary thromboprophylaxis in patients with antiphospholipid antibodies. Arthritis Rheum 2007;57:1487-1495.

4

Deep Venous Thrombosis in Children with Musculoskeletal Infection

Lawson A. B. Copley and Ngozi Okoro
Orthpaedic Surgery, University of Texas Southwestern
USA

1. Introduction

Deep venous thrombosis (DVT) is rarely identified in children. However, there has been an increase in the reported association of DVT with pediatric musculoskeletal infection.[1-13] The relationship appears to be tied to the rise of community-acquired, Methicillin-resistant *Staphylococcus aureus* (CA-MRSA).[5-13] Children who are affected by musculoskeletal infection and deep venous thrombosis appear to share similar clinical features. They often require intensive care, surgical intervention, and prolonged hospitalization.[5,6,9] Pulmonary involvement, including pneumonia and septic pulmonary emboli, is frequent.[9,11] It is possible that the causative organisms have an underlying genetic makeup, such as Panton Valentine leukocidin, that potentiates the cascade of clinical features seen in these children.[6,8,10] This chapter explores the relationship of DVT and pediatric musculoskeletal infection through meta-analysis of the medical literature from the past forty years. To the extent possible, risk factors and clinical characteristics are evaluated and evaluation and treatment strategies are discussed.

2. Review of literature

The earliest case report of DVT associated with osteomyelitis was by Horvath et al. in 1971.[14] Including that original case, 58 cases of pediatric DVT associated with musculoskeletal infection have surfaced in the medical literature (see table 1).[1-19] A decade by decade review of the case occurrence reveals an exponential increase in the number of cases reported since 2000, during which time 51 new cases have been identified. This is compared to one case from the 1970s and 3 cases from each decade of the 1980s and 1990s. The largest series, to the present, was reported at a single institution, Children's Medical Center of Dallas, compiled from two separate reports with overlapping study periods and included 15 unique cases of children with DVT.[5,9] Of the four studies that report the incidence of DVT within a series of children with musculoskeletal infection, the total number of children with DVT is 32 among a total of 430 children reviewed giving an estimated incidence of DVT associated with musculoskeletal infection of 7.4%.[3,6,8,9]

3. Gender, age, type, and site of infection

Several trends can be derived from the reported cases in a descriptive manner. Children with DVT were noted to be male 34 times out of the 46 cases in which gender was identified

Source	Year	Series	DVT	Age (y)	Sex	Type	Location	Organism	DVT Site	Pulmonary Findings	Features
Horvath[14]	1971		1	9	m	Osteo.	R proximal tibia	MSSA	R femoral; popliteal	L lower lobe infiltrate	
Jupiter[15]	1982		2	12	m	Osteo.	L humerus	MSSA	L arm deep	Multiple infiltrates	
				12	f	Osteo.	L femur, R tibia	MSSA	L femoral; popliteal	Diffuse infiltrates	
Muhlendahl[16]	1988		1	12	f	Osteo.	R distal femur	MSSA	R femoral	Multiple lung emboli	
Smith[17]	1997		2	4	f	Osteo.	L femur	S aureus	IVC and femoral	Pneumatoceles	Death
				2.5	f	Osteo.	L ilium	S aureus	IVC and common iliac	Pneumonia	
Letts[18]	1999		1	11.5	m	Osteo.	Sacrum	MSSA	R popliteal; R femoral; R atrium	R middle lobe SPE	
Gorenstein[19]	2000		3	11	m	Osteo.	L proximal femur	MSSA	L femoral	Pneumatoceles	Death
				10	m	Osteo.	L femoral head	MSSA	L femoral	Pneumonia, empyema	PneumoT.
				10	m	Osteo.	L femoral neck	S aureus	L iliac	Multiple infiltrates	
Walsh[2]	2002		4	11	m	Osteo.	L distal fibula	MSSA	L femoral; popliteal	Bil. patchy infiltrates	ICU
				4	f	Osteo.	L femur, R tibia	S aureus	IVC; L common femoral	patchy infiltrates	Death
				2.5	f	Osteo.	L ilium	S aureus	IVC; common iliac	Pneumonia	ICU
				6	f	Pyom.	L soleus	GABHS	L popliteal; peroneal	Unknown	Comp. sy.
Newgard[1]	2002		1	12	m	Osteo.	Sacroiliac	MSSA	R common iliac	SPE	
Martinez-Aguilar[3]	2004	59	5	U	U	Osteo.	Unkown	MRSA	Unkown	Unknown	PVL
				U	U	Osteo.	Unkown	MRSA	Unkown	Unknown	PVL
				U	U	Osteo.	Unkown	MRSA	Unkown	Unknown	PVL
				U	U	Osteo.	Unkown	MRSA	Unkown	Unknown	PVL
				U	U	Osteo.	Unkown	MSSA	Unkown	Unknown	PVL
Yuksel[4]	2004		1	3	m	Osteo.	R distal fibula	S aureus	R external iliac	Bil. Densities; cavities	
Gonzalez[6]	2006	116	9	12	m	Osteo.	R ilium	MSSA	R deep pelvic	Clear	
				3	m	Osteo.	R femur	MRSA	R common femoral; external iliac	Clear	PVL
				3	m	Osteo.	R tibia	MSSA	R femoral; popliteal	Clear	
				10	m	Osteo.	L ischium, pubis & ilium	MRSA	L common iliac	Bilateral infiltrates	PVL; CVC
				14	m	Osteo.	R femur and tibia	MRSA	R femoral; popliteal	SPE	PVL; CVC
				13	m	Osteo.	L femur and tibia	MRSA	L saphenous	Pleural effusions	PVL; CVC
				14	m	Osteo.	L tibia	MRSA	L popliteal; saphenous	SPE	PVL
				11	m	Osteo.	L femur	MRSA	L femoral vein	SPE	PVL; CVC
				14	m	Osteo.	R femur	MRSA	R common femoral; popliteal	SPE	PVL; CVC
Crary[5]; Hollmig[9]	2006/7	352	15	13	m	Osteo.	R distal femur	MRSA	SVC	Clear	CVC
				13	m	Osteo.	R proximal fibula	MRSA	R femoral; popliteal	Clear	CVC
				9	m	Osteo.	R proximal tibia	MRSA	R femoral; popliteal	SPE	CVC
				11	f	Osteo.	L distal femur	MRSA	L femoral; popliteal	SPE	CVC
				12	m	Osteo.	R proximal tibia	MRSA	SVC; L internal jugular; subclavian	Clear	CVC
				10	f	Osteo.	L sacrum	MRSA	L common iliac; L external iliac	Bil. opacities; effusions	CVC
				13	m	Osteo.	R distal femur	MSSA	R femoral; popliteal	Unknown	CVC
				7	m	Osteo.	Thoracic spine	MRSA	Azygous; IVC	SPE	CVC

Source	Year	Series	DVT	Age (y)	Sex	Type	Location	Organism	DVT Site	Pulmonary Findings	Features
				10	m	Osteo.	R proximal femur	MRSA	R femoral	SPE	CVC
				2	m	Osteo.	R proximal tibia	MRSA	R femoral; external iliac; saphenous	SPE	CVC
				14	m	Osteo.	L distal femur	MSSA	L popliteal	SPE	CVC
				4	m	Osteo.	L proximal tibia	C. Tropicalis	L popliteal	Unknown	CVC
				6	f	Osteo.	L distal tibia, L distal femur	MRSA	IVC and SVC	Unknown	CVC
				8	f	Pyom.	L calf	Strep. Milleri	L posterior tibial	Clear	
				6	f	Sep. Art.	L hip	GABHS	R IJ; Sigmoid; transverse sinues	Clear	
Castaldo[7]	2007		1	U	U	Sep. Art.	Hip	MRSA	Unkown	Necrotizing pneumonia	
Dohin[8]	2007	39	3	U	U	U	Unknown	S aureus	Unkown	Unknown	PVL
				U	U	U	Unknown	S aureus	Unkown	Unknown	PVL
				U	U	U	Unknown	S aureus	Unkown	Unknown	PVL
Mitchell[10]	2007		3	9	m	Osteo.	R proximal femur	MSSA	L femoral; bilateral IJs; R brachial	Unknown	ICU; PVL
				9	m	Osteo.	R proximal femur	S aureus	R femoral	Bilateral infiltrates	ICU; PVL
				13	m	Osteo.	R femur and tibia	S aureus	Unkown	SPE	PVL
Nourse[11]	2007		2	1	m	Osteo.	L femur	MRSA	L superficial/common femoral; iliac	SPE	PVL
				13	m	Osteo.	L proximal femur	MRSA	L superficial/common femoral	SPE	PVL
Gite[12]	2008		3	8	U	Osteo.	R femur	No growth	Unkown	Unknown	
				6	U	Osteo.	L femur	Enterococcus	Unkown	Unknown	
				13	U	Osteo.	L femur	S aureus	Unkown	Unknown	
McDonald[13]	2010		1	5	m	Osteo.	R proximal humerus	MRSA	R subclavian; brachial; cephalic	SPE	ICU

DVT-Deep vein thrombosis; y-years; m-Male; f-Female; U-Unknown; Osteo.-Osteomyelitis; R-Right; L-Left; MSSA-Methicillin Senstive Staph Aureus; Bil.-Bilateral;
MRSA-Methicillin Resistant Staph Aureus; S-staphyloccocus; GABHS-Group A beta hemolytic streptoccocci; IVC-Inferior vena cava; SVC-Superior vena cava;
SPE-Septic pulmonary emboli; PneumoT-Pneumothorax; ICU-Intensive care unit; Comp. sy.-Compartment syndrome; PVL-Panton-Valentine Leukocidin; C. Candida;
CVC-Central venous catheters; Sep. Art.- Septic Arthritis; Strep.- Streptoccocus; IJ-Internal jugular

Table 1. Summary of Published Cases of DVT in Patients with Musculoskeletal Infection

(73.9%).[1-19] The average age of the children with DVT in the reviewed studies was 9 years with only six children under the age of 4 years among the 49 children with a recorded age (12.2%).[1-19] The type of infection was found to be osteomyelitis in 51 out of the 55 cases (92.7%) in which the musculoskeletal infection type was delineated. [1-19] However, two cases of septic arthritis and two cases of pyomyositis were also noted.[2,7,9] The location of the infection was reported in 46 out of the 54 children with osteomyelitis and noted to be unifocal in 40 children and multifocal in the remaining six (see table 2). The site of osteomyelitis was most commonly reported in the femur (26 occurrences), and specifically reported in the proximal femur on 7 occasions and the distal femur on 6 occasions. The tibia was the second most common location of osteomyelitis (13 occurrences) with the proximal tibia specified in 5 cases and the distal tibia specified in one case. Overall, the location of the musculoskeletal infection was found to be in the pelvis (ilium, ischium, pubis, or sacrum) or lower extremities in 48 out of the 51 cases in which the site of infection was reported (94.1%), with the three remaining cases identified in the upper extremities (humerus in two children) and thoracic spine.

Location		Recorded occurrence	Percent
Thoracic spine		1	2%
Pelvis			
	Ilium	5	9%
	Ischium	1	2%
	Pubis	1	2%
	Sacrum	3	6%
	Total	10	
Femur	Unspecified	13	25%
	Proximal	7	13%
	Distal	6	11%
	Total	26	
Tibia	Unspecified	7	13%
	Proximal	5	9%
	Distal	1	2%
	Total	13	
Fibula			
	Proximal	1	2%
	Distal	2	4%
	Total	3	
Total		53	100%
Multifocal		6	12%

Table 2. Frequency Distribution of Osteomyelitis Site

4. Causative organism

Staphylococcus aureus was found to be the causative organism in 38 of 43 culture positive cases (88.4%) and, of those isolates, 18 (47.4%) were identified as Methicillin-resistant *Staphylococcus aureus*. In one series, the rise in recognition of DVT in their practice appeared to coincide with the establishment of USA 300 ST8 as the predominant clone of CA-MRSA in their community.[6]

5. Panton-Valentine leukocidin

The identification of Panton-Valentine leukocidin (PVL) genes in the isolates of *Staphylococcus* aureus in children with DVT has been reported in several studies.[3,6,8,10,11] These reports suggest that PVL may be associated with enhanced inflammatory response in cases of musculoskeletal infection including pneumonia, multifocal osteomyelitis, bacteremia, and concurrent pyomyositis, subperiosteal abscesses or intra-osseous abscesses requiring surgical debridment.[3,6,8,10,11] The advent of rapid PCR technology as a tool to identify the presence of PVL may prove valuable in identifying potentially "silent" cases of DVT that would otherwise go unrecognized. To this point, however, the technology to perform rapid testing to identify the bacterial genetics of the *S. aureus* isolates is not readily available at most institutions. Our meta-analysis identified 20 children out of the 58 reported cases with DVT who were found to be PVL positive (34.5%).[3,6,8,10,11]

6. Location of DVT

Among the 58 children with DVT, the location of occurrence of the DVT was recorded in 45 cases and was noted to be multi-focal in 22 (48.9%) children (see table 3). 79 specific locations of the DVT were recorded with the most common being femoral (25 or 32%); popliteal (14 or 18%); iliac (12 or 15%); and inferior vena cava (6 or 8%). Overall, the reported incidence of DVT involving a location inclusive of the inferior vena cava, pelvis, or lower extremities was 62 of the 79 occurrences (78.5%).

Location of DVT	Occurrence	
Sigmoid Sinus	1	1%
Transverse Sinus	1	1%
Internal Jugular	4	5%
Superior Vena Cava	3	4%
Subclavian	2	3%
Arm	4	5%
Atrium	1	1%
Azygous	1	1%
Inferior Vena Cava	6	8%
Iliac	12	15%
Femoral	25	32%
Popliteal	14	18%
Posterior Tibial	1	1%
Peroneal	1	1%
Saphenous	3	4%
Total	79	100%
Multiple locations reported	22	
Location not reported	13	

Table 3. Frequency Distribution of DVT Location

7. Clinical features

Several studies have suggested that children with DVT- associated osteomyelitis demonstrate a more severe clinical course when compared to children who do not have deep venous thrombosis.[3,5,6,8,9,10,11] Specifically, children with DVT are more likely to be admitted to the intensive care unit (ICU), require more surgical procedures, and have a longer hospitalization than their counterparts who do not have DVT but who do have similar forms of musculoskeletal infection.[2,5,9,10,13,17,19] One study found that children with DVT required an average of 2.6 surgical procedures per child and had a mean duration of hospitalization of 30.6 days, compared to children without DVT who underwent an average of 0.9 surgical procedures per child and were hospitalized an average of 9.5 days.[9] The same study determined that children with DVT presented with higher inflammatory indices in comparison to children who did not have DVT.[9] The mean C-reactive protein (CRP) in children with DVT was 16.9 mg/dL , compared with only 6.8 mg/dL in children without DVT.[9] While intuitively it might be thought that children with DVT would have a delay in clinical presentation to a healthcare facility, the authors found that there was in fact a shorter duration between the onset of admission for children with DVT compared to those without. (5.6 days versus 14.4 days).[9] This lends further support to the possibility that children with musculoskeletal infection and DVT have a more abrupt onset and rapid clinical decline to the point where medical attention is sought. Pulmonary involvement with a variety of manifestations including pneumonia, septic pulmonary emboli, cavitary pneumatoceles, empyema, and various infiltrates was recorded in 36 of the 58 children with DVT (62.1%).[1,2,4-7,9-11,13-19]

8. Central venous catheters

The use of central venous catheters (CVCs) in the treatment of children with musculoskeletal infection has raised the concern that these catheters may be associated with risk including DVT development. Our review noted the concurrent presence of CVLs in several children with DVT, but the conclusions were generally that there was no clear relationship.[5,6,9] Hollmig et al. found that CVCs were used in all eleven children with osteomyelitis and DVT in their series.[9] However, there did not appear to be a relationship between the location or temporal onset of the DVT to the CVC in their experience.[9]

9. Statistical analysis

We reviewed 19 articles (15 case reports[1,2,4,5,7,10-19], three studies pertaining to musculoskeletal infection in general[3,8,9], and one study focused on an osteomyelitis population[6]). In estimating the heterogeneity of the three musculoskeletal infection papers (k = 3), we measured the I^2 index as our test of heterogeneity and found the I^2 index to be 7.7%. The Cochran's Q value was found to be 2.153 ($p = 0.3407$). This statistic signifies a degree of heterogeneity between the three papers which makes it difficult to derive meaningful conclusions from the summary data from these studies. However, this level of heterogeneity is expected considering several factors such as different study methodology, different timing of the onset of disease, different disease severity and different patient groups.

The incidence rate of DVT was calculated to compare the difference between an incidence rate specific to osteomyelitis and the incidence related to musculoskeletal infection in general. From our results, the number of DVTs in the three musculoskeletal infection papers was 23 with a sample size of 450.[3,8,9] Therefore the incidence of DVT in children with musculoskeletal infection was 5.1%. However, in the one paper in which osteomyelitis alone was considered, the number of DVTs was 9 with a sample size of 116.[6] Hence, the incidence of DVT with osteomyelitis was 7.8%. Although the differences in incidence could be due to different populations being studied, there does appear to be a higher incidence of DVT specifically with pediatric osteomyelitis as compared to pediatric musculoskeletal infection in general. Further research is required in this area.

10. Evaluation recommendations

Any child with deep musculoskeletal infection, particularly osteomyelitis caused by *Staphylococcus* aureus should be considered at risk for DVT. However, in light of the medical literature, a higher index of suspicion should be held for those children with severe clinical presentation, including: intensive care unit admission, markedly elevated inflammatory indices, lower extremity location of the musculoskeletal infection, need for repeated surgical debridement, and pulmonary involvement with infiltrates or septic pulmonary emboli. These

children should undergo screening with non-invasive Doppler ultrasound evaluation of the extremities in the region of the musculoskeletal infection to look for DVT. If the ability to assess the PVL status of the organism is present within any institution, then this should be considered whenever *Staphylococcus aureus* is isolated from bone, joint, or muscle specimens.
While stratification of the relative risk of DVT may increase the awareness of the treating physician of the child's potential for DVT, it is important not to overlook the rare cases of DVT that might occur in children who fall outside of this risk profile, such as those with upper extremity locations of infection, infection types other than osteomyelitis, causative organisms other than *Staphylococcus aureus*, or age under 4 years. Whenever the clinical suspicion of DVT exists, supplemental imaging should be considered.

11. Treatment

Children with DVT and osteomyelitis can be effectively managed with low molecular weight heparin. Resolution of the DVT occurs at an average of ten to twelve weeks.[5,9] Follow-up imaging is helpful to ensure resolution of the DVT. In cases refractory to low molecular-weight heparin, consideration may be given to placement of an intravascular filter. Warfarin is also an option, but requires additional effort in managing the prothrombin time (PT) and international normalized ratio (INR) effectively.
Because children with DVT and osteomyelitis may require repeat surgical procedures, care must be taken to appropriately withhold and resume the anticoagulant therapy around periods of surgery to avoid bleeding complications.

12. Conclusions

Pediatric musculoskleletal infection is associated with the risk for DVT. Risk factors include: osteomyelitis; lower extremity location of infection; *Staphylococcus aureus*, particularly MRSA, as the causative organism; age greater than 4 years; markedly elevated inflammatory indices; severe clinical illness often requiring intensive care unit admission, intubation, or inotrope support; and pulmonary involvement with infiltrates, pneumonia, or septic pulmonary emboli. A high index of suspicion should be maintained when risk factors are present and appropriate screening imaging should be obtained. One study demonstrated a 40% rate of DVT when the child was greater than 8 years of age with positive cultures for MRSA and an initial CRP of greater than 6 mg/dL.[9] Consideration may be given to evaluating for the presence of PVL within the bacterial genetics to help further stratify the risk of DVT. Whenever DVT is identified, appropriate treatment should be administered in a timely manner and the child should be monitored until the point of resolution. The anticipated outcome is good.

13. References

[1] Newgard C. D, Inkelis S. H, & Mink R. (2002). Septic thromboembolism from unrecognized deep venous thrombosis in a child. *Pediatric Emergency Care, 18*(3), 192-196.

[2] Walsh Stewart, & Philips Fredrick. (2002). Deep vein thrombosis associated withpediatric musculoskeletal sepsis. *Journal of Pediatrics Orthopedics, 22*, 329-332.

[3] Martinez-Aguilar G, Avalos-Mishaan A, Hulten K, Hammerman W, Mason E O, & Kaplan S L. (2004). Community acquired methicillin-resistant and methicillin-

susceptible staphylococcus aureus musculoskeletal infections in children. *The Pediatric Infectious Disease Journal, 23*, 701-706.

[4] Yuksel Hasan, Ozguven Ali Aykan, Akil Ipek, Erguder Isil, Yilmaz Dilek, & Cabuk Mine. (2004). Septic pulmonary emboli presenting with deep venous thrombosis secondary to acute osteomyelitis. *Pediatrics International, 46*, 621-623.

[5] Crary S E, Buchanan G R, Drake C E, & Journeycake J M. (2006). Venous thrombosis and thromboembolism in children with osteomyelitis. *The Journal of Pediatrics, 149*, 537-541.

[6] Gonzalez B E, Teruya J, Mahoney D H, Hulten K G, Edwards R, Lamberth L B, et al. (2006). Venous thrombosis associated with staphylococcal osteomyelitis in children. *Pediatrics, 117*, 1673-1679.

[7] Castaldo ET, & EY, Y. (2007). Severe sepsis attributable to community-acquired methicillin-resistant staphylococcus aureus: an emerging fatal problem. *The American Surgeon, 73*, 684-687.

[8] Dohin B, Gillet Y, Kohler R, Lina G, Vandenesch F, Vanhems P, et al. (2007). Pediatric bone and joint infections caused by panton-valentine leukocidin-positive staphlococcus aureus. *Pediatric Infectious Disease, 26*, 1042-1048.

[9] Hollmig S T, Copley L A, Browne R H, Grande L M, & Wilson P L. (2007). Deep venous thrombosis associated with osteomyelitis in children. *Journal of Bone and Joint Surgery, 89*, 1517-1523.

[10] Mitchell PD, Hunt DM, Lyall H, Nolan M, & Tudor-Williams G. (2007). Panton-valentine leukocidin-secreting staphylococcus aureus causing severe musculoskeletal sepsis in children. A new threat. *Journal of Bone and Joint Surgery, 89-B*(No. 9), 1239-1242.

[11] Nourse C, Starr M, & W, M. (2007). Community-acquired methicillin-resistant staphylococcus aureus causes severe disseminated infection and deep venous thrombosis in children: literature review and recommendations for management. *Journal of Pediatric Child Health, 43*, 656-661.

[12] Gite A, Trived R, & Ali U. S. (2008). Deep Vein Thrombosis Associated with Osteomyelitis. *Indian Pediatrics, 45*, 418-419.

[13] McDonald John E, & A, C. L. (2010). Upper extremity deep venous thrombosis associated with proximal humeral osteomyelitis in a child. *The Journal of Bone and Joint Surgery, America, 92*, 2121-2124.

[14] Horvath F. L, Brodeur A. E, & Cherry J. D. (1971). Deep thrombophlebitis associated with acute osteomyelitis. *Journal of Pediatric, 79*(5), 815-818.

[15] Jupiter J. B, Ehrlich M. G, Novelline R. A, Leeds H. C, & Keim D. (1982). The association of septic thrombophlebitis with subperiosteal abscesses in children. *Journal of Pediatric, 101*(5), 690-695.

[16] von Muhlendahl KE. (1988) Pelvic and femoral vein thrombosis in childhood [in German]. *Monatsschr Kinderheilkd*, 136: 397-399.

[17] Smith A. G, Cornblath W. T, & Deveikis J. P. (1997). Local thrombolytic therapy in deep cerebral venous thrombosis. *Neurology, 48*(6), 1613-1619.

[18] Letts Merv, Lalonde Francois, Davidson Darin, Hosking Martin, & Halton Jacqueline. (1999). Atrial and venous thrombosis secondary to septic arthritis of the sacroiliac joint in a child with hereditary protein c deficiency. *Journal of Pediatrics Orthopedics, 19(2)*(March/April 1999), 156-160.

[19] Gorenstein Arkadi, Gross Eitan, Houri Sion, Gewirts Gabriella, & Katz Schmuel. (2000). The pivotal role in deep vein thrombophlebitis in the development of acute disseminated staphylococcal disease in children. *Pediatrics, 106*(No. 6), 87-89.

Part 2

Management and Complications

5

Current Endovascular Treatments for Venous Thrombosis

Glenn W. Stambo
Vascular and Interventional Radiology
St. Josephs Hospital and Medical Center, Tampa
USA

1. Introduction

Venous disease continues to increase in number of patients throughout the 2000's. With continued use of venous access devices, dialysis and cancer on the increase and overall patient sedentary life style, we will continue to see more and more venous disease in our population. Overall, venous disease is far more prevalent in the population than arterial disease. However, it is less diagnosed than arterial disease due in part too less acute symptomatology. Patients tend to present later in their disease process due to a multitude of factors including lack of debilitating symptoms, non-life threatening presentation and manageable discomfort until later stages.

Symptoms like gradual leg swelling in DVT patients, arm swelling in Dialysis fistulas and facial edema in superior vena cava (SVC) syndrome are slowly progressive until symptoms become debilitating. Even pulmonary emboli can be sub clinical with only non-specific findings like dyspnea and chest discomfort. Coumadin and the other low molecular weight heparin products are used as outpatient therapies in oral or injection preparations. These are adequate therapies for further prevention of clot formation and help resolve clots outside the hospital setting. However, weekly blood draws and side effects of these drugs particularly in the elderly can be significant and are potential reasons for multiple readmissions to the hospitals related to complications from bleeding.

2. Treatment options

The standard treatment for deep venous thrombosis and pulmonary is anti-coagulation embolism. Intravenous heparin is used in the acute hospital setting. Coumadin and the other low molecular weight heparin products are used as outpatient therapies.

For those patients with significant clot burden within peripheral or pulmonary embolism, endovenous therapies can be used if not candidates for anticoagulation. These patients present emergently with significant morbidity. In fact, acute extensive DVT of the lower extremity can cause severe peripheral vascular arterial emergency called Phlegmasia Cereulens Dolans. This disorder needs rapid clot lysis to dissolve the massive clot burden. Thus, only catheter directed thrombolysis could provide this direct form of endovenous therapy. Whether it is acute, semi acute or chronic venous occlusive process, endovenous therapies have become the first line of therapy. If left untreated or inadequately treated with conventional means, patients may develop post thrombotic syndrome.

Various areas may be treated within the venous distribution. The treatable areas include extremity veins, superior venacava, portal vein, inferior venacava, mesenteric veins, renal veins, and pulmonary veins. These cases present in various different clinical scenarios based on acuity and severity of symptoms. Extremity swelling, pain and positive Doppler duplex venous ultrasound are the typical presenting clinical picture. For other venous thromboses, more severe clinical sequela are evident in the setting of portal vein and mesenteric vein thromboses. If not treated quickly, these can present with severe bowel compromise requiring emergent surgery. Computed tomographic angiographic images usually confirm the findings. Massive pulmonary emboli can also present as cardiovascular collapse if not treated emergently. Various scenarios from life threatening entities to outpatient treatments can be approached with endovascular means.

3. Available devices

There are many devices now on the market to treat vascular thromboses and in particular venous thrombosis. Various types of endovascular devices are now on the market for venous thrombolysis. These include the Unifuse and Speed-Lyser infusion catheters (Angiodynamics, Queensbury, New York), Possis AngioJet Ultra thrombectomy system (Medrad, Minneapolis, Minnesota), EKOS endowave endovascular system (EKOS Corporation, Bothell, WA), Trellis peripheral infusion system (Bacchus Vascular, Santa Clara, CA), Spectranetics Turbo Elite Laser Ablation catheter (Spectranetics, Colorado Springs, CO) and a pure aspiration catheter called the Pronto Extraction catheter (Vascular Solutions, Minneapolis, MN).
There are three different types of catheter systems. One catheter is just used for thrombolytic drug infusion (Speed-Lyser and Uni-Fuse). The second sets of catheter systems are combined devices using both mechanical and pharmacological thrombolysis (EKOS endowave, Possis angiojet, and Trellis thrombectomy) The third set of devices use only mechanical thrombectomy (Possis angiojet, Spectranectics laser ablation and Pronto extraction catheter).

4. Thrombolysis/Infusion catheters

These catheters systems are the original type for thrombolysis. The Uni fuse is a single catheter system with multiple side holes throughout its infusion length. (Fig 1) They infuse drug directly into the clot and allow the drug to act directly on the thrombus intraluminally. The catheters come in various sizes and lengths. The speed lyser catheter is unique short device with only 15 and 20cm lengths. This device is designed to be used during fistulalysis procedures for dialysis patients. Both catheter systems are excellent for clot dissolution due to their ease of use and ability to use any drug combination.

5. Combination mechanical and pharmacological thrombolysis catheters

These devices combine both mechanical dissolution and pharmacological thrombolysis to the clot. The devices include EKOS endowave system, Trellis peripheral infusion system and the Possis Angiojet system. The EKOS system is the newest of the devices. EKOS uses ultrasonic agitation of the clot with drug infusion to speed the clot lysis. This helps clear the large bulky clot typically seen in the venous system. (Fig 2) (Fig 3) The large clot burden in the legs and pulmonary arteries are ideal for this device. Theoretically, there is less drug used and less infusion time resulting in less intensive care monitoring and lessening the cost of the hospital stay. (Fig 4)

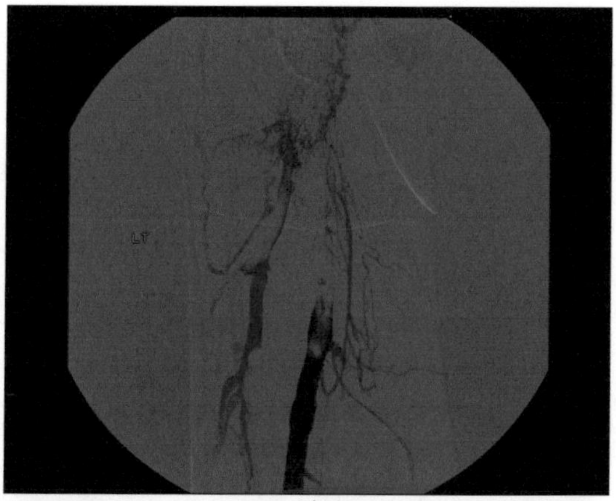

A)

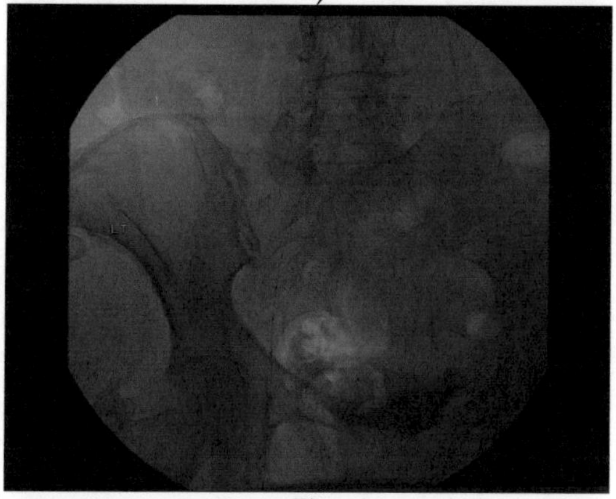

B)

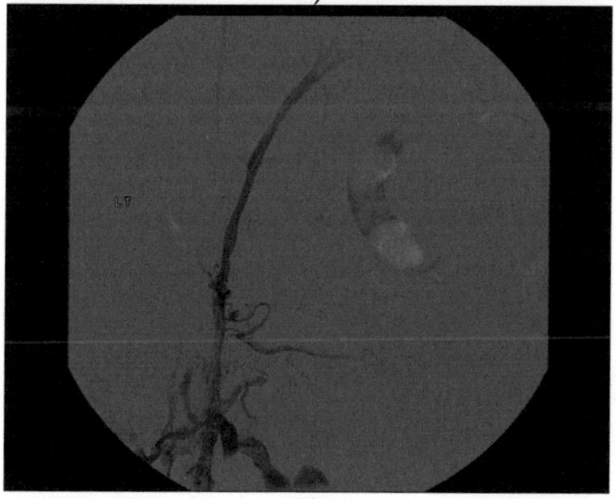

C)

Fig. 1. 64 y/o female with left leg swelling and pain and a positive U/S for DVT A) Extensive DVT Left SFV extending into iliac system B) EKOS Endowave combination thrombolysis catheter in place with TNK infusion overnight C) Widely patent ilio-femoral venous system following thrombolysis

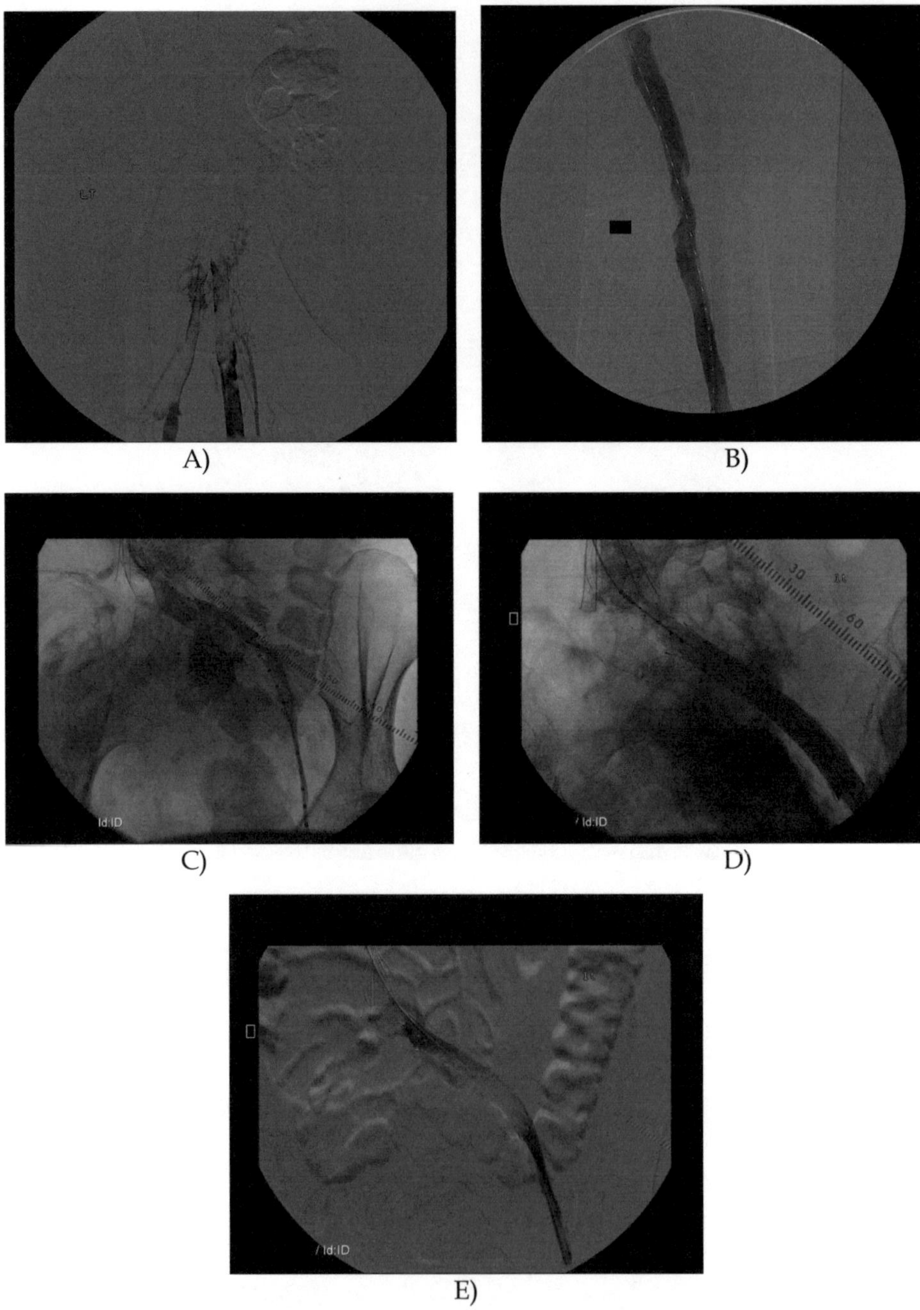

Fig. 2. 39 y/o female with May-Thurner Syndrome presents with left leg swelling, pain and + DVT A) Extensive DVT left leg B) Pure thrombolytic therapy performed with Unifuse catheter system and TNK for overnight infusion C) Uncovered irregular stenosis Left iliac vein D) Balloon venoplasty performed with improved appearance but residual stenosis remains E) Iliac venous stent placed now with widely patent venous flow through iliac veins

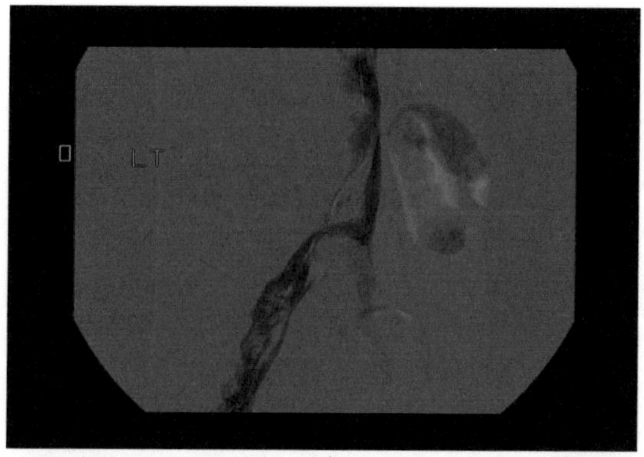

A)

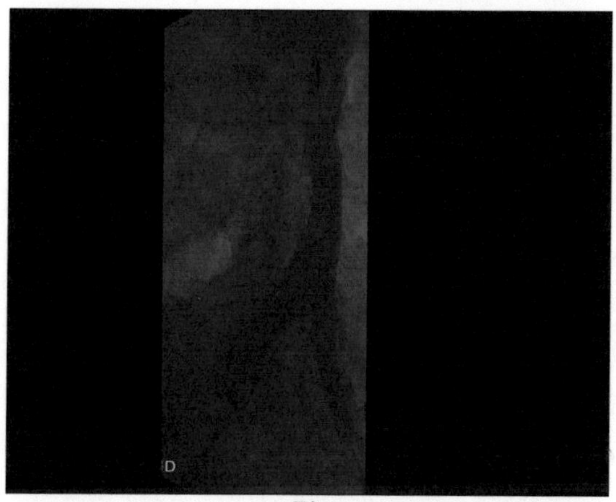

B)

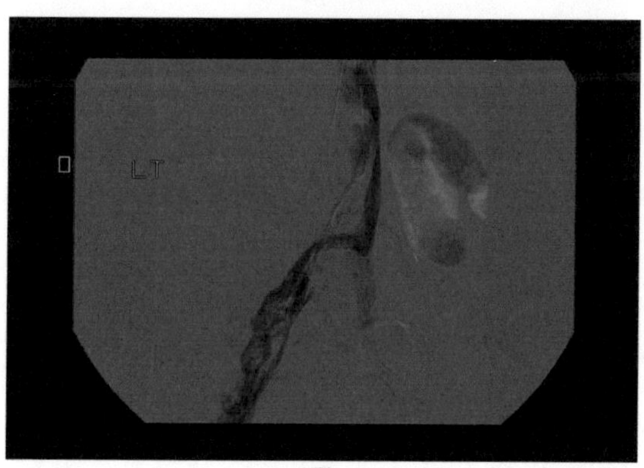

C)

Fig. 3. 54 y/o male with bilateral leg DVT and ilio-caval DVT
A) Extensive ilio-caval thrombus B) and C) Kissing EKOS catheters placed simultaneously with TNK initiated for overnight infusion now with widely patent iliac veins and venacava on final images

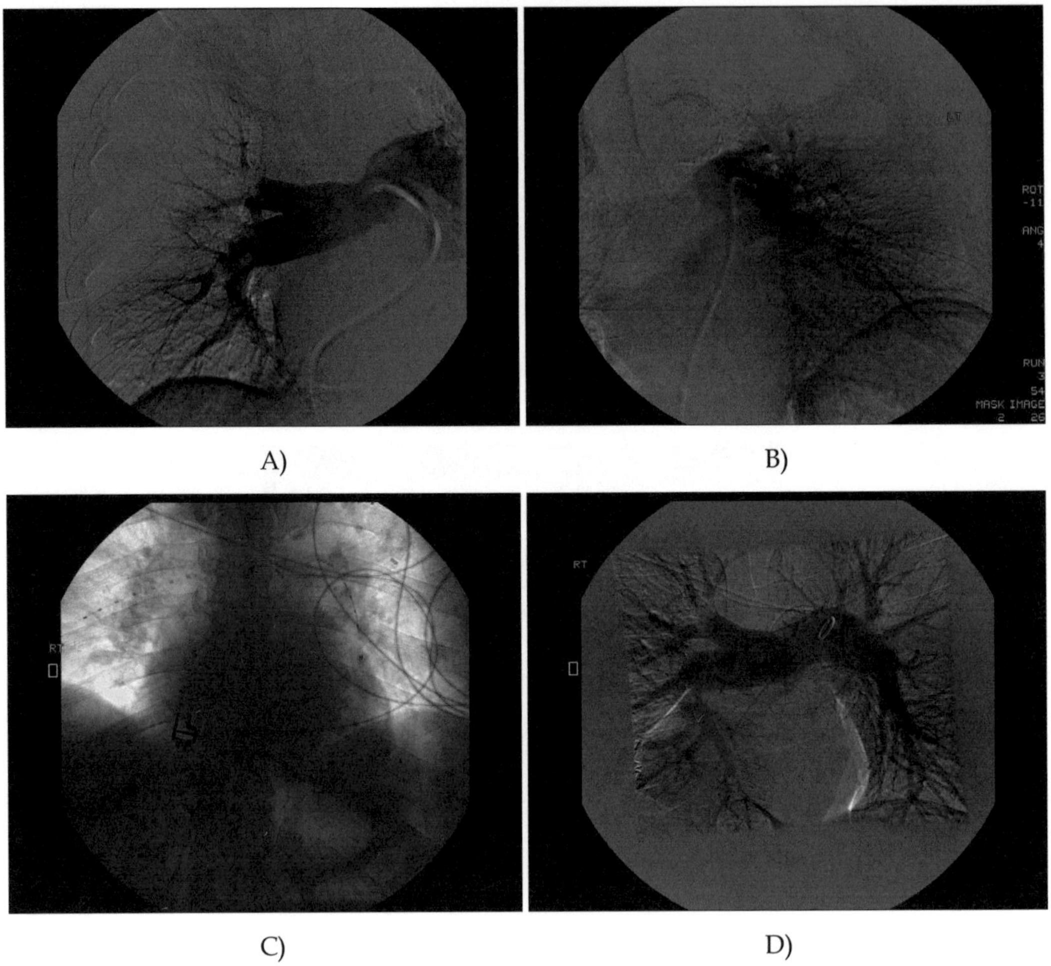

Fig. 4. 71 y/o male with cardiopulmonary collapse/shock with bilateral pulmonary embolism A) and B) Bilateral extensive pulmonary embolism C) Bilateral simultaneous EKOS/TNK combination thrombolysis catheters in place D) Widely patent pulmonary arteries following 12 hour infusion

The Trellis device also combines mechanical and pharmacological thrombolysis. This device comes in various lengths and uses balloon occlusion technique to focus on the segmental clot burden. The "whip like" mechanical disruption breaks up the clot allowing the drug to act more effectively. (Fig 5) This is a useful device for isolated clot and can be performed as an outpatient with need for hospital admission.

The Possis AngioJet system can be both a pure mechanical and combination mechanical and pharmacological thrombolytic system. For combined systems, the Possis catheter is used in a "power pulse spray mode" where the thrombolytic drug is pulse sprayed directly into the clot. It is then allowed to sit in the vessel and dissolve the clot and then is removed by the standard angiojet thrombectomy fashion. This device can be used in many venous distributions with its various lengths and catheter treatment diameters. (Fig 6)

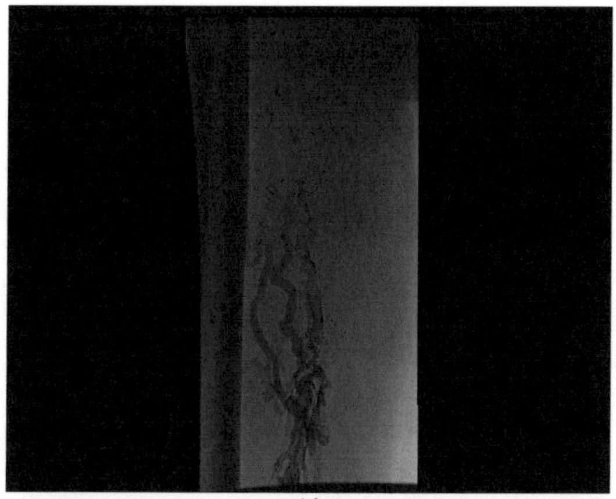

A)

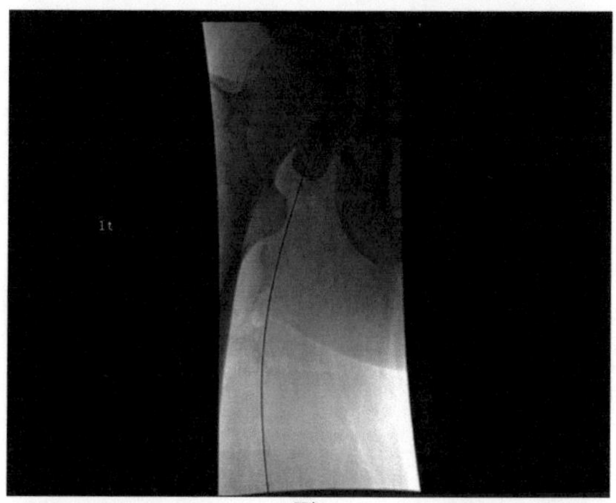

B)

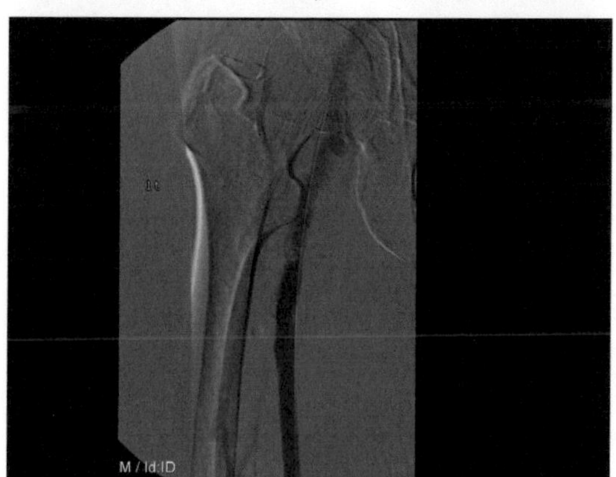

C)

Fig. 5. 59 y/o male with extensive DVT left leg swelling and pain
A) Extensive DVT identified B) Trellis thrombectomy device in SFV with balloon occlusion and mixed mechanical and pharmacological thrombolysis C) Marked improvement following Trellis device

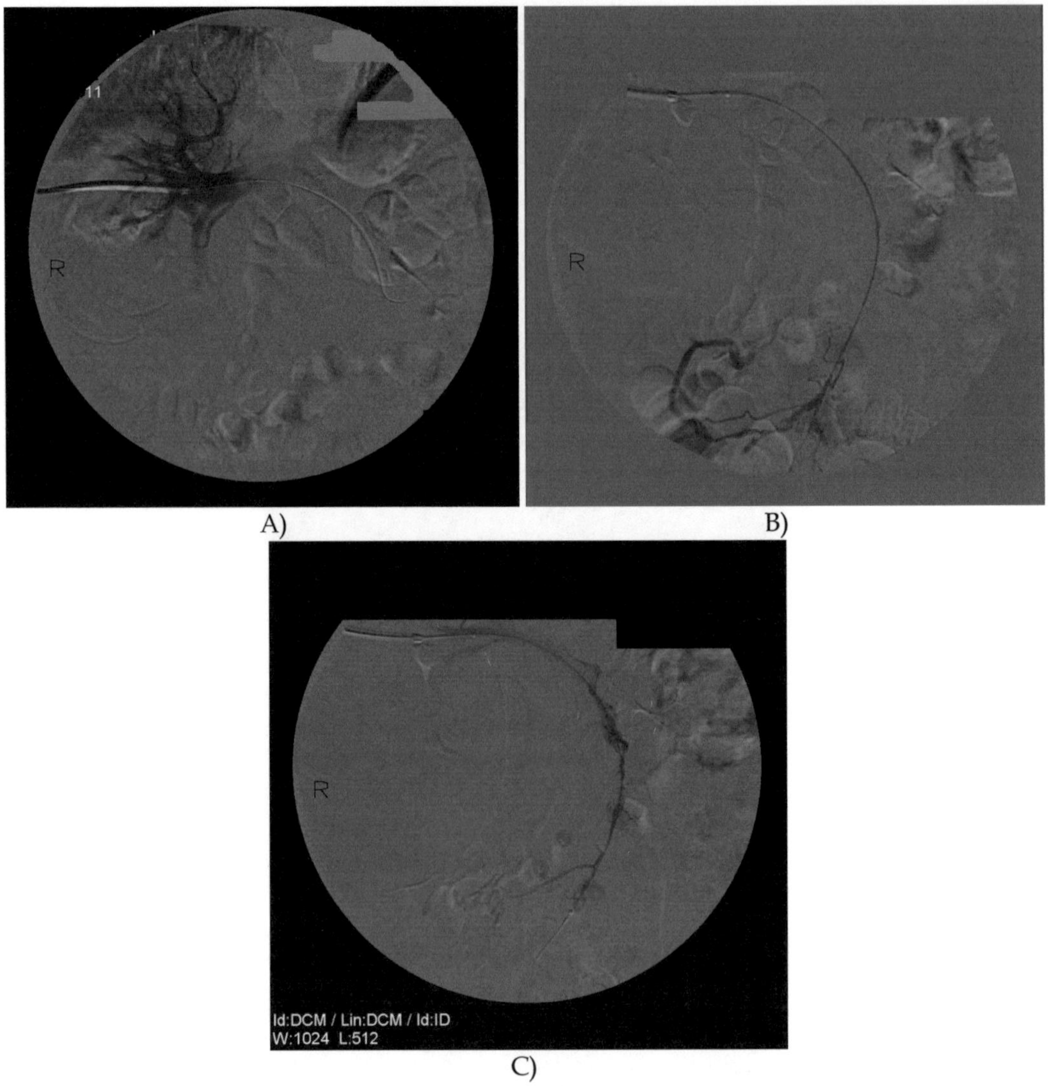

Fig. 6. 61 y/o male with chronic pancreatitis with portal vein thrombosis A) Extensive portal vein thrombosis as seen on this transhepatic portogram B) Power pulse spray possis angiojet and TPA thrombolysis of the portal vein C) Improved patency of portal vein

6. Pure mechanical devices

These devices require no thrombolytic agent to be infused into the vessel. The devices are the Possis angiojet catheter, Spectranectics laser catheter and Pronto extraction catheter. The Possis system uses saline jet through its distal side holes to create a Bernoulli effect thereby removing clot without need for drug therapy. (Fig 7) The Spectranectic device uses laser technology to vaporize the clot and thereby clear the vessel of clot quickly without chance of distal embolic phenomenon. They also come in various sizes for different vessel territories. This device can also be used as an outpatient without need for overnight stay.

The Pronto catheter (Pronto .035 extraction catheter, Vascular Solutions, Inc., Minneapolis, MN) is the newest pure mechanical device. Previously, developed from coronary interventions, it is now made for venous interventions. Pure aspiration catheters with large 8 French end hole-guiding catheters are used for cases with large clot burden such as massive pulmonary embolism and extensive deep venous thrombosis.

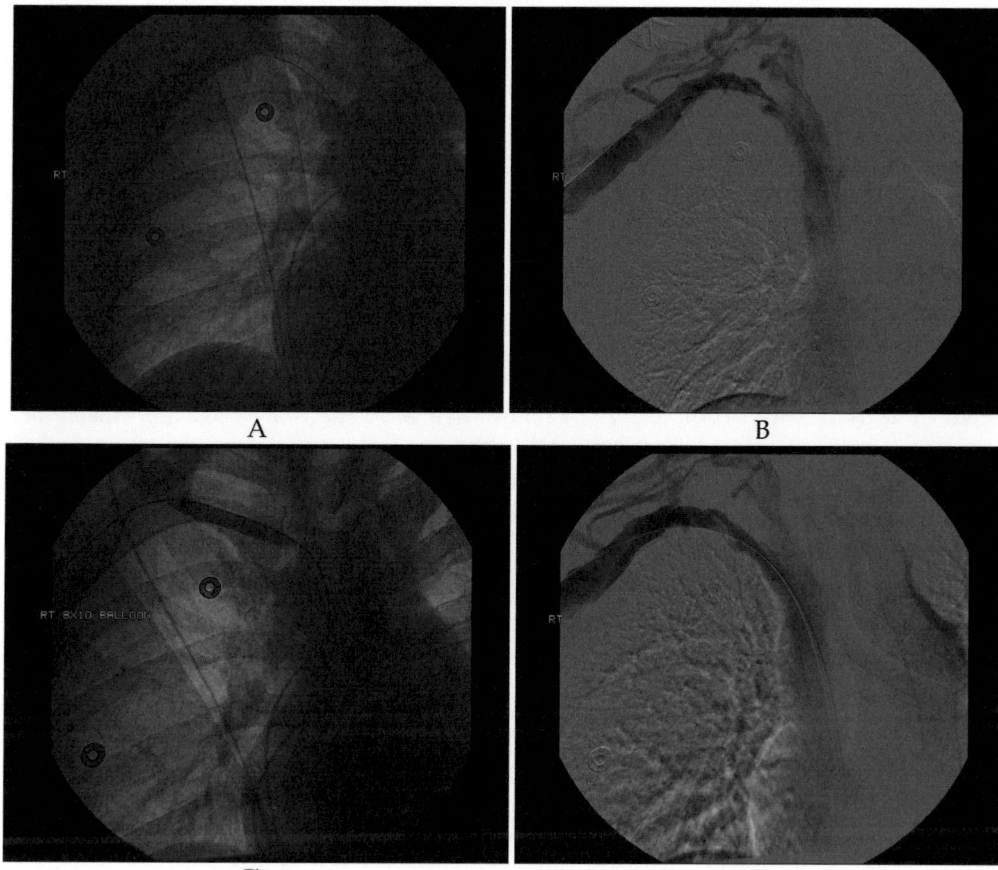

A B C) D)

Fig. 7. 31 y/o body building male with dominant right arm swelling and pain c/w Paget Schroetter syndrome A) Possis angiojet pure thrombectomy device cleared clot from subclavian vein B) Uncovered focal irregular stenosis in subclavian vein which is worse with adduction arm motion C) Balloon Venoplasty of right subclavian vein D) Patent right subclavian vein with all degrees of motion the right arm on final images

7. Additional venous interventions

Following mechanical or pharmacological thrombolysis for acute venous thrombolysis, additional endovascular interventions are usually necessary. Whether, there are focal stenoses uncovered following intervention as in Paget Schroetter syndrome, May -Thurner syndrome or fistula anastomoses in dialysis graft, there is typically some element of recoil in the vein, fixed stenosis or some chronic residual thrombus. Further interventions are required involving balloon venoplasty, stent placement or filter placement.

8. Balloon venoplasty

Balloon venoplasty can be performed after the bulky thrombus has been removed uncovering an underlying venous stenosis. This can be treated with venoplasty to improve the diameter of the vessel thus improving its flow. It is the gold standard for venous stenosis in various distributions including subclavian, iliac or venacava corresponding to the various syndromes described previously. Typically, these interventions treat the underlying venous stenosis resulting in venous patency. The more central the venous stenosis, the better the result following venoplasty. Recurrent or residual venous stenosis following balloon venoplasty occurs frequently especially in those patients with chronic central venous catheters. Despite venoplasty, these venous lesions are very difficult to treat and recurrent venous stenosis may require stenting

9. Venous stenting

Stents can be used in any venous distribution from peripheral to central veins. Covered and uncovered metal stents can be used for recurrent stenosis. Central venous stenosis as in the SVC and IVC require the largest available stents. Covered stents and the newest Flair covered stent (CR Bard, Tempe, AZ) are now available for dialysis fistula anastomoses where by a smaller fistula graft enters into the larger native venous outflow resulting in a smooth transition and improve flow dynamics. Venous stenting can also be performed following suboptimal balloon venoplasty result. Venous stenting is not performed on thrombus alone but is used as an adjunct to suboptimal venoplasty and venous thrombolysis.

10. Thrombolytic agents

Activase (TPA) (Genenetech, South San Francisco, CA) and Tenecteplase (TNK) (Genenetech, South San Francisco, CA) are the most common thrombolytic agents currently available. These drugs are fibrinolytic agents which break down fibrin into split products thus allowing clot to lyse within the vascular system. In the veins, both work similarly but TNK seems to lyse clot faster with less bleeding complications due to its exquisite fibrin specificity. Tenecteplase is the newer of the two agents. It has a 14 fold higher fibrin binding specificity than TPA. Due to the larger volume of clot within veins, a larger dose of drug is necessary to lyse the clot burden. This is one of the reasons for combining mechanical with thrombolytic agents. With combination therapy, less drug can be used in these larger capacitance vessels if combined with one of the above-mentioned mechanical devices.

11. Dialysis Interventions

Dialysis fistulas grafts are increasing in number, as renal failure becomes an epidemic. Failure of these grafts is frequent and accounts for most of the morbidity associated with these grafts. Immediate graft malfunction due to surgical causes is quickly identified during placement. Acute thrombosis within these grafts can occur at any time following placement. This is a constant problem for nephrologists due to the nature of hemodialysis itself. Chronic needle punctures within the graft 3-4 times a week results in numerous chances for thrombus formation. Also, heparinization during hemodialysis and then reversing the coagulation during and after dialysis catheter removal results in thrombosis of the graft. If unable to open the graft within a reasonable time, then other means of vascular access are required. Typically, another central venous dialysis catheter is needed until a new graft is created or the present one is cleaned out.

Interventional doctors are well adapted to lysis of dialysis graft using both pure pharmacological and mechanical thrombectomy. These grafts can be cleared of their thrombus burden in the interventional lab without requiring further surgery. Pure thrombolysis catheters like Speed Lyser delivers drug directly to the clot through multi-side holes via one micro catheter system. The drug is allowed to sit within the graft and dwell for a period of time called "lyse and wait" technique. Over this period of time, the clot is lysed and the graft is cleared of thrombus. TPA is used for this purpose. It can be injected directly into a graft. TPA can be given as a 6mg bolus within the dialysis grafts for this treatment. Following lysis, other interventions may be necessary to alleviate the source of the underlying graft malfunction.

12. Inferior venacava filter placement

Caval thrombosis can be acute or chronic. Filters can be used for the treatment of acute caval thrombosis, prophylaxis of pulmonary embolism and also be the source of caval thrombosis. Both treatment and cause of caval thrombosis makes interruption filters a double-edged sword. Either way, endovenous means are used exclusively for caval thrombosis.

Furthermore, most of the patients undergoing venous thrombolysis receive retrieval Inferior Vena Cava filter before the intervention. This is usually placed at the same setting. This idea is to reduce the risk of an iatrogenic fatal pulmonary embolism during the procedure. This filter can then be removed if indicated up to six months following implantation. Prior to removing the filter, a duplex venous ultrasound of the lower extremities is obtained to document clot resolution.

13. References

Parikh S, Motarjeme A, McNamara T, Raabe R, Hagspiel K, Benenati J, Sterling K, Comerota A."Ultrasound-accelerated Thrombolysis for the Treatment of Deep Vein Thrombosis: Initial Clinical Experience". Journal of Vascular and Interventional Radiology, 2008; 19(4) 521-528.

Marchigiano G, Riendeau D, Morse CJ. "Thrombolysis of Acute Deep Vein Thrombosis". Critical Care Nursing Quarterly, 2006; 29:312-323.

Chamsuddin A, Nazzal L, Kang B, Best I, Peters G, Panah S, Martin L, Lewis C, Zeinati C, Ho H, Venbrux A. "Catheter-directed Thrombolysis with the Endowave System in the Treatment of Acute Massive Pulmonary Embolism: A retrospective Multicenter Case Series". Journal of Vascular and Interventional Radiology, 2008; 19(3):372-376.

Comerota AJ, Aldridge SE. Thrombolytic therapy for acute deep vein thrombosis. Semin Vasc Surg 1992;5:76–84.

Plate G, Eklof B, Norgren L, et al. Venous thrombectomy for iliofemoral vein thrombosis – 10-year results of a prospective randomised study. Eur J Vasc Endovasc Surg 1997;14:367–374.

Mewissen MW, Seabrook GR, Meissner MH, et al. Catheter-directed thrombolysis for lower extremity deep venous thrombosis: Report of a national multicenter registry. Radiology 1999;211:39–49.

Comerota AJ, Throm RC, Mathias SD, et al. Catheter-directed thrombolysis for iliofemoral deep venous thrombosis improves health-related quality of life. J Vasc Surg 2000;32:130–137.

Vedantham S, Vesely TM, Sicard GA, et al. Pharmacomechanical thrombolysis and early stent placement for iliofemoral deep vein thrombosis. J Vasc Interv Radiol 2004;15:565–574

Stambo GW, Montague B. Bilateral EKOS(R) EndoWave(TM) Catheter Thrombolysis of Acute Bilateral Pulmonary Embolism in a Hemodynamically Unstable Patient. Southern Medical Journal: May 2010 - Volume 103 - Issue 5 - pp 455-457

6

Late Complications of Deep Venous Thrombosis: Painful Swollen Extremities and Non Healing Ulcers

Daniel Link
Davis School of Medicine University of California, USA

1. Introduction

Patients with complications of deep vein thrombosis (DVT) experience a "life changing event" stemming from their DVT. Constant swelling, pain and discoloration of the involved lower extremity are common. These symptoms result from "venous hypertension secondary to reflux, obstruction, or insufficiency of muscle pumps" (Kearon 2003; Labropoulos 2004). Although the symptoms are well described, patients often have no plan for long term follow up after the acute DVT event. The venous system adjusts to impaired valvular function and obstructed outflow venous channels in the first year following the DVT. A life long commitment to compression hose therapy (Franks, Moffatt et al. 1995) with ambulation and extremity elevation at rest will minimize swelling and pain. Unfortunately, in the acute phase patients often cannot tolerate compression hose but they should be "coached" into compression hose as soon as possible. "60% of patients post DVT develop post thrombotic syndrome (Ashrani, Silverstein et al. 2009); fitted, graded compression hose reduce the rate in half" (Kahn ; Brandjes, Buller et al. 1997; Pirard, Bellens et al. 2008). Following a course of anticoagulation and advice for compression hose therapy, DVT patients usually are followed by their primary care provider. Recently there has been increasing interest in more closely following DVT patients. A duplex supervised by a vascular/vein specialist should be performed to assess the "pumping" capacity, available venous channels and valvular competence a few weeks to months after a DVT event (van Ramshorst, van Bemmelen et al. 1994; Caps, Manzo et al. 1995; Salcuni, Fiorentino et al. 1996; Nicolaides 2000). This is especially indicated if patients experience persistent pain and swelling, or if a change occurs in the status of the limb swelling and pain after a long stable period, or if there is continued increase in pigmentation in the pressurized area. Chronic complications, post thrombotic syndrome (PTS), can present clinically depending on the initial severity of the deep venous abnormality, but may also develop abnormalities in the years following a DVT (Bradbury 2010). The overwhelming goal of the treatment of complicated post DVT patients is to preserve skin integrity and to prevent or heal ulceration (Kearon 2004; Bradbury 2010). Pain, infection, and loss of function result in a significant cost to the patient and the community as a whole.

2. Anatomy

Veins are substantially different from arteries and exist as a network of thin channels with little intrinsic muscular wall. Large intramuscular veins like the gastrocnemius vein can dilate with the muscle relaxed and empty with calf muscular contraction. The veins in the calf muscles (May 1975) and the plantar venous plexus (Corley, Broderick et al. 2010) are major components of the muscular pump but all muscular veins contribute as do the superficial systems to the return of extremity venous blood. Obstruction leads to dilation of these deep muscular veins and perforating vein connections to the subdermal veins.

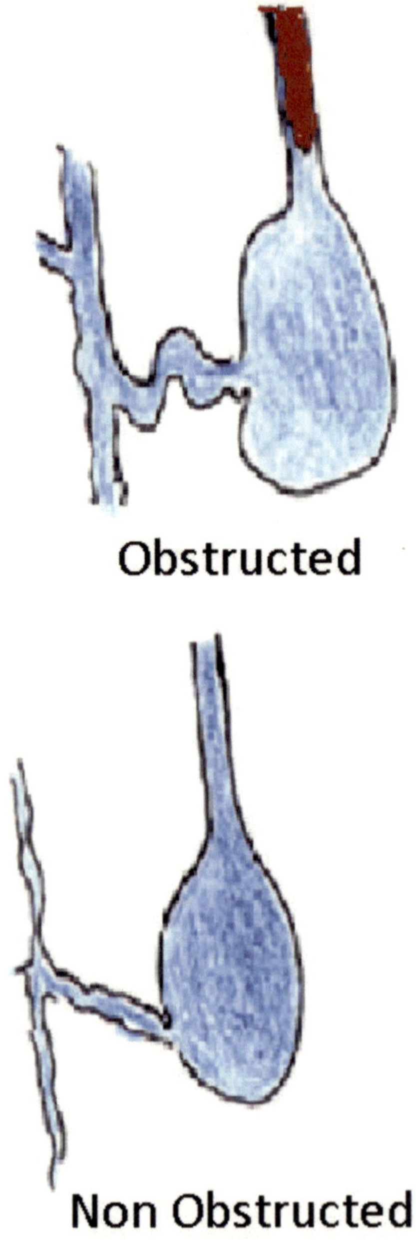

Fig. 1. Diagram of muscular pump with and without obstructing venous thrombosis. Note, bulging sub dermal veins.

Veins that connect the subdermal veins and saphenous veins to the deep vein are called perforating veins. The muscular vascular pedicle usually enters the proximal portion of the muscle with the distal muscle and tendons are relatively less vascular. The perforating veins usually follow the cutaneous nerves in a neurovascular bundle. The increased volume and eventually pressure to the subdermal (reticular) veins leads to expansion of the subcutaneous vascular space. The actual distribution of venous blood and pressure is distributed through this system and related to the configuration of each pressurized subdermal vein complex. Three different complexities have been described as the perforating vein (P) exits the deep fascia to enter a sub dermal vein (Hern and Mortimer 1999; Schaverien, Saint-Cyr et al. 2008).

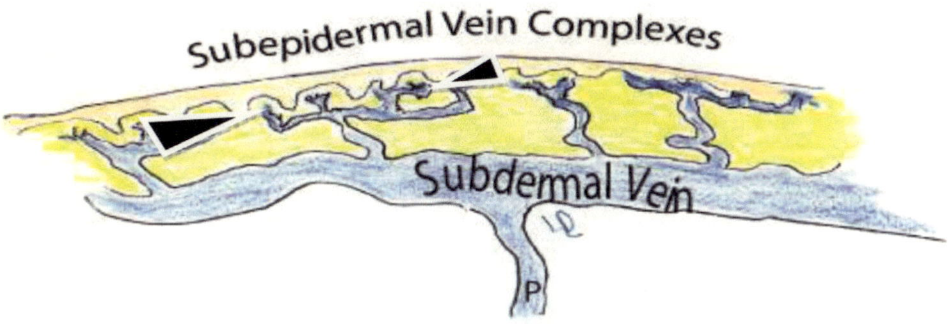

Fig. 2. Diagram of perforating vein, subdermal vein and subepidermal vein complexes.

Terminal Branches distribute the pressurized blood over this distribution. This increased pressure leads to dilation and increased tortuosity of the distal arterioles and capillaries That associated edema of the epidermal papillae, impaired skin nutrition and eventual ulceration (Hern and Mortimer 1999). The figures below show a normal venogram demonstrating venous filling and pumping for an injection of a vein in the foot. Varicose veins and abnormal perforating veins are also visualized on venography (figure 4). The resultant dilation of the subdermal veins also can be documented in the clinic with duplex imaging (Hanrahan, Araki et al. 1991; Stuart, Lee et al. 2001). This anatomy is complex and pressurization can affect the viability of the overlying dermis. Plastic surgeons have recognized and studied this venous anatomy (Schaverien, Saint-Cyr et al. 2008). In this work there are excellent figures with the anatomy of the epidermal and subdermal venous anatomy and emphasizes the role of the perforating vein and the complex of subdermal veins in the outcome of "anterolateral thigh perforator flap".

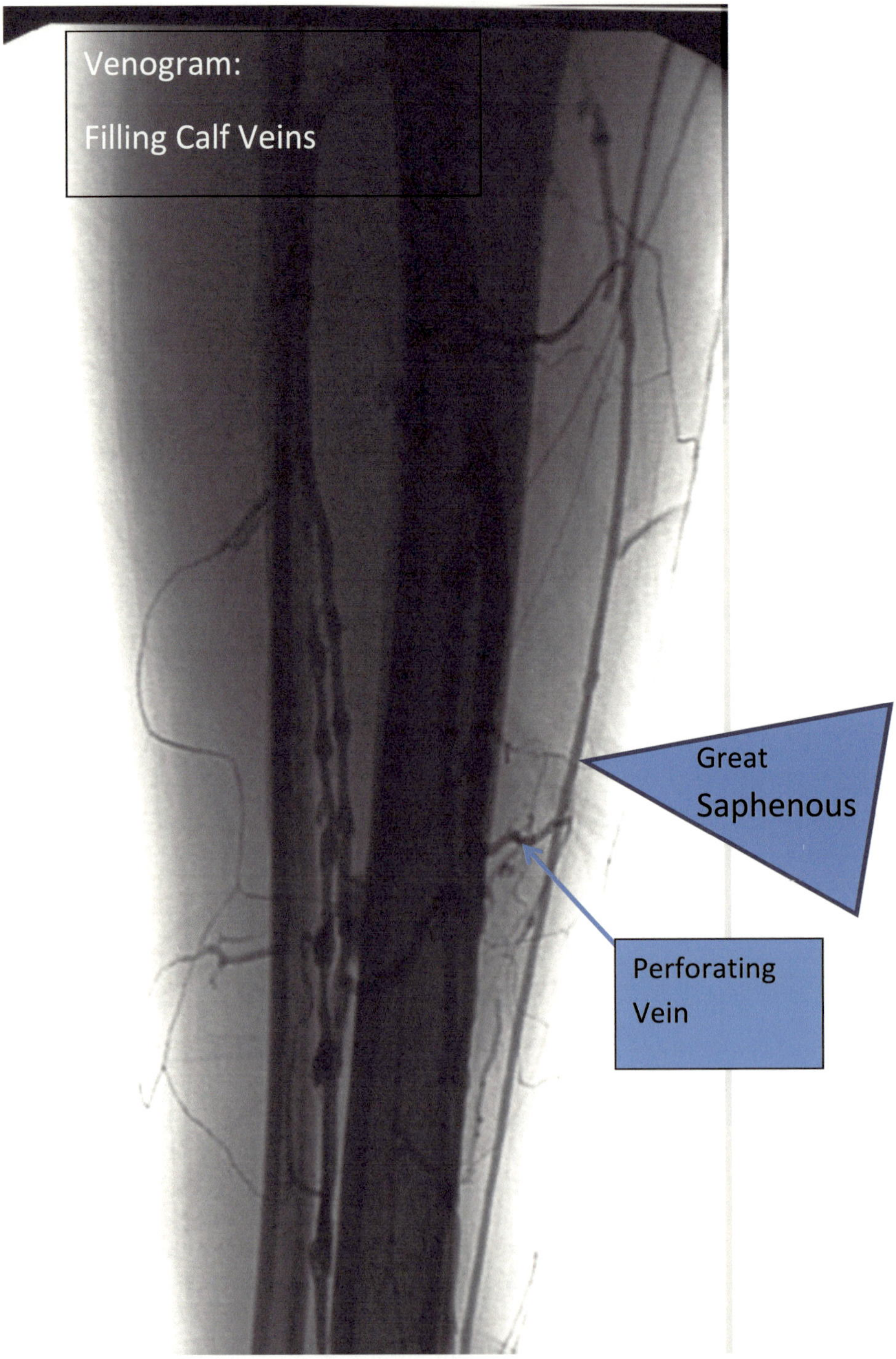

Fig. 3A. A foot veins has been injected with the patient at rest and the standing at 60 degree tilt. The extremity is non-weight bearing. The deep system fills preferentially. The great saphenous vein is small and perforating veins are demonstrated.

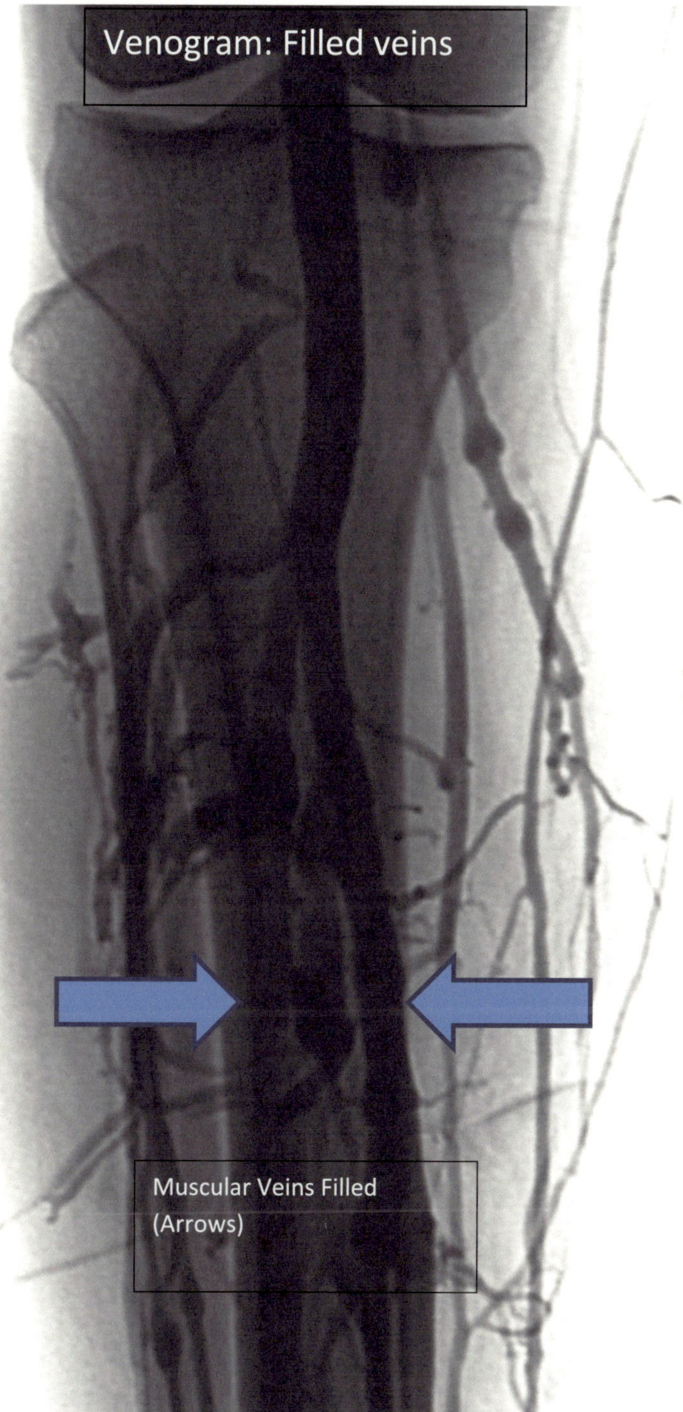

Fig. 3B. The deep veins of the calf fill and enlarge with the great saphenous vein remaining small. Normal perforating vein function.

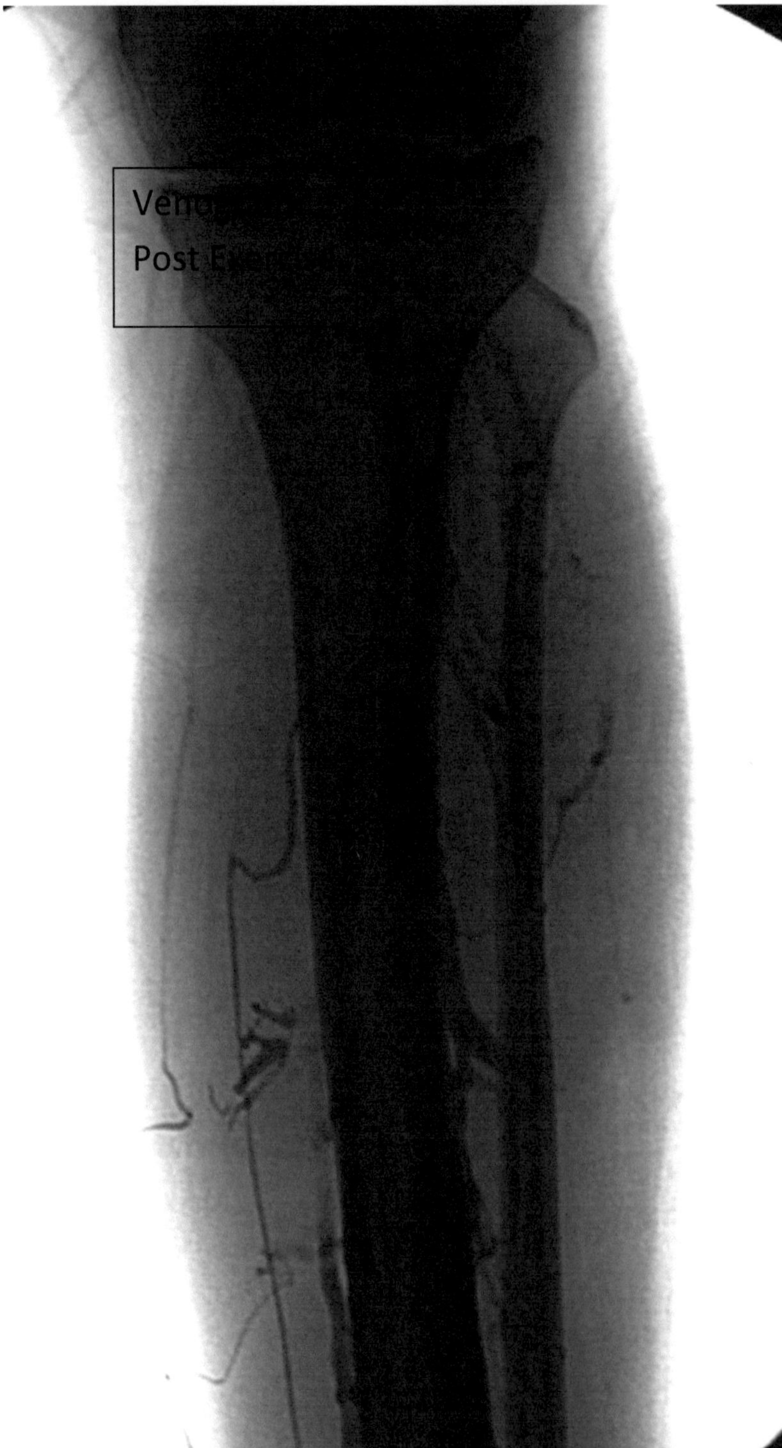

Fig. 3C. Following muscular contraction, the deep and superficial calf veins empty

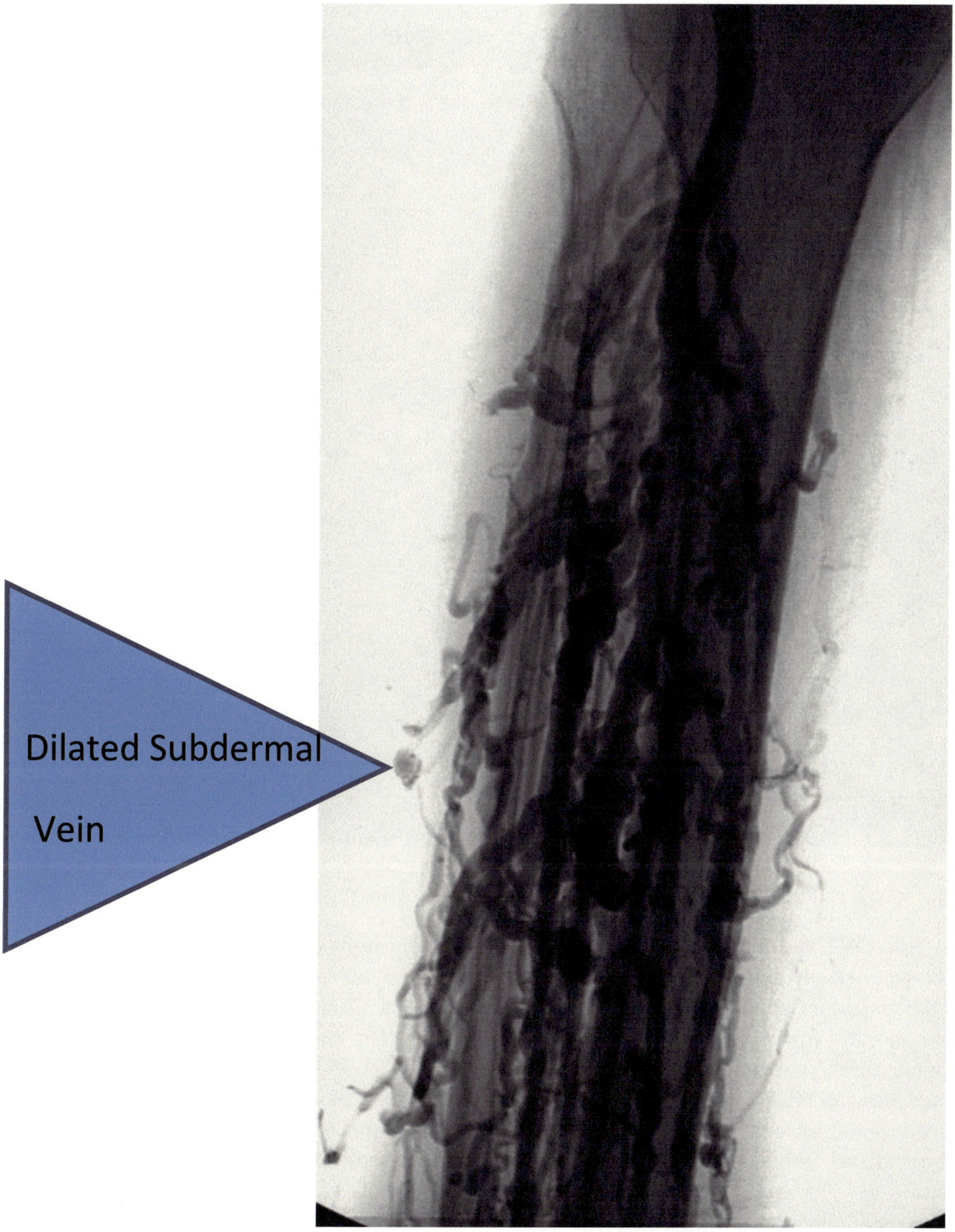

Fig. 4. Patient with proximal venous obstruction. Demonstrating dilation of subdermal vein complexes.

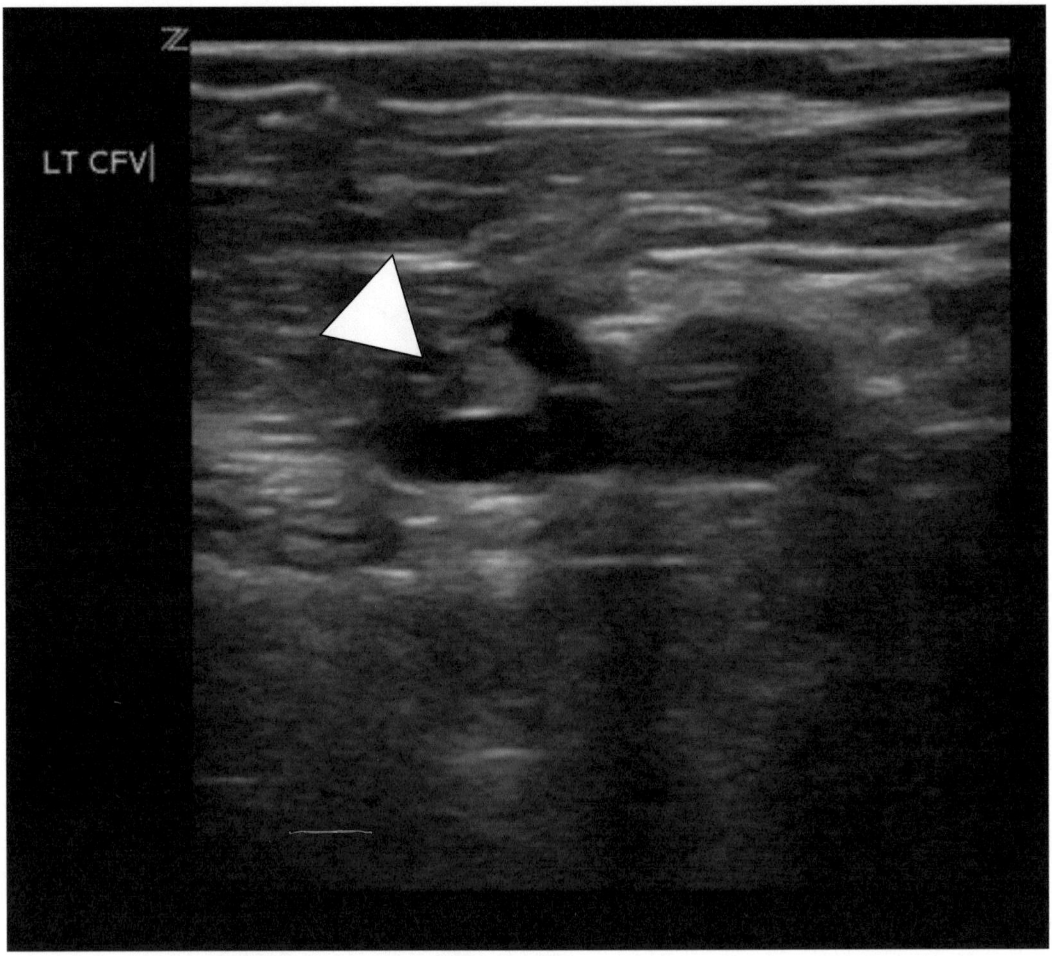

Fig. 5. Venous thrombosis left common femoral vein after 6 months, arrowhead.

After a DVT, the clinician should be aware of the early signs of a post thrombotic syndrome. At every stage following DVT there is a role for follow up in a center for vascular care and DVT patients should be alerted to the symptoms of venous hypertension, so that progression of the disease can be minimized early. The progression from increased skin pigmentation to non-healing ulceration can be prevented. Most patients cannot wear graded compression hose acutely, but as the swelling and tenderness subside the patients should be encouraged to wear compression before skin changes develop. Local venous hypertension from distal reflux leads to the skin changes and are usually associated with pain and swelling. The venous hypertension can persist and develop increasing pain and skin abnormalities including ulceration despite optimum compression hose therapy (Felty and Rooke 2005). In addition to pressurization of the subdermal veins patient develop tense swelling of the affected lower extremity, lymph edema (Shrubb and Mason 2006). Figure 5 shows thrombus in the femoral vein that is chronic and non-occluding. The patient, though

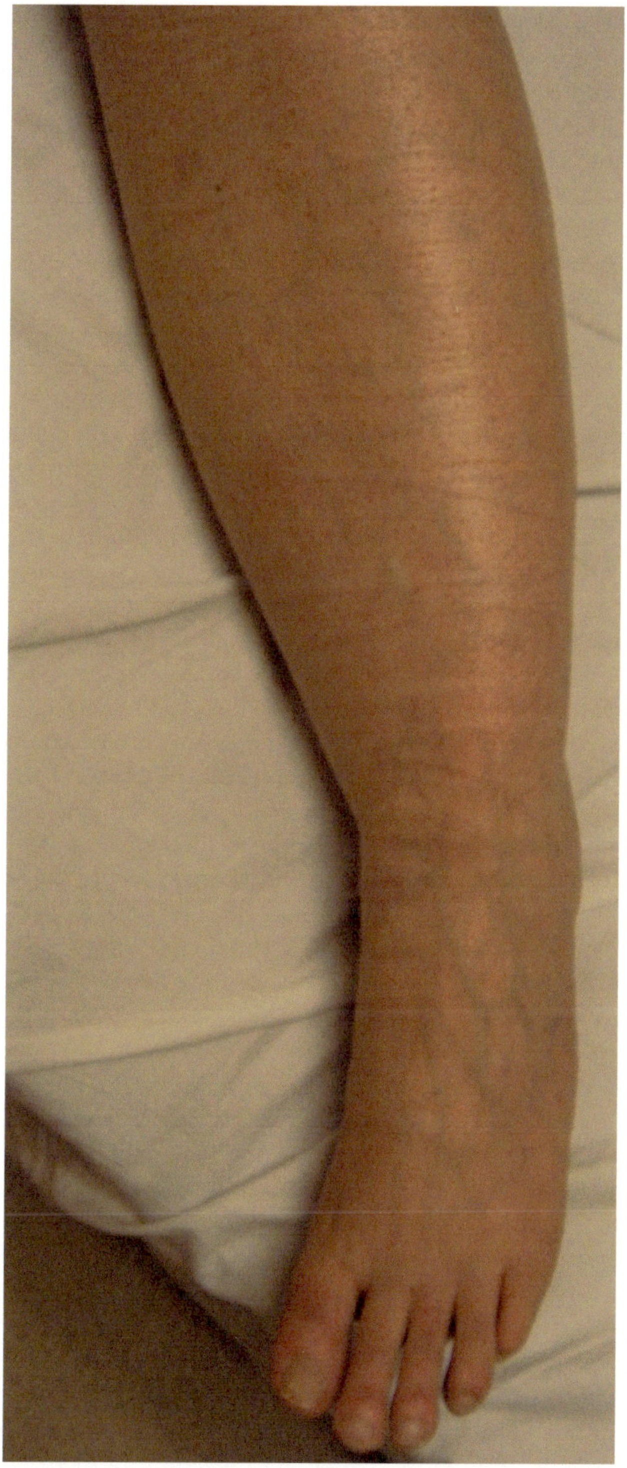

Fig. 6. Lymph edema 6 months following DVT in left femoral vein (figure 5).

wearing compression dressings as much as possible showed tense swelling of the leg to the ankle. 4 months following her initial visit and 7 months following the DVT the femoral vein thrombus had resolved by duplex, the only residual thrombus was a partially occluding thrombus in the popliteal vein. The gastrocnemius veins cleared with exercise and no reflux could be demonstrated in the femoral or common femoral veins by duplex. Lymph edema can persist following DVT despite resolution of deep venous reflux and obstruction. This patient had skin thickening and pitting edema, which is classified as Stage II lymph edema. Evaluating these patients require a clinical examination and duplex. Occasionally, unusual conditions may arise compressing the venous return (Bekou, Galis et al. 2011). The value of an evaluation of patients with suspected DVT is emphasized by a group studied where DVT (the thrombosis in the outflow veins) was found in "213 (28.6%) of 745 suspected cased". The clinical examination including sonography revealed, chronic vein thrombosis and superficial vein thrombosis, 122 patients (28%, and 76 patients with lymph edema (13.3%)(Taute, Melnyk et al. 2010). In acute venous hypertension may obstruct the lymphatic in the acute phase leading to the lymph edema seen as a result of gynecologic surgery where rich protein fluid absorption from the interstitium results (Bollinger, Isenring et al. 1982; Shrubb and Mason 2006; Ohba, Todo et al. 2011) . "In severe CVI leading to tropical changes of the skin lymphatic microangiopathy was detected. Obliterations of parts of the superficial capillary network, phenomena of cutaneous reflux and increased permeability of capillary fragments occurred. These findings contrast to primary lymph edema where the rete remains intact.."(Bollinger, Isenring et al. 1982). Imbalances between extracellular matrix synthesis and degradation has been found associated with chronic non healing ulcers(Moor, Vachon et al. 2009). Compression therapy is often painful. Physical therapy with massage and mechanical lymph edema pumps may be helpful but remain controversial; level one efficacy studies are not available. The patient in the example responded to the lymph edema pump, Flexitouch, Tactile Systems Technology, Inc Minneapolis, MN, USA).

Symptom severity and CEAP grade increase can be correlated to Perforating vein reflux. Perforating vein reflux is found in less than 10% of patients with CEAP grade 0 but there is an increase from 46% with Grade 2/3, 82% at with grade 4 and 90% with grade 5/6 (healed/open ulcers) (Stuart, Lee et al. 2001; Raju and Neglen 2009)

2.1 Ulcers with pain not responding to compression dressings

Evaluation of such patients by duplex can reveal large venous complexes deep the ulcers that impede healing and contribute to the pain. Sclerotherapy and Ablation (Radiofrequency Ablation(Marsh, Price et al. 2010) and Endovascular Laser(Proebstle and Herdemann 2007)) procedure can enhance healing.

Sclerotherapy has been used for many years, but targeting the subepidermal veins by ultrasound imaging can improve outcomes. Sodium Tetracyl sulfate (Sotradecol, 1 & 3 %, Angiodynamics, NJ) has been used. Other sclerosants included Pilodocanol, Asclera, and Aethoxysklerol approved only for small varicose veins, and hypertonic saline. Recently, steam has been used in a few patients with non healing ulcer. Steam would have the advantage of "percolating" into the target subepidermal vein complexes. Steam scalds the veins and coagulates the luminal contents. Further development studies are ongoing (Milleret 2011).

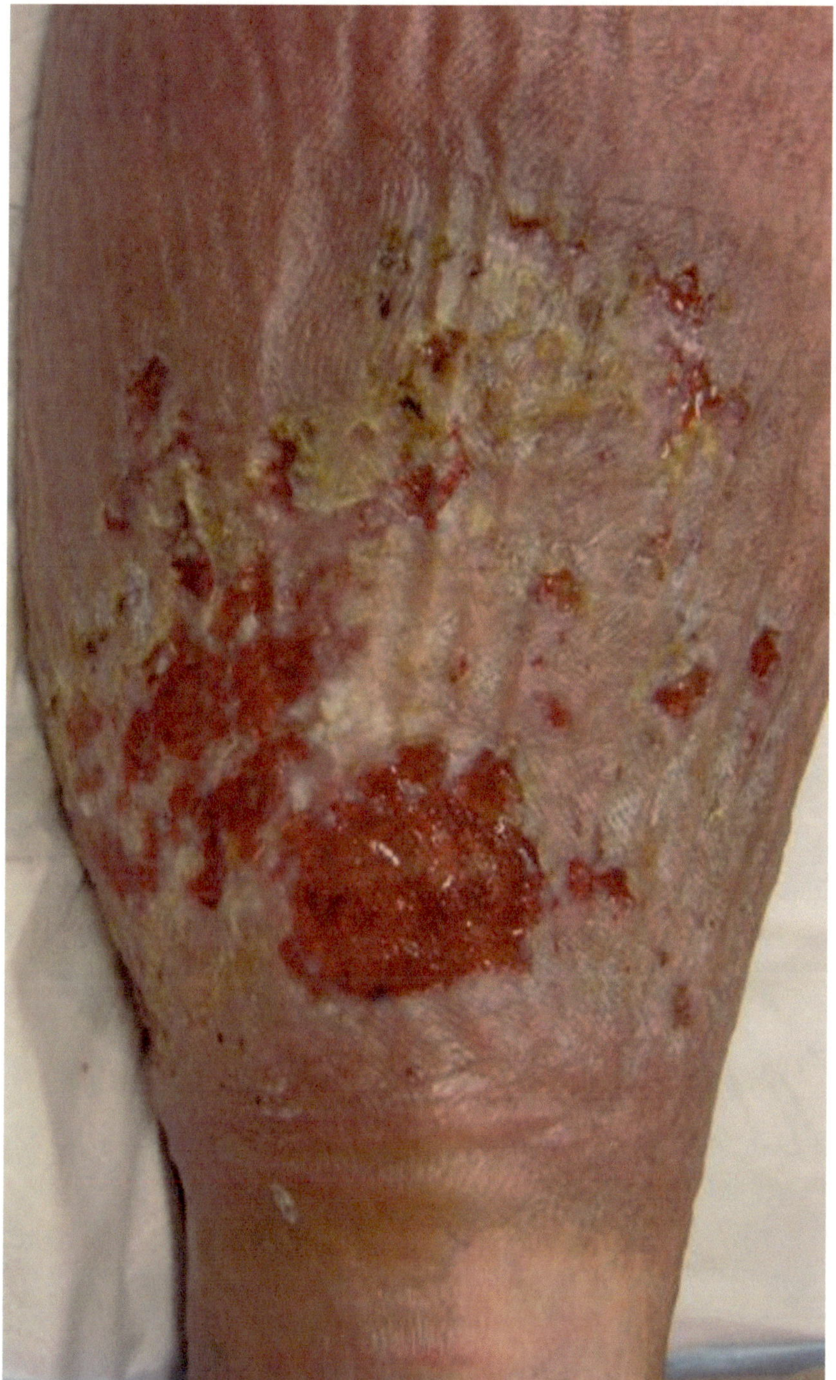

Fig. 7A. Patient with non healing ulcers years after DVT despite compression therapy.

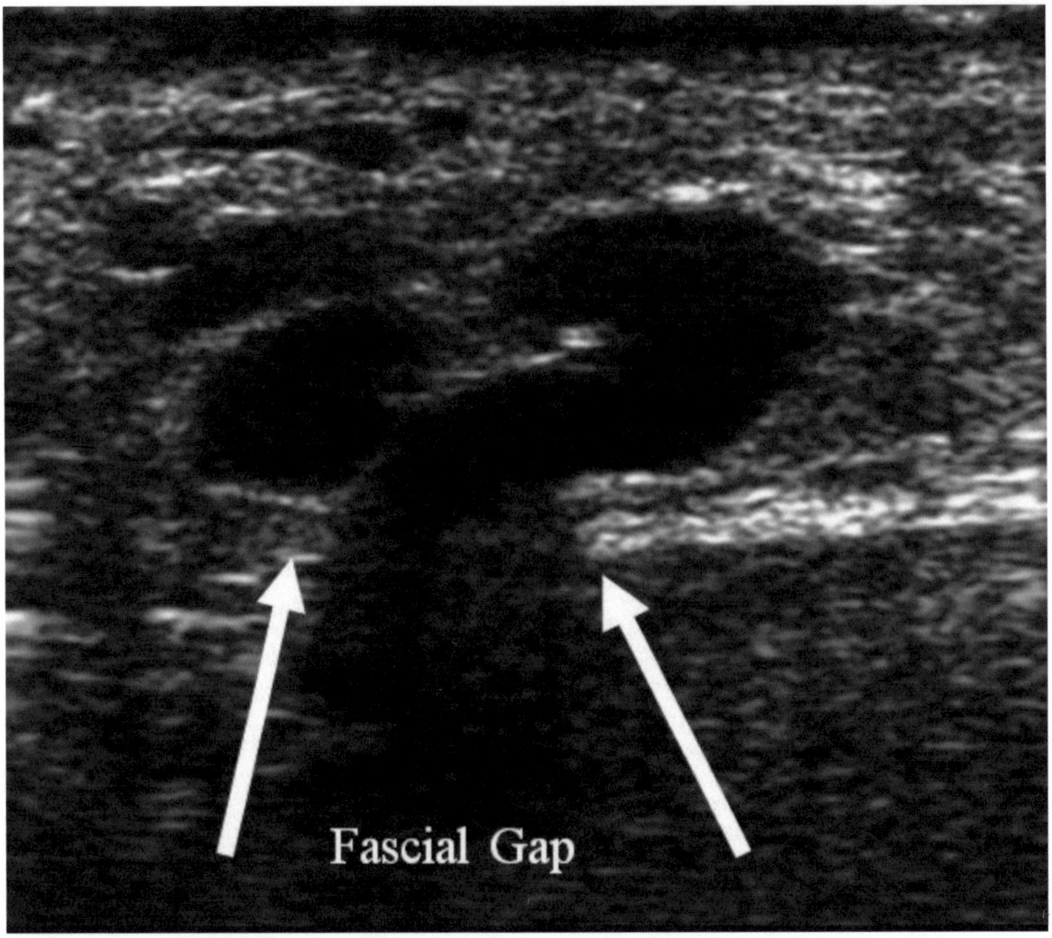

Fig. 7B. Pressuring perforating vein with incompetence by duplex.

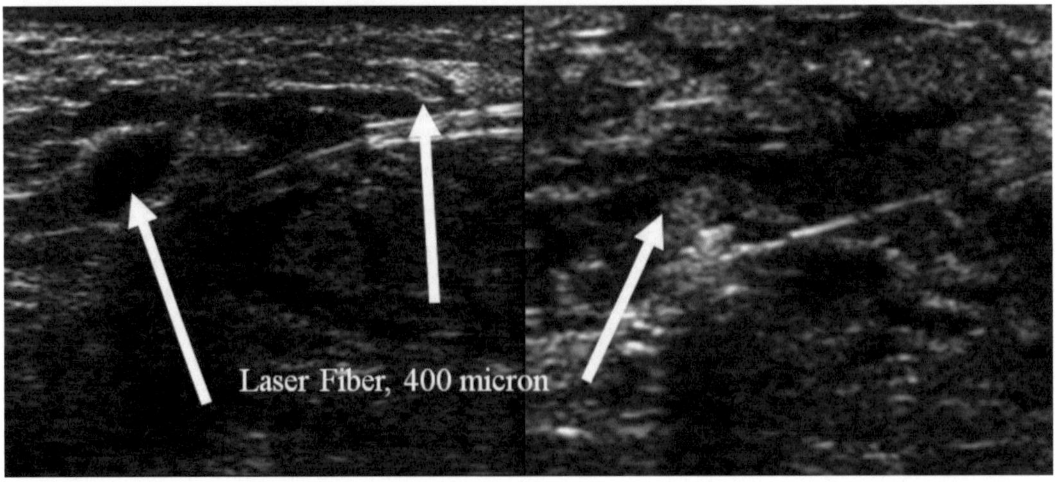

Fig. 7C. Intra procedural imaging of laser closure.

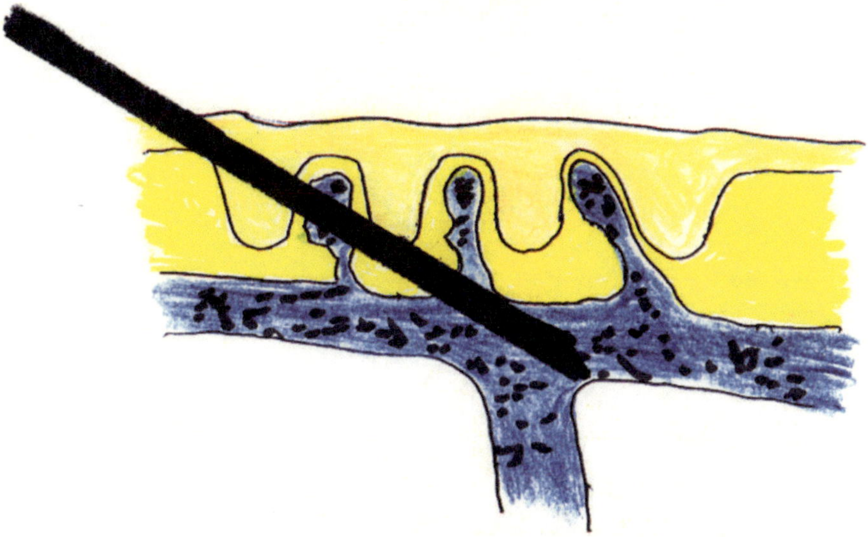

Fig. 8A. Diagram of foam sclerotherapy.

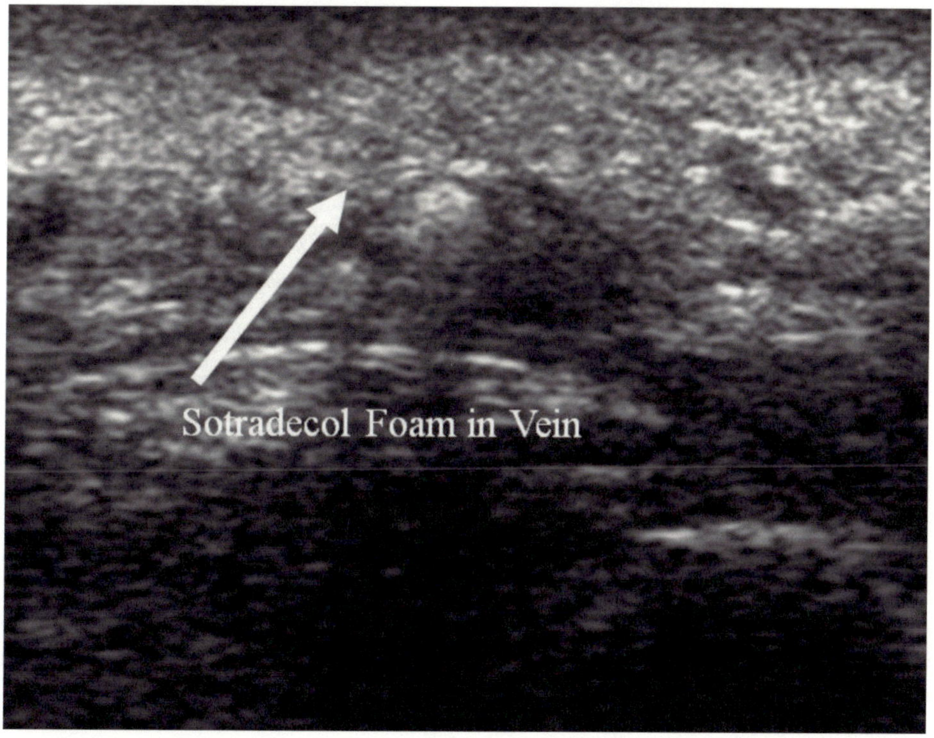

Fig. 8B. Intra procedural imaging of foam sclerotherapy.

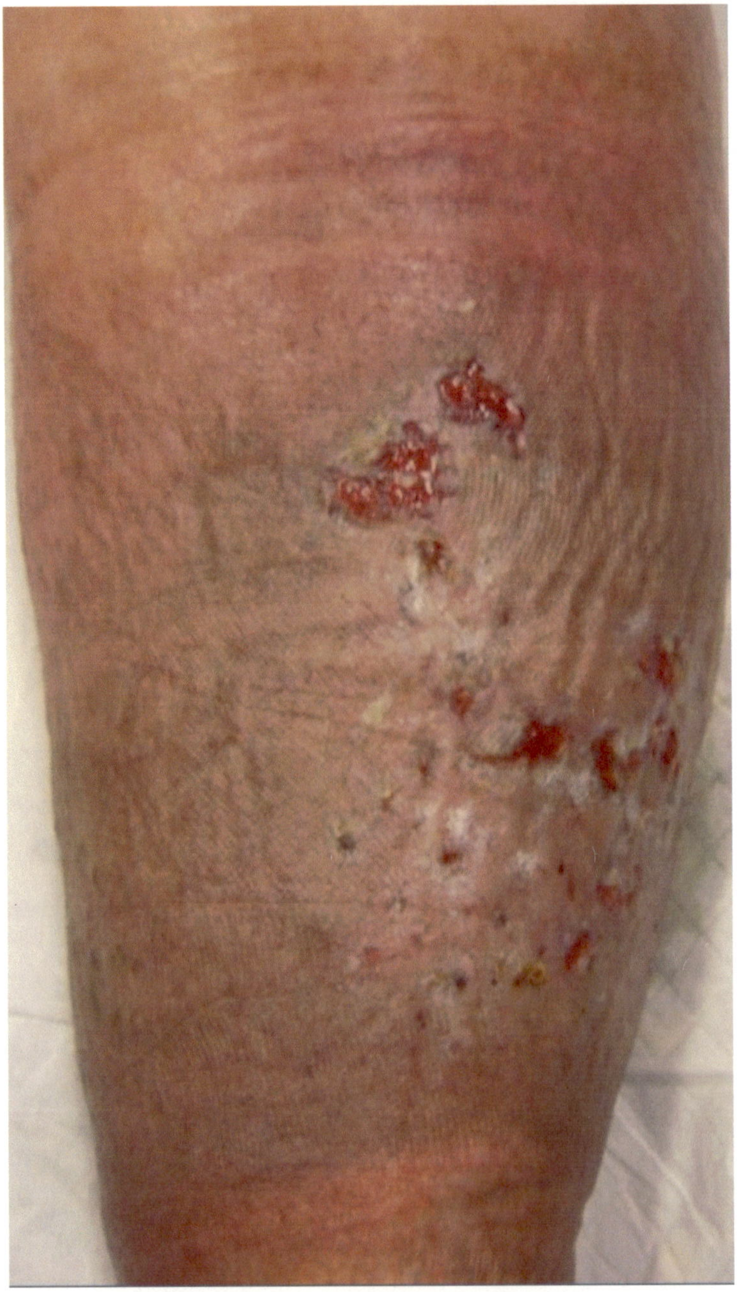

Fig. 9. Photograph of above patient after few weeks of foam and laser therapy.

Figures 7, 8 and 9 demonstrates an obese patient that has been in compression dressings, una boot or dynaflex for the last several years. Large non healing ulcers Figure 7A, Pressurizing perforating vein demonstrated, not seen incompetent by duplex, Figure 7B, Closure of perforating vein with laser fiber, Figure 7C. Diagram of foam sclerotherapy, Figure 8A Foam seen in veins deep to ulcer Figure 8B.

2.2 Arteriovenous malformations post venous thrombosis

Patients who start to develop lower extremity pain post DVT that is not controlled by compression therapy should be evaluated. Some patients will show arterial signals on duplex distal to venous occlusions. The high flow inflow from the AVM can be found with duplex. The natural history of the neovasularity in the thrombus in unknown but has been described in the cerebral sinus post thrombosis and in the peripheral veins (Link, Garza et al. ; Chikamatsu, Nagashima et al. 2001; Aboian, Daniels et al. 2009). Many of these patients have been found to be factor V Leiden positive (Link, Garza et al.). There is evidence that the veins are not passive and may play a significant and dynamic role in revascularization through angiogenesis (Aboian, Daniels et al. 2009). It is unclear whether the AVF/AVM in thrombus is transitory or may remain permanent. Figure 10A shows a chronic occlusion of the left internal iliac vein (presumably May-Thurner Syndrome (May R 1957; Fazel, Froehlich et al. 2007) in a patient followed by her primary care physician for many years without a specific, etiologic diagnosis. She developed large open and painful ulcers. The large collateral veins on her abdomen were unsightly but was not her concern, Figure 10. (Link 2011)

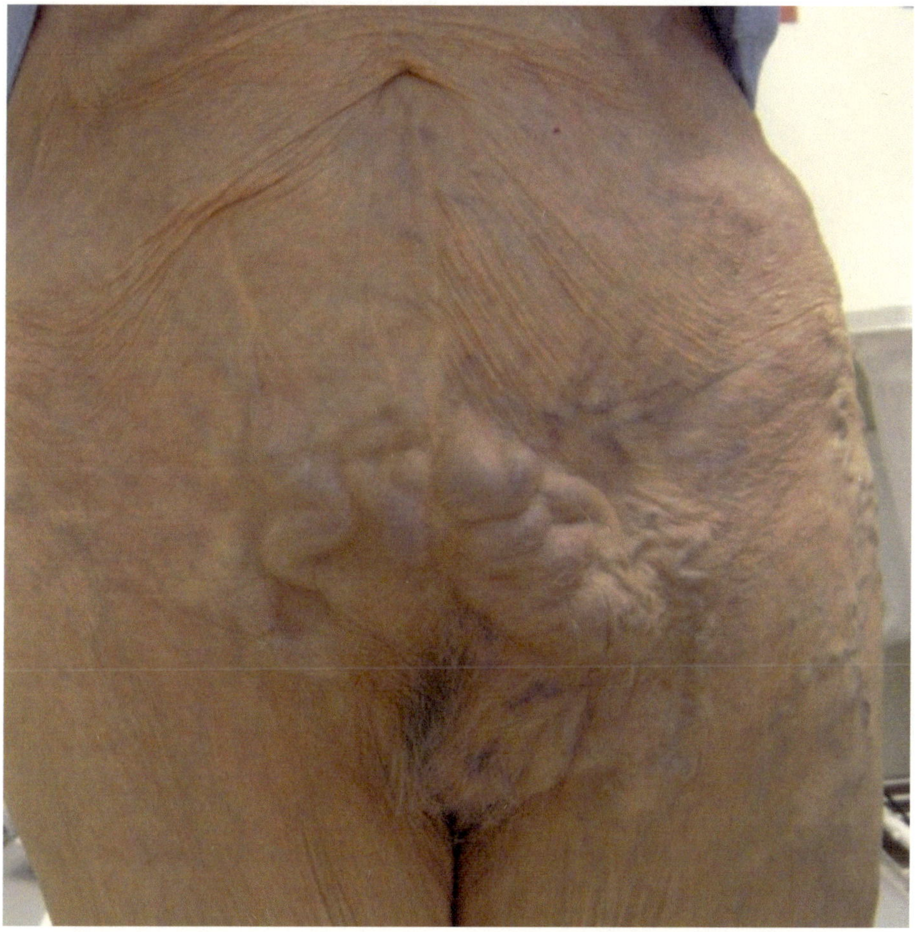

Fig. 10A. Patient with chronic left iliac vein occlusion after more than 20 years.

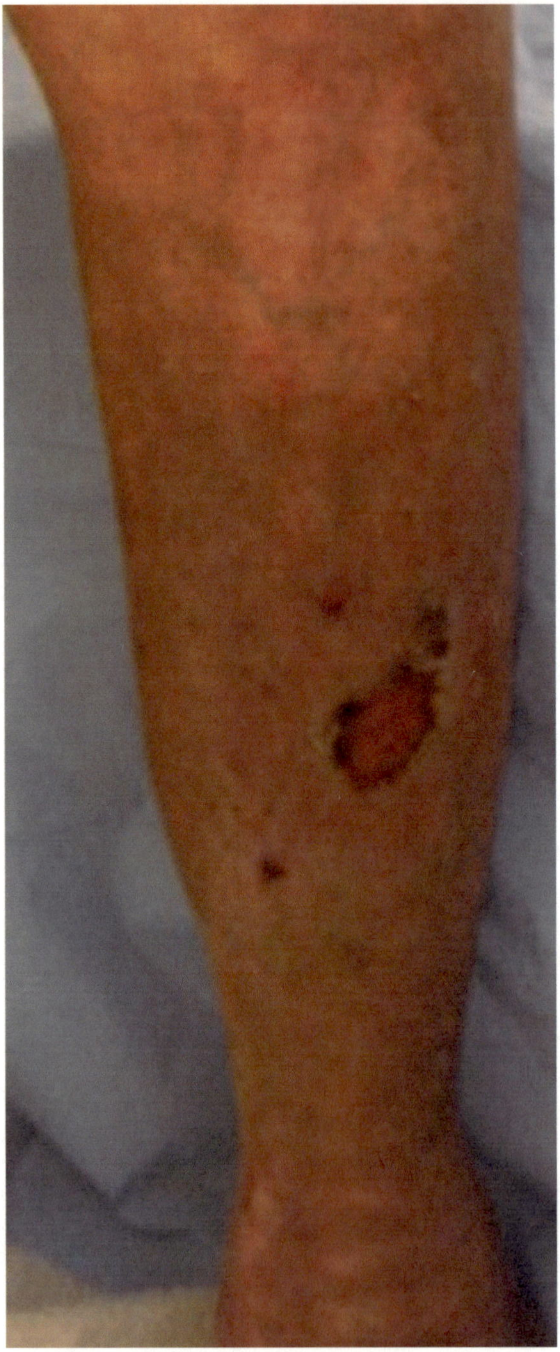

Fig. 10B. Non healing ulcers, extremely painful, patient's main compliant.

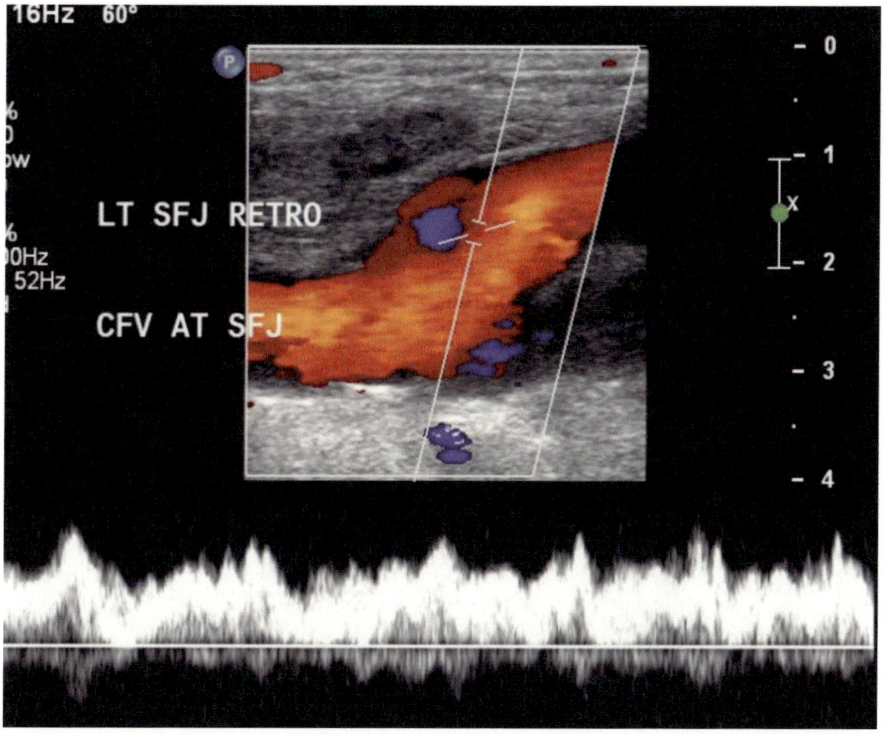

Fig. 10C. Duplex of left common femoral vein showing high flow with arterial pulses.

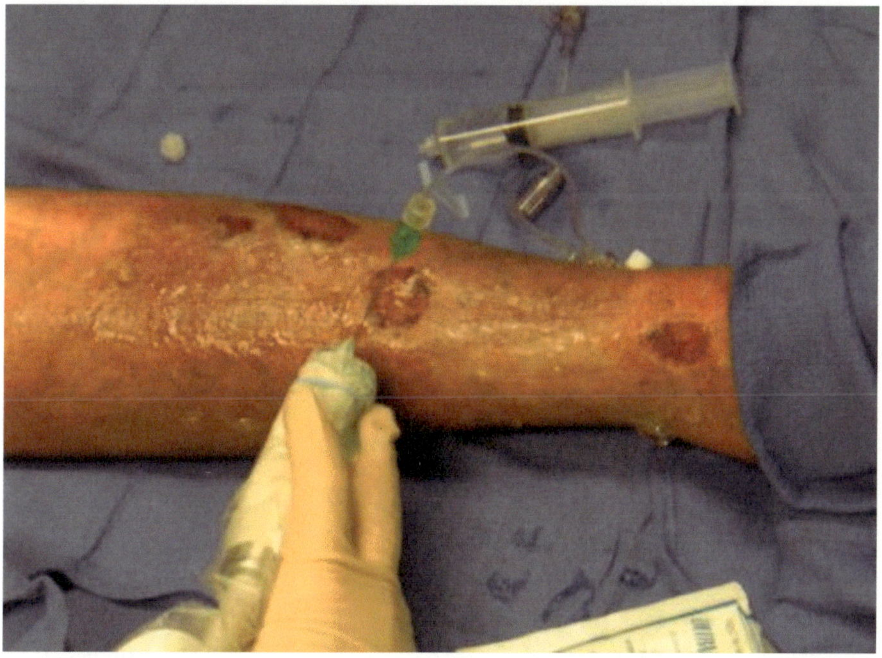

Fig. 11. Foam Sclerotherapy procedure in above patient (Figure 10).

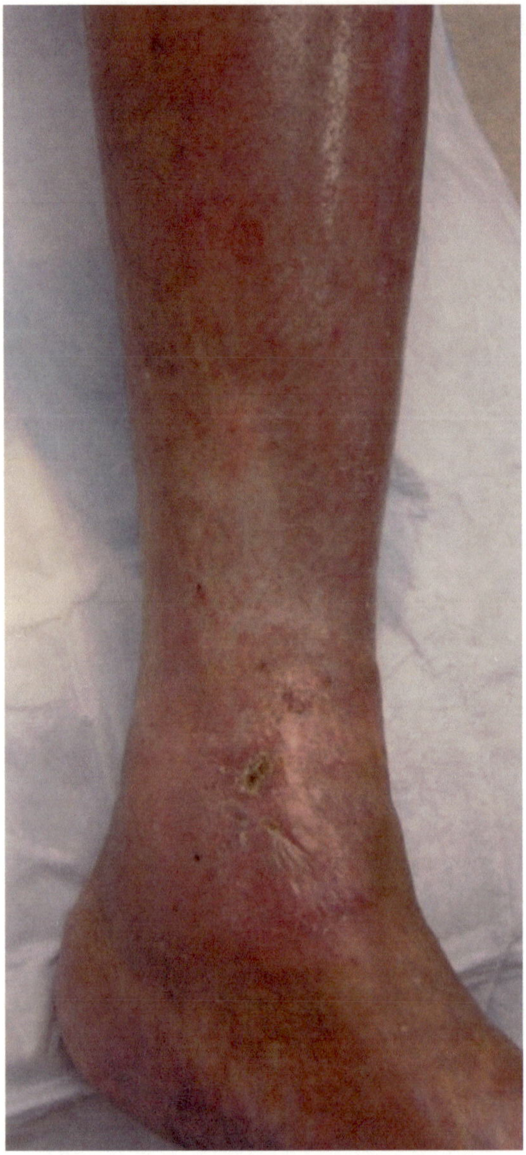

Fig. 11B. Photograph showing complete healing of ulcers; patient now pain free.

Duplex examination Figure 10C showed high velocity flow in the patient's femoral vein distal to the occluded external iliac vein. An arteriogram showed a large pelvic AVM with outflow to the deep pelvic veins and to the distal veins in the left lower extremity. Occlusion of the AVM was performed with injectable ethyl vinyl alcohol polymer dissolved in DMSO (Onyx, EV3 Neurovascular, Irvine, CA) (Link 2011). The pain in the ulcerated areas improved but persisted despite compression dressings being applied weekly. Endovenous Laser Ablation (EVLT) of the veins deep to the ulcers and foam sclerotherapy (0.5% Sodium tetradecyl *Sotradecol*, angiodynamics, Queensbury, NY was then performed on this patient). Following the procedures the ulcers healed and the patient was pain free. Interventions for this condition have included an outflow procedure to reduce the venous

hypertension with transcatheter embolization of the arteriovenous channels from the feeding arteries (Chikamatsu, Nagashima et al. 2001). Successful treatment of the pain has been achieved in localized femoral vein AVM lesions by transcatheter injection of the feeding arteries with anhydrous alcohol combined with tissue adhesive (n-Butyl Cyanoacylate, nbca, Trufill, Cordis neurovascular, Miami Lakes, Florida)(Link, Garza et al.). Non healing painful ulcers can be seen in end stage renal disease patients as a result of venous hypertension from their arteriovenous access,(George, Jhawar et al. 2008).
Patients who develop DVT should be followed for complications during and after the period of anticoagulation. Emphasis on compression and lymph edema treatment should lead to improved outcomes. Severe post thrombotic syndrome patients should be managed in a vascular group and some will respond to ablative and injection therapies.

3. References

Aboian, M. S., D. J. Daniels, et al. (2009). "The putative role of the venous system in the genesis of vascular malformations." Neurosurg Focus 27(5): E9.

Ashrani, A. A., M. D. Silverstein, et al. (2009). "Risk factors and underlying mechanisms for venous stasis syndrome: a population-based case-control study." Vasc Med 14(4): 339-349.

Bekou, V., D. Galis, et al. (2011). "Unilateral leg swelling: deep vein thrombosis?" Phlebology 26(1): 8-13.

Bollinger, A., G. Isenring, et al. (1982). "Lymphatic microangiopathy: a complication of severe chronic venous incompetence (CVI)." Lymphology 15(2): 60-65.

Bradbury, A. W. (2010). "Epidemiology and aetiology of C4-6 disease." Phlebology 25 Suppl 1: 2-8.

Brandjes, D. P., H. R. Buller, et al. (1997). "Randomised trial of effect of compression stockings in patients with symptomatic proximal-vein thrombosis." Lancet 349(9054): 759-762.

Caps, M. T., R. A. Manzo, et al. (1995). "Venous valvular reflux in veins not involved at the time of acute deep vein thrombosis." J Vasc Surg 22(5): 524-531.

Chikamatsu, E., T. Nagashima, et al. (2001). "Pelvic arteriovenous malformation with iliac vein thrombosis. A case report." J Cardiovasc Surg (Torino) 42(1): 115-118.

Corley, G. J., B. J. Broderick, et al. (2010). "The anatomy and physiology of the venous foot pump." Anat Rec (Hoboken) 293(3): 370-378.

Fazel, R., J. B. Froehlich, et al. (2007). "Clinical problem-solving. A sinister development--a 35-year-old woman presented to the emergency department with a 2-day history of progressive swelling and pain in her left leg, without antecedent trauma." N Engl J Med 357(1): 53-59.

Felty, C. L. and T. W. Rooke (2005). "Compression therapy for chronic venous insufficiency." Semin Vasc Surg 18(1): 36-40.

Franks, P. J., C. J. Moffatt, et al. (1995). "Factors associated with healing leg ulceration with high compression." Age Ageing 24(5): 407-410.

George, P., M. S. Jhawar, et al. (2008). "All that is swollen and red is not infection!" Indian J Nephrol 18(4): 162-165.

Hanrahan, L. M., C. T. Araki, et al. (1991). "Evaluation of the perforating veins of the lower extremity using high resolution duplex imaging." J Cardiovasc Surg (Torino) 32(1): 87-97.

Hern, S. and P. S. Mortimer (1999). "Visualization of dermal blood vessels--capillaroscopy." Clin Exp Dermatol 24(6): 473-478.

Kahn, S. R. "The post-thrombotic syndrome." Hematology Am Soc Hematol Educ Program 2010: 216-220.
Kearon, C. (2003). "Natural history of venous thromboembolism." Circulation 107(23 Suppl 1): I22-30.
Kearon, C. (2004). "Long-term management of patients after venous thromboembolism." Circulation 110(9 Suppl 1): I10-18.
Labropoulos, N. (2004). "Deep venous reflux and incompetent perforators: significance and implicaitons for therapy." Phebology 19: 22-27.
Link, D. P. (2011). Chronic Iliac Vein Occlussion and Painful Non Healing Ulcer Induced by High Venous Pressures from an Arterio-venous Malformation. Case Reports in Radiology.
Link, D. P., A. S. Garza, et al. "Acquired peripheral arteriovenous malformations in patients with venous thrombosis: report of two cases." J Vasc Interv Radiol 21(3): 387-391.
Marsh, P., B. A. Price, et al. (2010). "One-year outcomes of radiofrequency ablation of incompetent perforator veins using the radiofrequency stylet device." Phlebology 25(2): 79-84.
May, R. (1975). "[Disturbances of venous flow (author's transl)]." Langenbecks Arch Chir 339: 489-492.
May R, T. J. (1957). "the cause of the predominantly sinistral occurrence of thrombosis of the pelvic veins." Angiology 8(5): 419-427.
Milleret, R. (2011).
Moor, A. N., D. J. Vachon, et al. (2009). "Proteolytic activity in wound fluids and tissues derived from chronic venous leg ulcers." Wound Repair Regen 17(6): 832-839.
Nicolaides, A. N. (2000). "Investigation of chronic venous insufficiency: A consensus statement (France, March 5-9, 1997)." Circulation 102(20): E126-163.
Ohba, Y., Y. Todo, et al. (2011). "Risk factors for lower-limb lymphedema after surgery for cervical cancer." Int J Clin Oncol 16(3): 238-243.
Pirard, D., B. Bellens, et al. (2008). "The post-thrombotic syndrome - a condition to prevent." Dermatol Online J 14(3): 13.
Proebstle, T. M. and S. Herdemann (2007). "Early results and feasibility of incompetent perforator vein ablation by endovenous laser treatment." Dermatol Surg 33(2): 162-168.
Raju, S. and P. Neglen (2009). "Clinical practice. Chronic venous insufficiency and varicose veins." N Engl J Med 360(22): 2319-2327.
Salcuni, M., P. Fiorentino, et al. (1996). "Diagnostic imaging in deep vein thrombosis of the limbs." Rays 21(3): 328-339.
Schaverien, M., M. Saint-Cyr, et al. (2008). "Three- and four-dimensional computed tomographic angiography and venography of the anterolateral thigh perforator flap." Plast Reconstr Surg 121(5): 1685-1696.
Shrubb, D. and W. Mason (2006). "The management of deep vein thrombosis in lymphoedema: a review." Br J Community Nurs 11(7): 292-297.
Stuart, W. P., A. J. Lee, et al. (2001). "Most incompetent calf perforating veins are found in association with superficial venous reflux." J Vasc Surg 34(5): 774-778.
Taute, B. M., H. Melnyk, et al. (2010). "[Alternative sonographic diagnoses in patients with clinical suspicion of deep vein thrombosis]." Med Klin (Munich) 105(9): 619-626.
van Ramshorst, B., P. S. van Bemmelen, et al. (1994). "The development of valvular incompetence after deep vein thrombosis: a follow-up study with duplex scanning." J Vasc Surg 19(6): 1059-1066.

Part 3

Cerebral Venous Thrombosis and Venous Thrombosis of the Eye

Cerebral Venous Thrombosis in Patients Using Oral Contraceptives

Procházka Václav[1], Procházka Martin[2], Ľubušký Marek[2], Procházková Jana[3] and Hrbáč Tomáš[4]
[1]*Radiodiagnostic Institute FN Ostrava-Poruba*
[2]*Gynaecology and Obstetrics Department FN and LF UP Olomouc*
[3]*Haemato-oncology Department FN and LF UP Olomouc*
[4]*Neurosurgery Department FN Ostrava-Poruba*
Czech Republic

1. Introduction

Cerebral venous thrombosis is a relatively rare, however life-threatening condition. Current studies show that around 10% of the patients die. Earlier works proved that most of the thromboses originated secondarily, as a consequence of local or systemic infection, more than 30% of the cases were considered to be idiopathic. More recent studies also mention other risk factors, which may contribute to the onset of thrombosis. These include thrombophilic states or use of oral contraceptives. A number of hypercoagulation states or thrombophilic conditions, which contribute to the onset of thromboembolic disease, have been discovered and described in the recent years.

Thrombophilia is a congenital or acquired disorder of the haemostatic mechanism, characterized with an increased tendency towards blood clotting and thrombotization. Typical manifestations of the condition include frequent occurrence of lower extremities thromboses in young age, with frequent recurrence, or localization in unusual places. Congenital forms of the disorder are characterized with family occurrence. The most frequent conditions associated with congenital form of the disease are mutation of genes coding V^{Leiden} factor (Leiden mutation), prothrombin ^{G20210A}, hyperhomocysteinemia and furthermore also autosomal inheritance of antithrombin III (AT III), protein C and protein S deficit.

The point mutation of the factor V gene usually occurs in the place of protein C binding, which results in its cleavage and inactivation. The changes are associated with substitution of guanine with adenine at the 1691st nucleotide of the factor V, this substitution results in further substitution of glutamine with arginine on the 506th position of the factor V chain (FV Q506). The mutation is also known as "Leiden mutation", based on the place of its discovery (Leiden, Holland). Substitution of amino acids in the factor V chain causes resistance against the activated protein C, resulting in a higher tendency towards thrombosis. The mutation is considered to be autosomal dominant hereditary. It affects 5-9% of the European population. The mechanism of resistance against the activated protein C (APC resistance) was first described by Dahlbäck in 1993 in Sweden.

Another possible predisposition factor of venous thrombosis is a mutation of gene for prothrombin - G20210A variant. It is present in about 2% of the population. The mutation

causes an increase of the prothrombin level and contributes to elevation of the risk of thrombosis up to threefold level.
Deficit of the antithrombin III is a disorder with most prothrombotic effects. The risk of developing a thromboembolic disease during life is 70-80% in carriers in the heterozygous form (homozygous carriers suffer from a lethal thromboembolic event usually already during childhood). AT III is a polypeptide synthetized in hepatocytes with an increased half-time (65 hours). Apart from its effect on thrombin, AT III is also able to activate factors Xa, IXa, VIIa and plasmin. The activation of antithrombin III is increased up to 40 000 times with heparin binding. The deficit of AT III is caused by numerous point mutations, deletion and insertion, and the inheritance is mostly autosomally dominant.
Homocysteine is contained in plasma at concentrations of 5 - 16 μmol/l. Congenital hyperhomocysteinemia may be caused by a number of enzymatic defects. Clinical manifestations may be strengthened with a deficit of B6 and B12 vitamins, folic acid or during a treatment with methotrexate. Thrombophilia caused by hyperfibrinogenemia and dysfibrinogenemia is observed significantly less frequently.
Large population studies aimed at the relations between hormonal contraceptives and deep vein thrombosis have been performed. The increased risk was described mainly in patients using third-generation gestagens. Moreover, the identified risk of thrombosis in patients using hormonal contraceptives with thrombophilia is higher than what would correspond with a simple addition of risks. This finding confirms the theory that the procoagulation mechanisms are mutually strengthened in these women.
The problems of cerebral venous thrombosis in women in fertile age, who are the users of hormonal contraceptives have been studied in several trials including only a small number of patients. The results are in many cases misleading and inconsistent.
The aim of our study was to analyse cases of CVT in relation to sex, age, use of hormonal contraceptives and thrombophilic states, in correlation with CT, MRI and DSA findings and with clinical neurological findings.

2. Clinical study

We present a set of eight cases of women with a diagnosed cerebral venous thrombosis. The age scope of the group was 18.7 - 39.3 years of age, with mean of 28.1 years. The patients were hospitalized between April 2004 and October 2005. All patients were referred to CT / MRI and DSA venography examinations. Five of the women were treated with a therapeutic dose of low-molecular heparins (LMWH) only, with a transfer to warfarin treatment, other three patients underwent an interventional treatment with local thrombolysis with Actilyse® (rt-PA), following an ineffective LMWH application.
We have evaluated all medical records of the patients, the patients were examined physically and we have taken a detailed history record. Seven patients were using third-generation hormonal contraceptives with gestagens, one patient was using purely gestagen contraceptives, none of the patients smoked.

3. Laboratory examinations

All patients were referred for blood tests in order to define the presence of thrombophilic states. The blood samples were collected and tested prior to the onset of an anticoagulation treatment, and 3-6 months following a thrombotic event.

APC resistance was tested with the use of factor V deficient plasma (Coatest® APC resistance Chromogenix). The test presents almost 100% sensitivity and specificity in detection of factor V mutations (Leiden). Patients with APC ratio below 1.86 were tested with PCR analysis for the presence of FV:Q^{506} allele. We have also chromatogenously determined the levels of protein C, antithrombin III (AT III), prothrombin, heparin II cofactor and plasminogen. Protein S was determined immunologically, as a free form of protein S.
In order to determine the complex mutations of FV 1691 G-A, prothrombin 20210 G-A and MTHFR 677 C-T, we used specific, polymerase chain reaction (MS PCR), according to the works of Austrian authors Endler et al. This method is a single-tube PCR technique based upon the use of allele-specific primers, differing mutually in 8-10 pairs of bases (bp). The subsequent amplification was carried out in accordance with the protocol, which was optimised for thermocycler Perkin Elmer 2400. Following the initial 10-minute denaturation at 95°C, 34 cycles follow, consisting of separation of DNA chains for 1 min at 95°C , annealing primers for 2 min at 56°C and DNA synthesis for 1 min at 72°C. After completion, final elongation was carried out for 7 min at 72°C, followed with cooling to 4°C. To separate the PCR products we used electrophoresis on Spreadex 400 gel (Elchrom Scientific), which enables separation of products up to 400 pb, with high resolution. The results were reviewed on UV review table at 254 nm, the photo documentation was obtained using a yellow filter with Mitsubishi camera enabling digital recording.

3.1 Case Report of CVT – Application of local fibrinolysis in 24-year patient using HAK

24-year-old female patient with a negative history, including pregnancy or thromboembolism used third-generation gestagen as oral contraceptives. The patient was admitted to Neurology ICU, suffering from a strong headache, localized retroaurically, lasting for the period of one week. During the previous two days, the pain was associated with vomiting. Neurological findings included IV-degree somnolence, apathy, dysarthria, nuchal rigidity with 12 points on the GCS (Glasgow Coma Scale) on admission. A CT examination and conventional DSA were carried out in the evening. Angiography showed a partial thrombotic closure of the superior sagittal sinus and complete closure of right-hand lateral and sigmoid sinus, Galen's vein and direct sinus with stagnation of venous drainage in thalamus and basal ganglia. CT examination confirmed hypodensity in the right side of the thalamus and basal ganglia, oedema in right-hand temporal-occipital area and a minor haemorrhage in the area of right lateral and sigmoid sinus.

Neurological examination

The examination showed left-hand hemiparesis, divergent strabismus, bilateral miosis, nuchal rigidity and tachycardia 120/min. Oedema of the papillae was not present. Considering the progreding disorder of consciousness gradating into coma, the patient was intubated and left on artificial ventilation. Consequently, the patient was taken to Anaesthesiology-Resuscitation Department. We introduced anticoagulation treatment with dalteparine 1000 IU/hr and antibiotic therapy with amoxyciline with clavulanic acid 1,2 g/ 8 hrs and ciprofloxacine 100 ml/12 hrs. The ventilation was maintained with FiO2 0,3, tidal volume (Vt) 550 ml and positive end-expiratory pressure (PEEP) of 5 cm H20. ECG was normal, without any ischemic signs, frequency 120/min. Magnetic resonance and magnetic resonance venography (MRV) confirmed vasogenic inflation, blood hypovolemia of the right mesencephalum, right thalamus and basal ganglia, as well as thrombosis of deep cerebral veins and venous sinuses.

Laboratory examination

Creatinine 63,6 umol/l, glucose 6,1 mmol/l, *coagulation*: INR 1,41, fibrinogen 4,69 g/l, D dimers elevated 6-fold, protein C 45%, free protein S 56%, APC resistance negative- 4,791, AT III- 74%, factor II 76%, factor VIII – 112% (% of the standard).

Despite the use of conventional anticoagulation treatment and anti-oedematous therapy according to the protocol, the serious brain stem symptoms progreded on the 5th day after admission, associated with a loss of vertical and horizontal oculocephalic reflexes. The patient was referred to interventional centre for endovascular treatment of cerebral venous thrombosis. After admission, a control DSA examination with three-dimensional venography (3D-XRV) was carried out, with reconstruction of the venous phase. We found an incomplete thrombotic closure of both venae cerebri internae, Galen's vein and direct sinus, as well as a complete thrombosis of the right transversal and sigmoid sinuses. On the basis of this imaging examination, we decided to proceed with a local thrombolysis with rt-PA.

Technique of the procedur

5F Terumo loader (Radiofocus, Tokyo) was inserted into the common femoral vein for the purpose of a venous approach, and another 5F Terumo loader was inserted retrogradely into common femoral artery for angiography imaging of the right-side carotid basin. Control position digital subtraction angiography was carried out with the 4F Vertebral Aqua - Tempo catheter (Cordis - Endovascular, JJ, Miami, FL), with 3D-Xra reconstruction of the venous phase, with the outcome of a complete thrombolysis of the basal Rosenthal's and Galen's veins, sinus rectus, sinus transversus, sinus sigmoideus and right jugular vein (Fig. 1). The patient received unfractionated Heparin in the dose of 5000 U i.a. Another 4F Vertebral Aqua – Tempo catheter was inserted into the right v. jugularis interna, using the Terumo 035´/260cm loader (Radiofocus, Tokyo, Japan), and subsequently smoothly through the thrombus up to the area of confluens sinuum (Fig. 2). We have initiated local continuous thrombolysis on the 5th day after admission, using the application of rtPA in the dose of 0,6mg/hr, with continuous application of UF Heparin in the dose of 700 IU/hr, to reach the therapeutic levels of anticoagulation therapy. Fibrinogen, aPTT, blood count and the count of thrombocytes were monitored in 6-hour intervals. The thrombolytic treatment lasted for a total of 48 hours.

Control angiography with 3D-XRA venography performed on the 7th day confirmed recanalization of both cerebri internae, basal Rosenthal's vein, Galen's vein, sinus rectus, transversal and sigmoid sinuses, as well as v. jugularis interna, with a rapid drainage into cortical collectors. Thrombolytic therapy was terminated after the restoration of venous flow. Control CT examination excluded bleeding complications, and subsequent MRI examination confirmed regression of hyperaemia in the area of thalamus and right basal ganglia.

During the following two days, the patient wakes from the comatose state, with further diminishing of clinical symptomatology in the following period. The NIHSS scale was scored at 4 points on the 7th day after the interventional procedure. During a follow-up check after one month, the patient is fully self-sufficient, with mRs – 0 points. The examination aimed at thrombophilic states verified heterozygous form of MTHFR: A/V 223 and homozygous form of PAI-I 4G/5G genotype mutation. The patient was introduced to anticoagulation treatment with warfarin, with periodical monthly INR check-ups. Subsequent neuro-psychological examination confirmed an excellent outcome: WAIS-R:IQ global test 141, verbal 128 and non-verbal 146 points, with Wechsler memory quotient MQ l0l, pointing towards high intellectual functions. The examination further confirmed a high psychomotor speed, optimal verbal expression and memory functions at three months after the treatment.

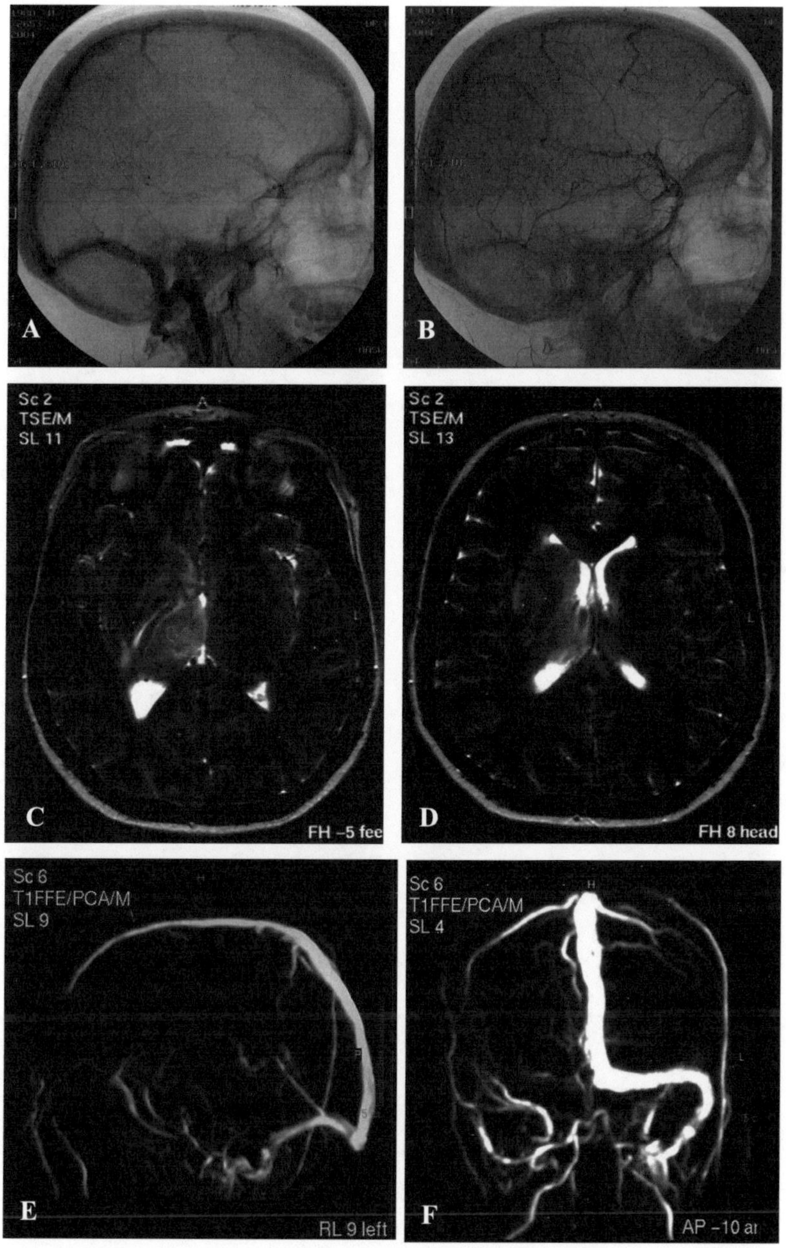

A, B, DSA (day 1) closure of sinus transversus, vena magna cerebri (Galen), vena cerebri interna and vena basalis Rosenthali. Drainage of cortical venous collectors preserved.
C,D, T2- weighted images (day 4)- hyperaemia, or cerebral turgescence of right-hand side basal ganglia and the thalamus, with an image of signal hypersensitivity, imitating cerebral ischemia.
E, MR venography – lateral image (day 4)- incomplete thrombosis of the sinus rectus, non-detectable flow in vena basalis Rosenthali.
F, Sagittal view on MR – venography – thrombosis of the right-hand side sinus transversus and sigmoideus and right vena jugularis interna.

Fig. 1. DSA, MRI + MR- venography- „Time of Flight-TOF"

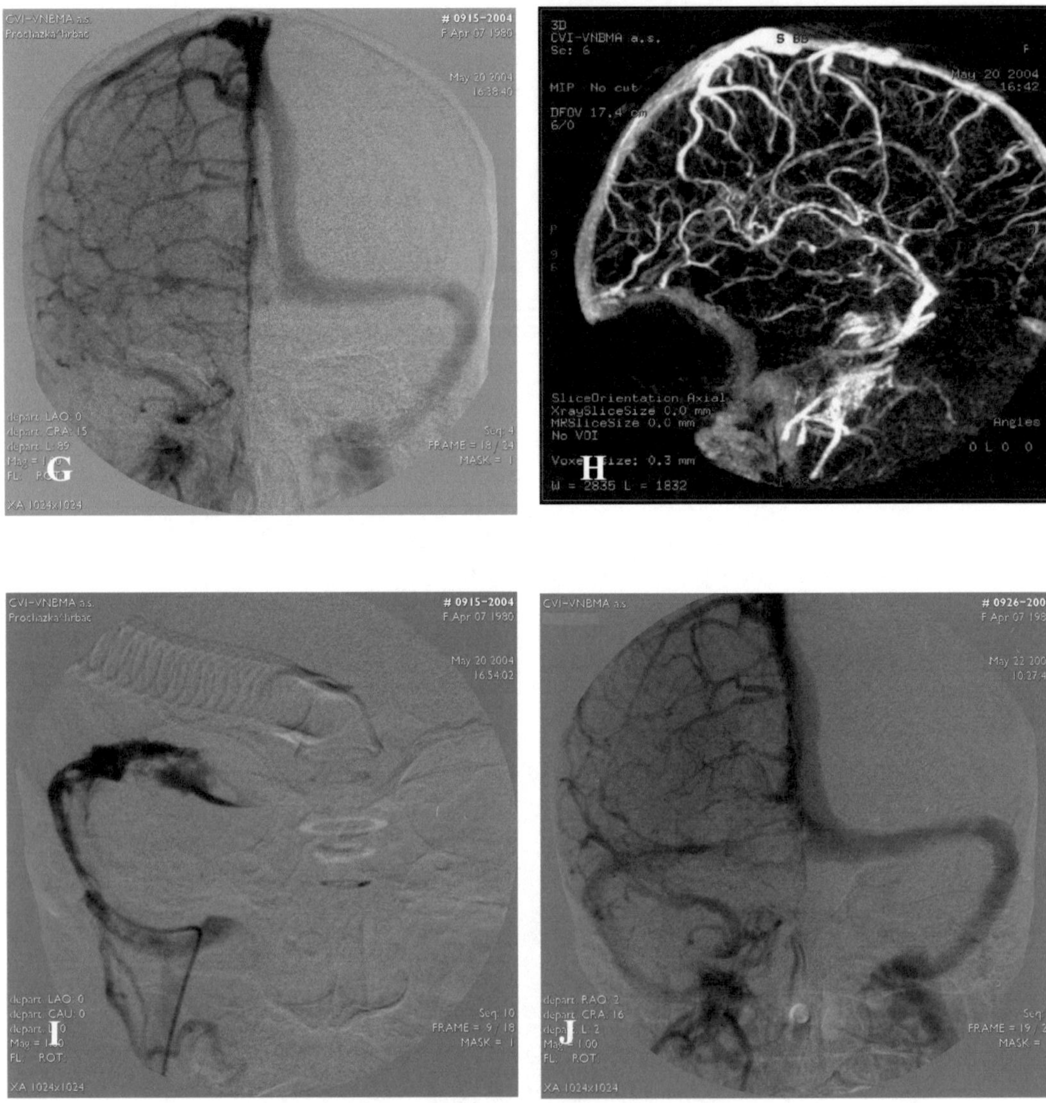

G, Sagittal view on DSA (day 5) – thrombosis of sinus transversus and sigmoid.
H, 3D-Xra digital rotational angiography, partial thrombosis, sinus rectus – "double railing" image, thrombosis of vena basalis Rosenthali. Closure of right sinus transversus and sigmoid.
I,4F-Vertebral Tempo Cordis JJ catheter inserted into right-hand sinus transversus, into the area of confluens sinuum, through a soft thrombus for introduction of local thrombolysis.
J, Sagittal view - DSA (day 7) – 48 hours of local thrombolysis - recanalization of the right-hand side sinus transversus and sigmoid.

Fig. 2. Interventional procedure + 3D-Xra control angiography and MRI after thrombolysis

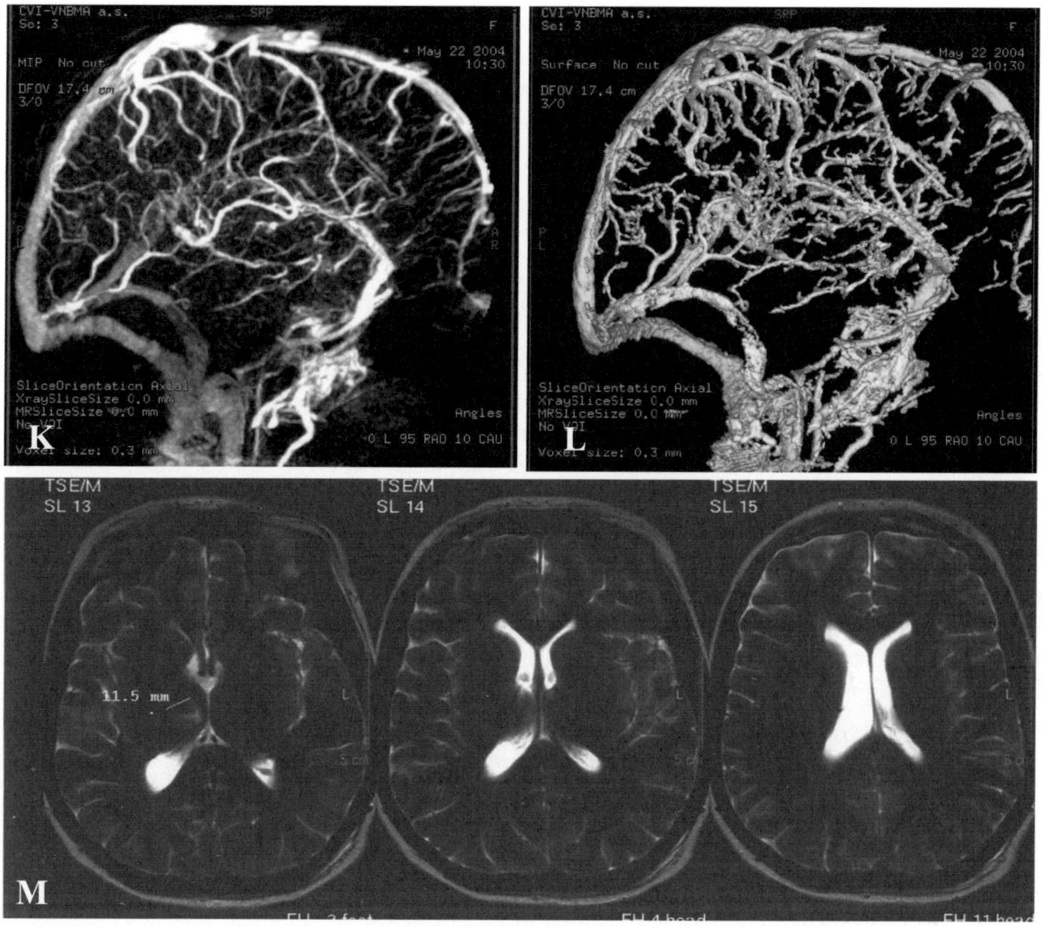

K, L, 3D-Xra digital rotational angiography with a complete recanalization of sinus rectus, vena magna cerebri, vena basalis Rosenthali and venae cerebri internae.
M, Control MRI - (1 month), with a minor venous infarction of pulvinar thalami on the right.

Fig. 2. Continues.

3.2 Case report – CVT with malignant course

Thirty-three-year-old female patient with a negative history and negative allergic history, using third-generation hormonal contraceptives for a short period of one month was examined for a headache localised in the right-hand side occipital area, accompanied with repeated vomiting. After five days of cephalgias, the patient observed worsening of the visual acuity, namely in the right eye. The patient was admitted at Neurology department due to an epileptic seizure. The subsequent CT examination was described as negative. On admission, the patient complained about inappetence and overall sickness after using individual tablets of the contraceptive. On the 8th hospitalisation day, the patient suddenly lost consciousness, tonic stiffening of the limbs and jaw appeared, accompanied with sweating, and, having regained consciousness, the patient showed signs of overall confusion. Control CT examination was performed, with the image of squalid cortical areas and suspected subarachnoidal haemorrhage in the occipital area on the right, around

sinuses. Within further two hours, the patient lost consciousness, accompanied with meningeal symptomatology and left-side hemiparesis.
The patient was referred for MRI examination, which revealed a massive cerebral venous thrombosis of all cerebral sinuses, with a closure of the deep vein system drainage in the diencephalic area and around basal ganglia (Fig. 3). After subsequently performed examinations, the patient was intubated in semi-comatose state and transferred to the interventional centre for an emergency endovascular procedure.

Interventional procedure

Under general anaesthesia, through a cannulation of right-hand side common femoral vein, we inserted 4F sheath Terumo and applied UF-Heparin 5000 U i.a.. Through the sheath we inserted 4F Vertebral Aqua - Tempo (Cordis - Endovascular, JJ, Miami, FL) diagnostic catheter and proceeded with diagnostic angiography of the cerebral arteries. The AG revealed a significantly delayed capillary filling, and venous drainage of both hemispheres, as well as a complete thrombosis of sinus sagitalis superior, sinus transversus and sigmoideus on the right side, a complete closure of deep venous drainage - v. basalis Rosenthali, v. cerebri internae, v. magna cerebri and sinus rectus. We inserted a second 5F Terumo loader into the common femoral vein, and through it a second diagnostic Vertebral catheter, on Terumo loader (Radiofocus, Tokyo, Japan) we penetrated into v. jugularis interna on the right, through foramen jugulare into sinus sigmoideus and transversus on the right, up to the confluens sinuum area. We initiated the application of local thrombolysis in the dose of 1mg rt-PA/hr per 24 hours.

Therapy at the Anaesthesiology-Resuscitation Department

Patient was left on controlled artificial lung ventilation, on antibiotics (amoxyciline with clavulanic acid i.v., at the dose of 1,2 g every 8 hours), parenteral infusion therapy with crystaloids, glucose, massive anti-oedematous therapy, continuous local thrombolysis.

Laboratory examination

Antithrombin III 88..67, Leukocytes 15,7; Erythrocytes 4,40; Haemoglobin 13,6, Haematocrit 0,357; Thrombocytes 291; APTT 180 vt., Quick 19,4; INR 1,62; Fibrinogen 3,0.

Control CT on the following day

Significant progression of the cerebral oedema, faded basal cisterns, clouded structures of the mesencephalon, smoothened gyrification, clouded structure of the right basal ganglia, medium line without deviation, faded lateral ventricles, high density in sinus sagitalis superior and sinus rectus with proven thrombosis. Conclusion – manifestation of a diffusive oedema, together with thrombosis of cerebral sinuses.

Neurological examination

Patient without attenuation, on artificial lung ventilation without any spontaneous activity, no reaction to painful stimuli, stem reflexes not manifested, generalized hypotonic state with C5-C8, L2-S2 areflexia. Conclusion: areactive coma, without manifestation of stem reflexes, corresponding to cerebral death. The patient dies on basal therapy after 11 days of hospitalization.

Pathology-anatomic finding

see Fig. 4. The image confirms extensive cerebral venous thrombosis, cerebral oedema, mainly in the area of brainstem, without manifestations of intracerebral haemorrhage.

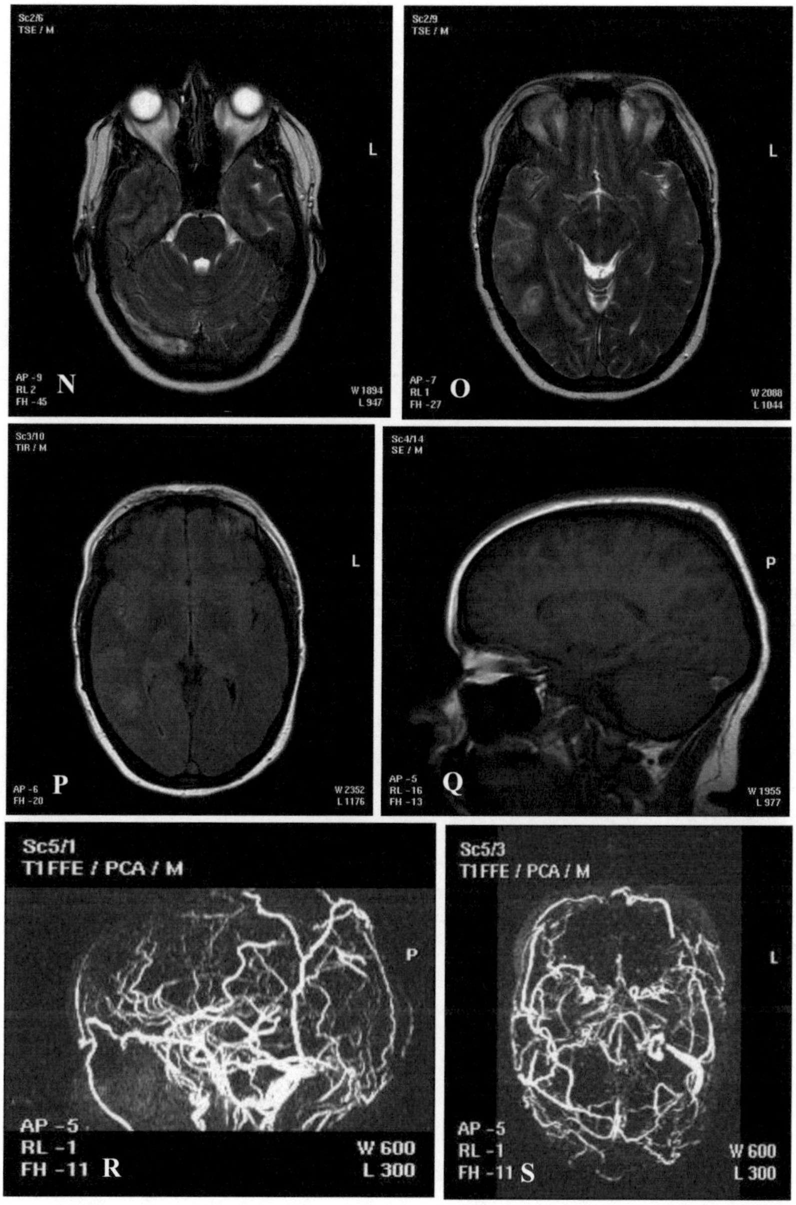

N, T1WI-MRI - axial scan with the image of hyperintense signal of sinus transversus thrombosis on the right and hyperaemia, or vasogenic dilatation of the right temporal lobe.
O,P T1WI-MRI axial scan with the image of hyperaemia, or vasogenic inflation of the right temporal lobe.
Q, T1WI-MRI – image of "analogous delta sign" at the thrombosis at the area of division of the transversal sinus from confluens sinuum.
R,S, TOF- MR venography with findings of sinus sagitalis superior, sinus transversus and sigmoideus thrombosis on the right, deep vein system - sinus rectus, v. magna cerebri, vv. cerebri internae, and v. basalis Rosenthali.

Fig. 3. MRI examination and MR venography - (TOF) – sub-acute stage

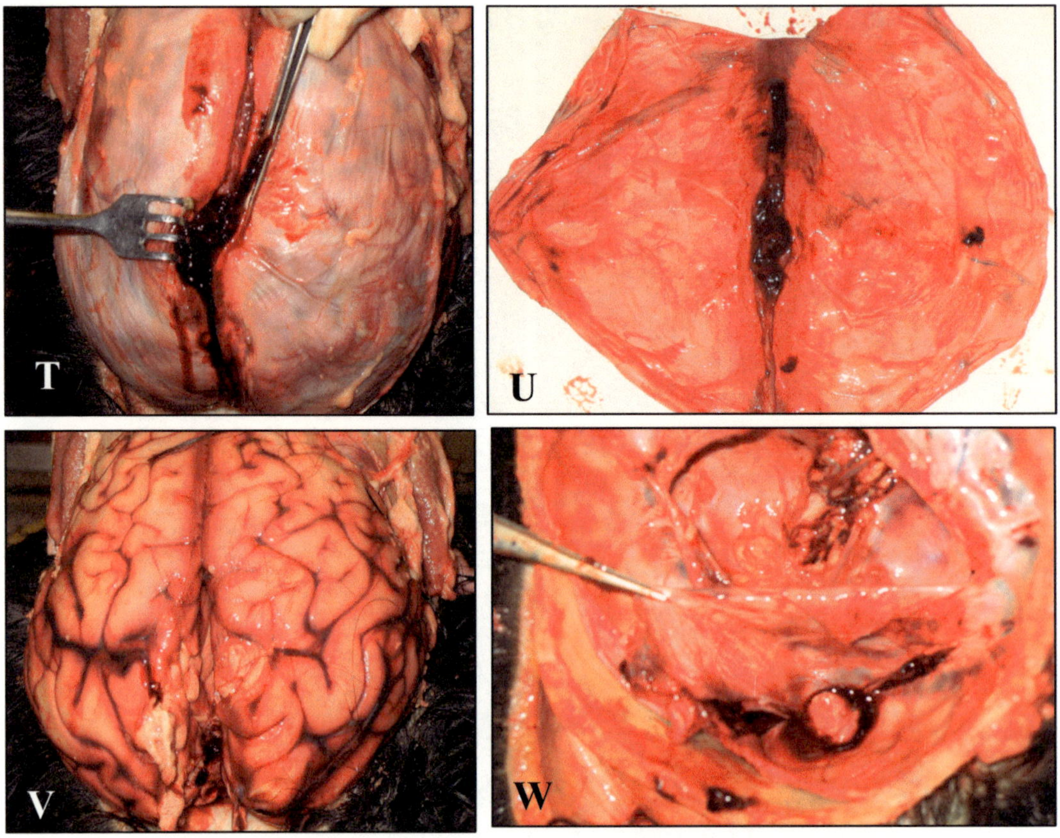

T,U Thrombosis of sinus sagitalis superior as seen after opening of the sinus and removal of the hard meninges

V Thrombosis of confluens sinuum and sinus rectus orifice, thrombosis of Labe collector on the right and cortical veins parietally on the left

W Thrombosis of perimesenphalic veins with hyperaemia in the area of medulla oblongata

Fig. 4. Pathology-anatomic finding

4. Results

We present eight cases of cerebral venous thrombosis in a group of young women (aged between 18.7 and 39.3 years, mean age 28.1 years), who were hospitalized between April 2004 and October 2005.

The most frequently observed manifestations of CVT (see Table 1) were headache (100%) and vertigo (87,5%). The most frequently detected objective findings were movement disorders - central hemiparesis or quadruparesis (75%), the same percentage applies to spasms, behavioural disorders, altered consciousness, sensoric disorders and aphasias (25%). CT and MRI examinations (see Table 3, 4) showed venous infarction or vasogenic inflation in 62.5% and presence of petechial haemorrhage in 25%. Digital subtraction 3D-XR venography most frequently confirmed a combination of occlusions of sinus transversus and sigmoideus (75%), sinus sagitalis superior (62,5%), cortical veins (62,5%) and deep venous system (50%).

The outcomes of the therapy were excellent in seven patients receiving the basic treatment. The treatment included administration of a combination of low weight molecular heparin in the treatment dose and subsequent coverage with warfarin. In three patients with insufficient effect of LMWH, we used local thrombolysis Actilyse ® (rt-PA). One of the women died, despite acute thrombolysis and complex therapy. The results of coagulation tests (see Table 6) showed the presence of several thrombophilic risk factors in all women in our group. Homozygous form of the MTHFR-C677T gene mutation was detected in three patients, two patients had a mutation of the gene for PAI-1 in homozygous form. A combination of both homozygous forms was detected in one patient, the combination was present in heterozygous forms in two patients. The tests further detected an elevated level of factor VIII in three patients, and five of the patients showed a deficit of protein S, always in combination with mutations of the gene responsible for MTHFR-C677T, three of these were present in homozygous form.

5. Discussion

The first clinical and pathological finding of cerebral venous thrombosis was described by Ribs in 1825 in a 45-year-old male patient with generalized malignant process. Without the possibility of angiography imaging, the diagnosis was determined on the basis of clinical findings - progreding headaches, oedema of the eye papilla, spasms, focal deficit, coma, and was most usually confirmed with pathology-anatomical findings of thrombosis in the area of dural sinuses, accompanied with haemorrhagic infarsation. In 2001, an important study "International Study of Cerebral Vein Thrombosis" - ISCVT was published; the study prospectively monitored data of 624 patients with this diagnosis. (2)

Deep vein system, including vv. cerebri internae, v. basalis Rosenthali, v. magna cerebri and sinus rectus, responsible for the drainage of diencephalon, basal ganglia and deep structures of the white matter of hemispheres, is usually affected in 10% of cerebral venous thromboses. More serious clinical cases, including hemipareses and quadrupareses are caused by compression of capsula interna, with unilateral of bilateral infliction of the thalami or basal ganglia, and can be diagnosed with non-invasive examinations, e.g. CT or MRI under the image of the oedema or haemorrhagic infarction. Limitations of venous outflow result in cerebral hyperaemia, mostly detected on MRI in patients with CVT (3,4,5).

The diagnosis of CVT in our group of patients was confirmed with MRI imaging, MR venography and subsequently also with digital subtraction angiography. Liang et al. confirm the importance of three-dimensional imaging of magnetic resonance MP-RAGE venography, supported with the use of contrast, in the diagnostics of thromboses in the area of dural sinuses. This method was also very useful in our patient group. (6) As an alternative diagnostic procedure for CVT it is also possible to perform CT venography, together with the subtraction of bone structures "Mathed Mask Bone Elimination" (MMBE). (7) 3D-Xra-digital rotation venography provides an excellent alternative, with the possibility of imaging the speed and direction of the flow in a normal section of the venous system, as well as in partially thrombotized parts of dural sinuses and deep vein system.

The treatment of patients with intracranial venous thrombosis depends on the timeliness of the clinical suspicion of CVT and subsequent confirmation of the diagnosis with imaging techniques. Purdon Martin and Sheehan (1941) were the first to recommend anticoagulation therapy for the treatment of CVT. The treatment with heparin is currently considered as a treatment of choice in patients with CVT. (2) However, the effect of heparin may be too

slow, especially in patients with rapidly progreding symptoms and involvement of most of the dural sinuses and deep venous system. This patient population should be referred for thrombolytic treatment, as the overall mortality of these patients reaches 10%. (8-11) Our current experiences also point towards the possibility of mechanical revascularization of the obstructed venous bed, using the techniques of rheolytic thrombectomy and mechanical disturbance of the thrombus with balloon catheters. (12,13)
Thrombophilic states are commonly observed in 25-35% of patients with venous thrombosis. (14,15) Hormonal contraceptives are currently used by more than 100 million women. Shortly after their introduction in 1960s, an increased incidence of thrombotic vascular complications was observed (16-18), together with an interaction of hormonal contraceptives and haemocoagulation system. Increased activity of coagulation factors VII, VIII, X and fibrinogen is a common finding in most cases. (19) Martinelli et al. in their work define the risk of onset of cerebral venous thrombosis in users of hormonal contraceptives OR 6,1 95% CI (3,3 - 11,00). This potential risk may be further intensified by congenital haemostatic disorders. (20)
Peroral contraceptives induce extensive changes in the fibrinolytic system. The levels of plasminogen and plazmin-alfa2-antiplazmin complex are elevated, also the activity of tissue activator of plasminogen (tPA) is increased, at the same time, the level of antigen inhibitor of the plasminogen-I activator (PAI-I) and the PAI-I activity are decreased, and many other changes occur. The fibrinolysis in the users of contraceptives is elevated, which is most probably caused by the response and compensation of the prothrombogenic state, caused by hormonal preparations. These changes are identical in preparations containing levonorgestrel, as well as third-generation gestagens. (21) Genetically conditioned thrombophilic states of the fibrinolytic system (PAI-I) increase the potential risk of the onset of thrombosis in HAK users. An increased activity and clustering of platelets was observed. (22)
Hormonal contraceptives with third-generation gestagens are connected with an increased risk of venous thromboses, in comparison with previous generations of contraceptives. This risk is also present in women without V Leiden factor mutation or a positive family history. (23)

6. Conclusion

Our experience points towards the possibility of CVT onset in young women using hormonal contraceptives. This condition needs to be taken into account in cases of intracranial difficulties. CVT is most commonly manifested with headaches, vertigo and visual disorders. That is why the diagnosis should be considered when a sudden onset of such manifestations occurs in otherwise healthy young woman. The CT or MRI examinations should be directed towards the possibility of affection of the venous intracranial system. MRI and MR-venography or 3DX-RA venography significantly decrease the diagnostic process in patients with disorders of the deep venous cerebral system and a rapid development of symptoms. Direct endovascular thrombolysis, with the possibility of mechanical revascularization may dramatically improve the clinical course of patients with thrombosis of cerebral veins in patients with insufficient effect of anticoagulation therapy, associated with rapidly progreding disorders of consciousness. Thrombolytic therapy also decreases the occurrence of secondary complications following thrombolyses of cerebral veins, such as chronic intracranial hypertension with visual disorders or onset of arterio-venous shunts. (24,25) Taking into account the incidence of these serious complications, we consider as essential, in compliance with recommendations of the Czech Society of

Gynaecology and Obstetrics JEP, prior to administration of HAK, to perform a detailed analysis of personal and family history, and in indicated cases also a detailed examination of the presence of thrombophilic states. The significance of individual thrombophile mutations is inconsistent. Absolute contraindications for HAK usage include deficit of the antithrombin III, protein C deficit, homozygous form of V Leiden factor and combination of other thrombophile mutations. Other thrombophile mutations present a relative contraindication only. Screening examination of women prior to administration of HAK is not indicated. (26) However, in our study group, although we performed a detailed retrospective analysis, the personal and family history were negative in all patients. Considering this fact there arises the question of a facultative possibility of thrombophile examination covered by the patient, based on the patient's request, prior to administration of HAK.

As a certain surprise we may mention the high incidence of homozygous form of C677T in out study group (37,5%), which may be in consistence with the findings of Martinelli et al., who proved the risk of CVT onset in users of hormonal contraceptives with hyperhomocysteinemia OR 19,5 95% CI (5,7 - 67,3). The levels of homocystein were not monitored in our patients. Other frequently observed findings included mutations of the plasminogen activator inhibitor gene (PAI-1) and deficit of protein S, which may be also present in combinations strengthening the prothrombogenic effect. On the other hand, we did not observe an incidence of V Leiden factor in patients with CVT, however this factor is frequently mentioned in literature as a significant thrombophilic risk factor.

7. Tables

	1.	**2.**	**3.**	**4.**	**5.**	**6.**	**7.**	**8.**	**Mean**
Age	32.0	32.5	24.1	18.7	33.3	24.8	39.3	20.2	28.1

Table 1. Age of patients included into the study

Symptoms	1.	2.	3.	4.	5.	6.	7.	8.	%
Headache	+	+	+	+	+	+	+	+	100
Vertigo		+	+	+	+	+	+	+	87.5
Central hemiparesis and quadruparesis		+	+		+	+	+		62,5
Sight disorders				+	+				25.0
Sensitivity disorder		+				+			25.0
Behavioural disorder							+	+	25.0
Aphasia		+					+		25.0
Spasms					+	+			25.0
Coma			+		+				25.0

Table 2. Subjective and objective manifestations on admission

CT/MR	1.	2.	3.	4.	5.	6.	7.	8.	%
Venous infarction, vasogenic inflation		+	+		+	+	+		62,5
Petechial haemorrhage					+		+		25,0

Table 3. Parenchymatous lesions on CT/MRI

	1.	2.	3.	4.	5.	6.	7.	8.	%
Sinus sagitalis superior	+		+	+	+		+		62.5
Sinus transversus, sigmoideus	+		+	+	+	+	+		75,0
Deep vein system			+	+	+	+			50,0
Cortical veins		+	+	+	+	+			62.5
V.jugularis interna	+		+					+	37.5
Cerebellar veins						+			12.5

Table 4. Occlusion of sinuses / cortical veins on DSA 3D- XR venography

	1.	2.	3.	4.	5.	6.	7.	8.
Contraceptives	+	+	+	+	+	+	+	+
Treatment	LMWH + Wa	LMWH + Wa	LKT + LMWH + Wa	LKT + LMWH + Wa	LKT + LMWH	LMWH + Wa	LMWH + Wa	LMWH + Wa
Outcome	Complete recovery	Complete recovery	Complete recovery	Complete recovery	Patient died	Complete recovery	Complete recovery	Complete recovery
Smoking	-	-	-	-	-	-	-	-

LMWH – Low Molecular Weight Heparin, Wa – warfarin, LKT - local continuous thrombolysis

Table 5. Therapy

	1.	2.	3.	4.	5.	6.	7.	8.
Factor V Leiden	-	-	-	-	-	-	-	-
MTHFR	++	++	+-	+-	-	++	+-	+-
PAI-1	-	-	++	-	-	++	+-	+-
Factor VIII	-	-	-	+	+	+	-	-
Hyperhomo-cysteinemia	+	-	-	-	-	-	-	-
Protein C deficit	+	-	+	-	-	-	-	-
Protein S deficit	+	+	-	+	-	+	-	+
Antithrombin deficit	-	-	+	-	-	-	-	-

Legend:- negative, +- heterozygous, ++ homozygous
-MTHFR- methylentetrahydrofolate reductase, PAI- plasminogen activator inhibitor

Table 6. Results of thrombophilic parameters

8. References

[1] Berenstein A, Lasjaunias P., Ter Brugge K.G: Venous Occlusive Disease. Surgical Neuroangiography vol. 2.1 Clinical and Endovascular Treatment Aspects in Adults. Second edition, Springer-Verlag Berlin Heidelberg, 135-152; 2004

[2] Ferro JM, Canhao P, Stam J, Bousser MG, for the ISCVT Investigators: Prognosis of cerebral vein and dural sinus thrombosis, results of the International Study on Cerebral Vein and Dural Sinus Thrombosis (ISCVT). Stroke 35; 664-670, March 2004

[3] Forbes P.N.K, Pipe JG, Heiserman JE: Evidence for cytotoxic edema in the pathogenesis of cerebral venous infarction. AJNR Am J Neuroradiology 22;450-455, March 2001

[4] Peeters E, Stadnik T, Bissay F, Schmedding E et Al.:Diffusion-weighted MR imaging of an acute venous stroke. AJNR Am J Neuroradiology 22;1949-1952,November 2001

[5] Ducreux D,Oppenheim C,Vandamme X et Al.:Diffusion-weighted imaging patterns of brain damage associated with cerebral venous thrombosis. AJNR Am J Neuro-radiology 22;261-268, February 2001

[6] Liang L, Korogi Y, Sugahara T et Al: Evaluation of the Intracranial Dural sinuses with a 3D contrast-enhanced MP-RAGE sequence: prospective comparison with 2D-TOF MR venography and digital subtraction angiography. AJNR Am J Neuro-radiology 22; 481-492, March 2001.

[7] Majoie CHB, van Straten M, Venema HW: Multisection CT Venography of the dural sinuses and cerebral veins by using matched mask bone elimination. AJNR Am J Neuroradiology 25; 787-791, May 2004.

[8] Rael JR, Orrison WW Jr., Baldwin N, Sell J: Direct thrombolysis of superior sagittal sinus thrombosis with coexisting intracranial hemorrhage. AJNR Am J Neuro-radiology 18;1238-1242, Aug 1997

[9] Spearman MP, Jungreis ChA,Wehner JJ, et Al: Endovascular thrombolysis in deep cerebral venous thrombosis. AJNR Am J Neuroradiology 18; 502-506, Mar 1997

[10] Ciccone A, Canhao P, Falcao F, Ferro JM, Sterzi R: Thrombolysis for cerebral vein and dural sinus thrombosis. Cochrane Corner .Stroke 35; 000-001, Aug 2004

[11] Frey JL, Murro GJ, McDougall CG, Dean BL, Jahnke HK: Cerebral venous thrombosis-combined intrathrombus rtPA and intravenous heparin. Stroke 30; 489-494, February 1999

[12] Opatowsky MJ , Morris PP, Regan JD et Al: Rapid thrombectomy of superior sagittal sinus and transverse sinus thrombosis with a rheolytic catheter device. AJNR Am J Neuroradiology 20;414-417, March 1999.

[13] Dowd ChF, Malek AM, Phatouros CC, et Al: Application of rheolytic thrombectomy device in the treatment od dural sinus thrombosis: A new technique. AJNR Am J Neuroradiology 20; 568-570, April 1999.

[14] Provenzale JM, Barboriak DP,Allen NB, et Al: Antiphospholipid Antibodies: Findings at Arteriography. AJNR Am J Neuroradiology 19; 611-616, April 1998.

[15] Reuner KH, Ruf A, Grau A, Rickmann H, et AL: Prothrombin Gene G20210→A transition is a risk factor for cerebral venous thrombosis. Stroke 29; 1765-1769, September 1998.

[16] Lüdemann P, Nabavi DG, Junker R, Wolff E, Papke K et AL: Factor V Leiden mutation is a risk factor for cerebral venous thrombosis, A Case –control study of 55 patients. Stroke 29; 2507-2510, December 1998.

[17] Cantu C, Alonso E, Jara A, Martínez Leticia et Al: Hyperhomocysteinemia, low folate and vitamin B12 concentrations, and methylene tetrahydrofolate reductase mutation in cerebral venous thrombosis. Stroke 35; 1790-1794, August 2004.

[18] Rosendaal, F.R., Helmerhorst, F.M., Vandenbroucke J.P. Oral contraceptives, hormone replacement therapy and thrombosis. Thromb Haemost 2001; 86: 112 –123.

[19] Bloemenkamp, K.W.M., Helmerhorst, F.M., Rosendaal, F.R., Vandenbroucke J.P., Thrombophilias and gynaecology. Best Practice&Research Clinical Obsterics & Gynaecology, vol.17, 3, 509-528, 2003.

[20] Martinelli I, Battaglioli T., Pedotti P. et al. Hyperhomocysteinemia in cerebral vein thrombosis. Blood, 2003; 102: 1363-1366.

[21] Norris, L.A, Bonnar, J., The effect of oestrogen dose and progesteron type on haemostatic changes in women taking oral contraceptives. Br J Obstet Gynaecol, 1996, 103: 261 - 267.

[22] Kunz, F., Pechlander, C., Taberelli, M. et al. Influence of oral contraceptives on coagulation tests in native blood and plasma.Am J Obstet Gynaecol,1990,163:417– 420.

[23] World Health Organization. Cardiovascular disease and steroid hormone contraception. Report of a WHO Scientific group. WHO Technical Report Series, no.877. World Health Organization, 1998, Geneva.

[24] Stolz E, Gerriets T, Bödeker RH, Penzel MH,Kaps M: Intracranial venous hemodynamics is a factor related to a favorable outcome in cerebral venous thrombosis. Stroke 33; 1645-1650, June 2002.

[25] Phatouros C, Halbach VV, Dowd ChF, Lempert TE, Malek AM et Al: Acquired pial arteriovenous fistula following cerebral vein thrombosis. Stroke 30; 2487-2490, November 1999.

[26] Čepický P., Cibula D., Dvořák K, et al. Doporučení k předpisu kombinované hormonální kontracepce (CC). Aktualizace 2005. Čes.Gynek. 70; 2005; 4, 320-324.

Cerebral Venous Sinus Thrombosis - Diagnostic Strategies and Prognostic Models: A Review

Penka A. Atanassova[1], Radka I. Massaldjieva[2],
Nedka T. Chalakova[1] and Borislav D. Dimitrov[3]
[1]*Department of Neurology,*
[2]*Clinic of Psychiatry, Medical University, Plovdiv,*
[3]*Department of General Practice, Division of Population Health Sciences,*
Royal College of Surgeons in Ireland, Dublin,
[1,2]*Bulgaria*
[3]*Republic of Ireland*

1. Introduction

In 1825, Ribes described a case of a 45-year old man who died after a 6-month history of epilepsy, seizures and delirium. The autopsy examination revealed thrombosis of the superior sagittal sinus, the left lateral sinus and a cortical vein in the parietal region. This was probably the first detailed description of extensive cerebral venous sinus thrombosis (CVST). Since then, the literature describing this disease has comprised of case reports, series and some newer prospective studies, including recent reviews and guidelines (statement) on the diagnosis and management of CVST (Siddiqui & Kamal, 2006; Stam, 2005; Saposnik et al, 2011; Brown & Thore, 2011).

The cerebral venous sinus thrombosis is a challenging condition and it is most common than previously thought. CVST accounts for 0.5% to 1.0% of all strokes and usually affects young individuals. Important advances have been made in the understanding of the pathophysiology of this vascular disorder. The diagnosis of CVST is still frequently overlooked or delayed as a result of the wide spectrum of clinical symptoms and the often sub-acute or lingering onset. Patients with CVST commonly present with headache, although some develop a focal neurological deficit, decreased level of consciousness, seizures, or intracranial hypertension without focal neurological signs. Uncommonly, an insidious onset may create a diagnostic challenge. The main problem of this disorder is that it is very often unrecognised at initial presentation. In particular, a prothrombotic factor or a direct cause is identified in approximately 66% of the CVST patients (a list of most important causal and risk factors are listed in **Table 1**).

Cerebral venous thrombosis is more common in women than men, with a female to male ratio of 3:1 (cited in Ferro & Canhao, 2011). The imbalance may be due to the increased risk of CVST associated with pregnancy and puerperium and with oral contraceptives. The female predominance in CVST is found in young adults, but not in children or older adults.

Genetic prothrombotic conditions
- Antithrombin deficiency[5]
- Protein C and protein S deficiency[6-8]
- Factor V Leiden mutation[9-11]
- Prothrombin mutation (the substitution of A for G at position 20210)[9,11,12]
- Homocysteinemia caused by gene mutations in methylenetetrahydrofolate reductase[13,14]

Acquired prothrombotic states
- Nephrotic syndrome
- Antiphospholipid antibodies[7,15]
- Homocysteinemia[14]
- Pregnancy[16,17]
- Puerperium[17]

Infections
- Otitis, mastoiditis, sinusitis[6]
- Meningitis
- Systemic infectious disease[6]

Inflammatory disease
- Systemic lupus erythematosus[18]
- Wegener's granulomatosis[8]
- Sarcoidosis
- Inflammatory bowel disease
- Behçet's syndrome[19,20]

Hematologic conditions
- Polycythemia, primary and secondary
- Thrombocythemia
- Leukemia[21]
- Anemia, including paroxysmal nocturnal hemoglobinuria[22]

Drugs
- Oral contraceptives[9,23]
- Asparaginase[6,21]

Mechanical causes, trauma

Table 1. Most important causes of and risk factors associated with cerebral venous sinus thrombosis. *Reproduced with the written permission from the paper by Stam (2005).*

In the prospective International Study on Cerebral Vein and Dural Sinus Thrombosis (ISCVST) cohort of 624 adults with CVST, women comprised 465 (75%) of the patients. Compared with men, women had significantly lower mean age (42 vs 34 years). Furthermore, a gender specific risk factor — oral contraceptives, pregnancy, puerperium, and hormone replacement therapy — was identified in 65% of the women. CVST is more common in neonates than it is in infants, children or adults. In adults, CVST affects patients who are younger on average than those with arterial types of stroke. In the ISCVST, the mean age of patients with CVST was 39 years, and only 8% of them were older than 65 years (Ferro & Canhao, 2011). Topographically, the most frequent occurrence of CVST has been observed in the superior sagitral sinus (62%) followed by the transverse (lateral) sinus (41-45%) (**Figure 1**).

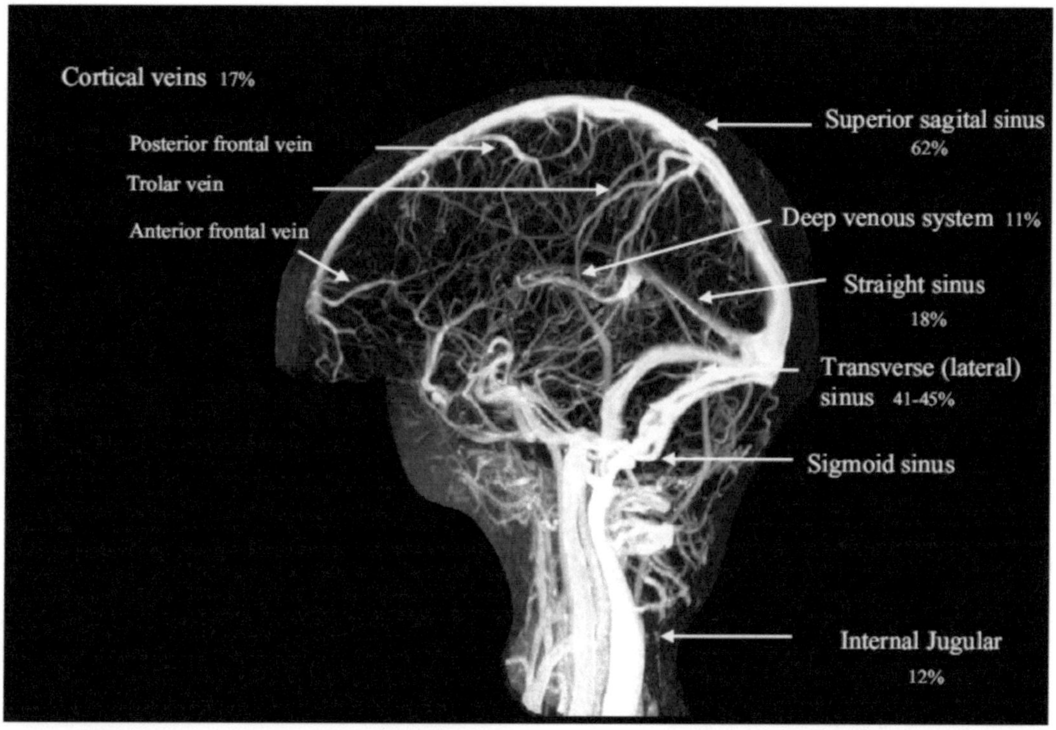

Fig. 1. MRI venogram of the cerebral venous system and most frequent location of CVST. *Reproduced with the written permission from the paper by Saposnik et al. (2011)* as derived from data on 624 patients in the International Study on Cerebral Venous and Dural Sinuses Thrombosis as reported by Manolidis & Kutz (2005).

The pathogenesis of CVST remains incompletely understood because of the high variability in the anatomy of the venous system, and the paucity of experiments in animal models of CVST. However, there are at least two different mechanisms that may contribute to the clinical features of CVST: a) *thrombosis of cerebral veins or dural sinus leading to cerebral parenchymal lesions or dysfunction*; and b) *occlusion of dural sinus resulting in decreased cerebrospinal fluid (CSF) absorption and elevated intracranial pressure*. (**Figure 2**). Obstruction of the venous structures may result in increased venous pressure, decreased capillary perfusion pressure, and increased cerebral blood volume. Dilatation of cerebral veins and recruitment of collateral pathways play an important role in the early phases of CVST and may initially compensate for changes in pressure. The increase in venous and capillary pressure leads to blood-brain barrier disruption, causing vasogenic edema, with leakage of blood plasma into the interstitial space. As intravenous pressure continues to increase, mild parenchymal changes, severe cerebral edema, and venous hemorrhage may occur due to venous or capillary rupture. The increased intravenous pressure may lead to an increase in intravascular pressure and a lowering of cerebral perfusion pressure, resulting in decreased cerebral blood flow (CBF) and failure of energy metabolism. In turn, this allows intracellular entry of water from failure of the Na+/K+ ATPase pump, and consequent cytotoxic edema (Ferro & Canhao, 2011).

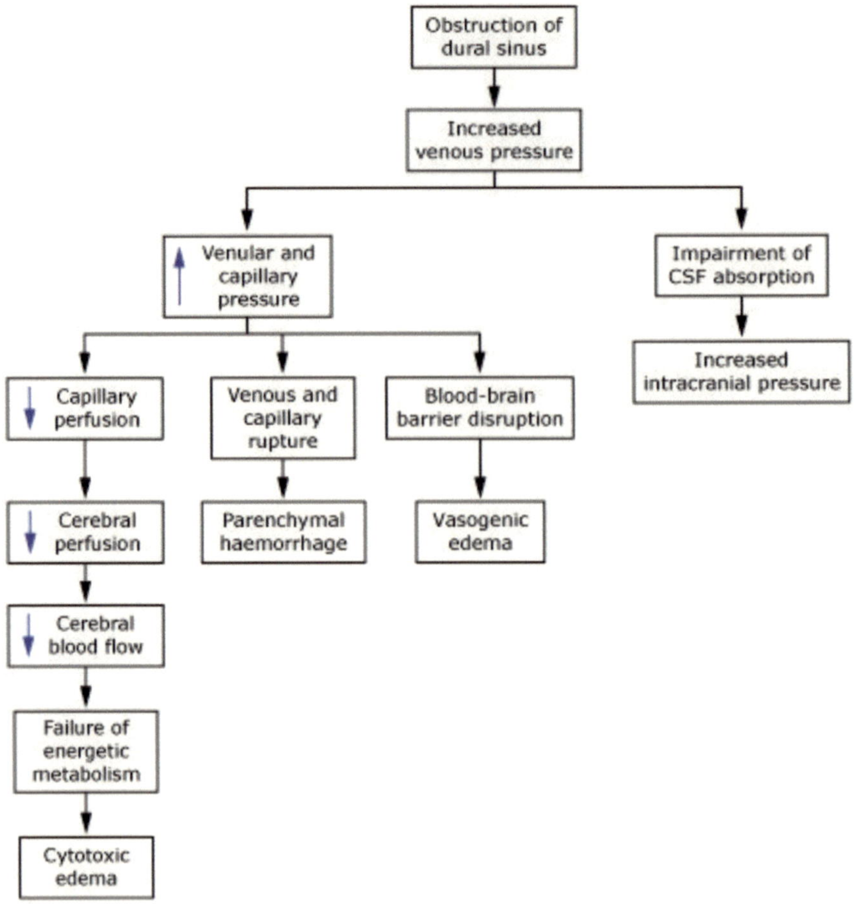

Fig. 2. Possible mechanisms of the development of CVST. *Reproduced with the written permission from the paper by Ferro & Canhao (2011).*

Advances in our understanding of the venous occlusion pathophysiology have been achieved by the use of newer magnetic resonance imaging (MRI) methods, mainly diffusion-weighted MRI (DWI) and perfusion-weighted MRI (PWI). These techniques have demonstrated the coexistence of both cytotoxic and vasogenic edema in patients with CVST. The other effect of venous thrombosis is impairment of CSF absorption. Normally, CSF absorption occurs in the arachnoid granulations (Leach et al, 2008), which drain CSF into the superior sagittal sinus. Thrombosis of the dural sinuses leads to increased venous pressure, impaired CSF absorption, and consequently elevated intracranial pressure. Elevated intracranial pressure is more frequent if superior sagittal sinus thrombosis is present, but it may also occur with thrombosis of the jugular or lateral sinus, producing a rise of pressure in the superior sagittal sinus.

As shown in Table 1, many causes or predisposing conditions are associated with CVST. The major risk factors for CVST in adults can be grouped in two classes: *transient* or *permanent* (**Table 2**) . In more than 85% of the adult patients, at least one risk factor for CVST can be identified, most often a prothrombotic condition as mentioned above. In the ISCVST cohort, a prothrombotic condition was found in 34%, and a genetic prothrombotic condition

was found in 22% of all patients. Although infectious causes of CVST were frequently reported in the past, they are responsible for only 6 to 12 percent of cases in modern-era studies of adults with CVST. As with venous thrombosis in other parts of the body, multiple risk factors may be found in about half of adult patients with CVST. No underlying etiology or risk factor for CVST is found in approximately 13% of adult patients. However, it is important to continue searching for a cause even after the acute phase of CVST, as some patients may have a condition such as the antiphospholipid syndrome (APS), polycythemia, thrombocythemia, or malignancy that is discovered weeks or months after the acute phase.
It should be noted that the risk for CVST is influenced by the individual's genetic background. In the presence of some prothrombotic conditions, patients are at an increased risk of developing CVST when exposed to a precipitant such a head trauma, lumbar puncture, jugular catheter placement, pregnancy, surgery, infection, and drugs. These prothrombotic conditions include the following: antithrombin deficiency, protein C deficiency or protein S deficiency, Factor V Leiden mutation or G20210 A prothrombin gene mutation.

Transient risk factors	Permanent risk factors
Infection	**Inflammatory diseases**
Central nervous system	Systemic lupus erythematosus
Ear, sinus, mouth, face, and neck	Behçet disease
Systemic infectious disease	Granulomatosis with polyangiitis (Wegener's)
Pregnancy and puerperium	Tromboangiitis obliterans
Other disorders	Inflammatory bowel disease
Dehydration	Sarcoidosis
Mechanical precipitants	**Malignancy**
Head injury	Central nervous system
Lumbar puncture	Solid tumour outside central nervous system
Neurosurgical procedures	Hematologic
Jugular catheter occlusion	**Hematologic condition**
Drugs	Polycythemia, thrombocythemia
Oral contraceptives	Anemia, including paroxysmal nocturnal hemoglobinuria
Hormone replacement therapy	**Central nervous system disorders**
Androgens	Dural fistulae
Asparaginase	**Other disorders**
Tamoxifen	Congenital heart disease
Glucocorticoids	Thyroid disease

Table 2. Classification of systemic and local conditions increasing the risk of cerebral venous thrombosis. *Reproduced with the written permission from the paper by Ferro & Canhao (2011).*

In particular, the most frequent risk factor in young women is the use of oral contraceptives. Two case-control studies have shown an increased risk of sinus thrombosis in women who use oral contraceptives. Furthermore, the risk for CVST in women using oral contraceptives is increased if they have a prothrombotic defect. In elderly CVST patients, the proportion of cases without identified risk factors is higher (37%) than it is in adults <65 years of age. The most common risk factors in those ≥65 years old are genetic or acquired thrombophilia, malignancy, and hematologic disorders such as polycythemia (Ferro & Canhao, 2011; Plata et al, 2002).

2. Methods

Search strategy. For the purpose of this review, a systematic search of the literature databases (e.g., PubMed) by the EndNote software as well as other reference and electronic databases (e.g., Cochrane Library) have been searched by specifically chosen MESH terms, back to 1960. In total, while using the main four single terms ("cerebral", "sinus", "venous", "thrombosis") and combinations thereof, 4049 peer-reviewed titles have been initially found which have been later reduced down to 43 titles, among which 25 review papers have been also identified. Many references for this review came from the authors' own archives. Two of us (PAA, BDD) independently reviewed all 43 titles for inclusion as retrieved as above and 35 of them were decided to be included. Additionally, through hand-searching the references of the selected articles and other relevant electronic sources (e.g., Google Scholar), several additional relevant titles were also reviewed for inclusion. Finally, out of the initially 4049 identified titles and all other relevant titles, 39 articles were studied and included in this review. Any disagreements between the original reviewers have been resolved by a third, blinded reviewer (NTC); any further discrepancies have been solved by an open consensus among all of the reviewers.

3. Results

Most of the articles that were identified were case reports or limited case series. Others were original articles and reviews or overviews. We were able to initially identify 4049 peer-reviewed titles in PubMed, including 25 review papers. To note, we were able to identify separately only 3 systematic reviews in the Cochrane Library (Ciccone et al, 2004; Kwan & Gunther, 2006; Stam et al, 2002 as cited in Stam, 2005). Finally, 39 articles were included for the purposes of this review.

3.1 Early clinical detection and diagnostic strategies with imaging in CVST

Clinical signs and symptoms and laboratory tests. The diagnosis of CVST is typically based on a clinical suspicion and imaging confirmation. Clinical findings in CVST usually fall into 2 major categories: a) *focal brain injury from venous ischemia/infarction or hemorrhage* and b) *increased intracranial pressure attributable to impaired venous drainage.* Headache, generally indicative of an increase in intracranial pressure, is the most common symptom in CVST (in 90% of the patients in the ISCVST). The headache of CVST is typically described as diffuse and often progresses in severity over days to weeks. A minority of patients may present with thunderclap headache (Saposnik et al, 2011), suggestive of subarachnoid hemorrhage (SAH) (Atanassova et al, 2006), and a migrainous type of headache has been described. Isolated headache without focal neurological findings or papilledema occurs in up to 25% of the patients with CVST and presents a significant diagnostic challenge. CVST is an important diagnostic consideration in patients with headache and papilledema or diplopia (caused by sixth nerve palsy) even without other neurological focal signs. When a focal brain injury occurs, most common are hemiparesis and aphasia, but other cortical signs and sensory symptoms may be also observed, together with psychosis in such cases. The clinical manifestations of CVST may also depend on the location of the thrombosis as mentioned above (Figure 1). The superior sagittal sinus is most commonly involved. For the lateral sinus thromboses, as a second prevalent location, the symptoms related to an underlying condition (middle ear infection) may be noted, including constitutional symptoms, fever, and ear discharge. Pain in the ear or mastoid region and headache are typical. On examination, an increased intracranial pressure and distention of the scalp veins may be noted (hemianopia, contralateral weakness, and aphasia may sometimes be seen owing to cortical involvement). Approximately 16% of the patients with CVST have thrombosis of the deep cerebral venous system (internal cerebral vein, vein of Galen, and straight sinus), which can lead to thalamic or basal ganglial infarction (van der Bergh et al, 2005). Most patients present with rapid neurological deterioration (Saposnik et al, 2011). Importantly, several principal clinical features distinguish CVST from other cerebrovascular diseases (CVD). Notably, the focal or generalized seizures are frequent, occurring in about 40% of patients; and, secondly, as a clinical correlate to the anatomy of cerebral venous drainage, the bilateral brain involvement is not infrequent. The latter is particularly notable in cases that involve the deep venous drainage system, when bilateral thalamic involvement may occur, causing alterations in level of consciousness without focal neurological findings. Bilateral motor signs, including paraparesis, may also be present due to sagittal sinus thrombosis and bihemispheric injury. Finally, patients with CVST often present with slowly progressive symptoms. It has to be underlined that very frequently the delays in diagnosis of CVST are common and significant. In the ISCVST, symptom onset was acute (<48 hours) in 37% of patients, subacute (>48 hours to 30 days) in 56% of patients, and chronic (>30 days) in 7% of the patients. The median delay from the onset of symptoms to the hospital admission was 4 days, and from symptom onset to the diagnosis - 7 days.

Specific diagnostic cues. About 40% of the patients with CVST present with *intracranial hemorrhage* (ICH). The features suggestive of CVST as a cause of ICH include prodromal headache (which is highly unusual with other causes of ICH), bilateral parenchymal abnormalities, and clinical evidence of a hypercoagulable state. These features may not be present, however, and a high index of clinical suspicion is necessary. An isolated subarachnoid hemorrhage may also occur due to CVST, although this is rare (0.8% of patients in ISCVST). A second specific occurrence is *isolated headache/idiopathic intracranial hypertension* – for example, 25% of the CVST patients may present with isolated headache, and another 25% - with headache in conjunction with papilledema or sixth nerve palsies suggestive of idiopathic intracranial hypertension. In a series of 131 patients who presented with papilledema and clinically suspected idiopathic intracranial hypertension, 10% had CVST at MRI/magnetic resonance venography (MRV). Imaging of the cerebral venous system has been recommended for all patients with the clinical picture of idiopathic intracranial hypertension. Regarding headache - it is an extremely common symptom, and most patients with isolated headache will not have CVST. The cost-effectiveness and yield of routine imaging are highly uncertain. Factors that may suggest the diagnosis, and thus prompt imaging evaluation, include a new, atypical headache; headache that progresses steadily over days to weeks despite conservative treatment; and thunderclap headache, especially if a hypercoagulable state is also present. A third difficult occurrence in CVST is when the patients present with *somnolence or a confusional* *state in the absence of obvious focal neurological abnormalities* (more common in the elderly and with thrombosis of the deep venous system). Although a number of mechanisms may underlie this clinical presentation, an important cause is bilateral thalamic lesions due to involvement of the deep venous system. Early CT scanning may not be useful; MRI will usually demonstrate abnormalities in such cases (Saposnik et al, 2011).

Laboratory and other biochemical tests. A complete blood count, chemistry panel, sedimentation rate, and measures of the prothrombin time and activated partial thromboplastin time are indicated for suspected CVST. These may be indicative of hidden hypercoagulable state, infectious process or inflammatory state as contributing factors to the CVST development. Further, the examination of the cerebrospinal fluid (CSF) is typically not helpful in cases with focal neurological abnormalities and radiographic confirmation of the diagnosis of CVST unless there might be a suspicion of meningitis. An elevated opening pressure may be a clue for diagnosing CVST in patients who present with headaches (i.e., such pressure may be present in >80% of the patients). Elevated cell counts may be present in about 50% of the patients and the increased protein levels - in about 35%, however, their absence should not exclude a consideration of CVST. Usually, there are no specific CSF abnormalities in CVST. Additionally to the above routine tests, the D-dimer, a product of fibrin degradation, has a diagnostic role in exclusion of DVT or pulmonary embolus when used with pre-test probability assessment. In a well-designed prospective, multicenter study of 343 patients presenting to the emergency department with symptoms that suggested CVST, a positive D-dimer level (defined as a level >500μg/l) was found in 34 of 35 patients with confirmed CVST and 27 of 308 patients without CVST (sensitivity >97% and specificity >90%). Having a negative predictive value of 99.6% a normal D-dimer level test may easily help identify patients with a low probability of CVST. Several factors may account for some of discrepant findings of the D-dimer test - first, D-dimer levels decline with time from onset of symptoms, which suggests that patients who present with subacute or chronic symptoms are more likely to have negative D-dimer levels; second, the anatomic extent of thrombosed sinuses may correlate with D-dimer levels, which suggests that patients with lesser clot burden may have false negative D-dimer testing results.

In the view of the above evidence, the following specific recommendations may be summarised (Saposnik et al, 2011):

- In patients with suspected CVST, routine blood studies consisting of a complete blood count, chemistry panel, prothrombin time, and activated partial thromboplastin time should be performed; screening for potential prothrombotic conditions that may predispose a person to CVST (eg, use of contraceptives, underlying inflammatory disease, infectious process) is recommended in the initial clinical assessment;
- A normal D-dimer level according to a sensitive immunoassay or rapid enzyme-linked immunosorbent assay (ELISA) may be considered to help identify patients with low probability of CVST - if there is a strong clinical suspicion of CVST, a normal D-dimer level should not preclude further evaluation;
- In patients with lobar ICH of otherwise unclear origin or with cerebral infarction that crosses typical arterial boundaries, imaging of the cerebral venous system should be performed;
- In patients with the clinical features of idiopathic intracranial hypertension, imaging of the cerebral venous system is recommended to exclude CVST; in patients with headache associated with atypical features, imaging of the cerebral venous system is reasonable to exclude CVST.

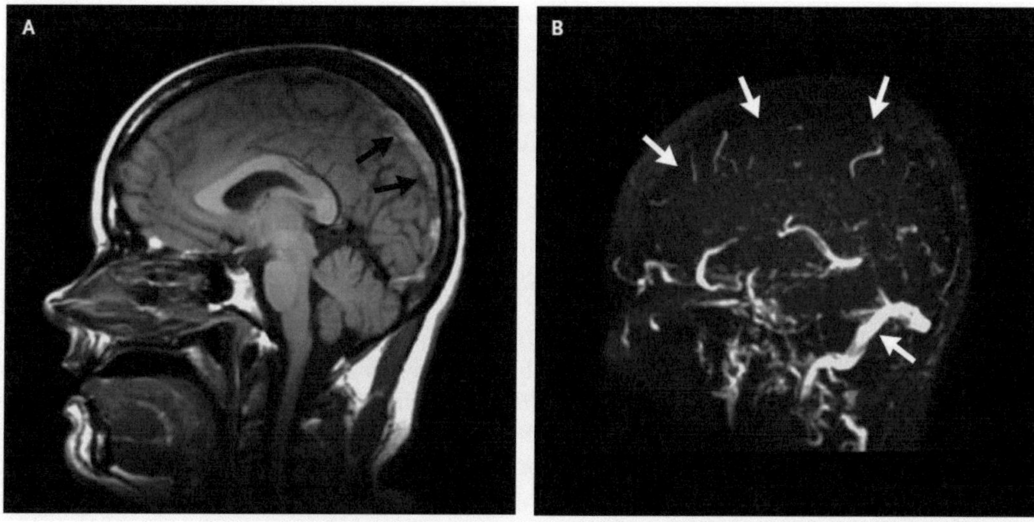

Fig. 3. MRI of Sinus Thrombosis.In Panel A, a T1-weighted MRI scan obtained with the spin–echo technique provides a sagittal view of a hyperintense signal in the thrombosed superior sagittal sinus (arrows). In Panel B, a magnetic resonance venogram obtained without the administration of contrast material reveals the absence of a signal in the superior sagittal sinus (upper arrows) and a normal flow signal in the transverse and sigmoid sinuses (lower arrow) as well as in a number of veins. *Reproduced with the written permission from the paper by Stam (2005).*

Diagnostic imaging in CVST. The diagnostic imaging has played an increasing role in the better diagnosis and management of CVST. The aim is to determine vascular and parenchymal changes associated with this medical condition (possibly, the diagnosis is made only with cerebral digital subtraction angiography).

Noninvasive diagnostic techniques: CT, MRI and ultrasound. *Computed tomography* (CT) is widely used as the initial neuroimaging test in patients who present with new-onset neurological symptoms such as headache, seizure, mental alteration, or focal neurological signs. CT without contrast is often normal but may demonstrate findings that suggest CVST. Anatomic variability of the venous sinuses makes CT diagnosis of CVST insensitive, with results on a plain CT being abnormal only in about 30% of CVST cases. The primary sign of acute CVST on a non-contrast CT is hyperdensity of a cortical vein or dural sinus. Acutely thrombosed cortical veins and dural sinuses appear as a homogenous hyperdensity that fills the vein or sinus and are most clearly visualized when CT slices are perpendicular to the dural sinus or vein. However, only approximately 30% of CVST demonstrates direct signs of hyperdense dural sinus. Thrombosis of the posterior portion of the superior sagittal sinus may appear as a dense triangle, the dense or filled delta sign. An ischemic infarction, sometimes with a hemorrhagic component, may be seen. An ischemic lesion that crosses usual arterial boundaries (with a hemorrhagic component) or in close proximity to a venous sinus is suggestive of CVST. Subarachnoid hemorrhage is not frequent - it is seen only in up to 0.8% of the CVST patients, and when present, it was localized in the convexity as opposed to the area of the circle of Willis usually observed in patients with aneurysmal rupture. Contrast-enhanced CT may show enhancement of the dural lining of the sinus with a filling defect within the vein or sinus. Contrast-enhanced CT may show the classic "empty delta" sign, in which a central hypointensity due to absent or very slow flow within the sinus is surrounded by contrast enhancement in the surrounding triangular shape in the posterior aspect of the superior sagittal sinus. This finding may not appear for several days after onset of symptoms but does persist for several weeks. Due to delays or overlooking, CVST may be seen only during the subacute or chronic stage. Compared with the density of adjacent brain tissue, thrombus may be isodense, hypodense, or of mixed density. In this situation, contrast CT or CT venography (CTV) may assist the imaging diagnosis. In general, the *magnetic resonance imaging* (MRI) is more sensitive for the detection of CVST than CT at each stage after thrombosis (**Figure 3**). CVST is diagnosed on MRI with the detection of thrombus in a venous sinus. Findings are variable but may include a "hyperintense vein sign". Isolated cortical venous thrombosis (Chang et al, 1995) is identified much less frequently than sinus thrombosis. The magnetic resonance signal intensity of venous thrombus varies according to the time of imaging from the onset of thrombus formation. Acute thrombus may be of low intensity. In the first week, venous thrombus frequently appears as isointense to brain tissue on T1-weighted images and hypointense on T2- weighted images owing to increased deoxyhemoglobin. By the second week, thrombus contains methemoglobin, which results in hyperintensity on T1- and T2-weighted images. With evolution of the thrombus, the paramagnetic products of deoxyhemoglobin and methemoglobin are present in the sinus. A thrombosed dural sinus or vein may then demonstrate low signal on gradient-echo and susceptibility-weighted images of magnetic resonance images. The principal early signs of CVST on non–contrast-enhanced MRI are the combination of absence of a flow void with alteration of signal intensity in the dural sinus. MRI of the brain is suggestive of CVST by the absence of a fluid void signal in the sinus, T2 hypointensity suggestive of a thrombus, or a central isodense lesion in a venous sinus with surrounding enhancement. This appearance is the MRI equivalent of the CT empty delta sign. An acute venous thrombus may have hypo-intense signal that mimics a normal flow void. The nature of the thrombus then evolves through a subacute and chronic phase.

Thus, a contrast-enhanced MRI and either CTV or MRV may be necessary to establish a definite diagnosis. The secondary signs of MRI may show similar patterns to CT, including cerebral swelling, edema, and/or hemorrhage. Occasionally, diffusion-weighted imaging (DWI) and perfusion-weighted MRI may assist in making the diagnosis. DWI may show high signal intensity as restricted diffusion- and perfusion-weighted MRI with prolonged transit time. Brain parenchymal lesions of CVST are better visualized and depicted on MRI than at CT. Focal edema without hemorrhage is visualized on CT in about 8% of cases and on MRI in 25% of cases. Focal parenchymal changes with edema and hemorrhage may be identified in up to 40% of patients. Petechial or confluent hemorrhage may also represent an underlying hemorrhagic venous infarction. This may include DWI abnormalities consistent with acute infarction, but the degree of DWI findings may be reduced in venous infarction compared with arterial infarction. An altered enhancement pattern suggestive of collateral flow or of venous congestion may be seen. There are some characteristic patterns of brain parenchymal changes that distinguish CVST from other entities. Also, to some extent, lesions related to specific sinuses are regionally distributed. Brain parenchymal changes in frontal, parietal, and occipital lobes usually correspond to superior sagittal sinus thrombosis. Temporal lobe parenchymal changes correspond to lateral (transverse) and sigmoid sinus thrombosis. Deep parenchymal abnormalities, including thalamic hemorrhage, edema, or intraventricular hemorrhage, correspond to thrombosis of the vein of Galen or straight sinus. MRI signal can also predict radiographic outcome to some extent, because DWI abnormality within veins or sinus predicts poor recanalization. The *CT venography* (CTV) can provide a rapid and reliable modality for detecting CVST. CTV is much more useful in subacute or chronic situations because of the varied density in thrombosed sinus. Because of the dense cortical bone adjacent to dural sinus, bone artifact may interfere with the visualization of enhanced dural sinus. CTV is at least equivalent to MRV in the diagnosis of CVST. However, drawbacks to CTV include concerns about radiation exposure, potential for iodine contrast material allergy, and issues related to use of contrast in the setting of poor renal function. In some settings, MRV is preferable to CTV because of these concerns. The most commonly used magnetic resonance venography (MRV) techniques are time-of-flight (TOF) MRV and contrast-enhanced magnetic resonance. Phase-contrast MRI is used less frequently, because defining the velocity of the encoding parameter is both difficult and operator-dependent. T2-weighted magnetic resonance image showing mixed hypointensity (white arrow) and isointensity (black arrow) signals representing an acute hemorrhage at left parietal lobe.

The 2D TOF technique is the most commonly used method currently for the diagnosis of CVST, because 2-dimensional TOF has excellent sensitivity to slow flow compared with 3-dimensional TOF. It does have several potential pitfalls in imaging interpretation Despite the challenges, other sequences such as gradient echo, susceptibility/weighted imaging, and contrast MRI/MRV may assist in these situations. Nonthrombosed hypoplastic sinus will not have abnormal low signal in the sinus on gradient echo or susceptibility-weighted images. The chronic thrombosed hypoplastic sinus will have marked enhanced sinus and no flow on 2-dimensional TOF venography. Contrast-enhanced MRI offers improved visualization of cerebral venous structures (**Figure 4**).

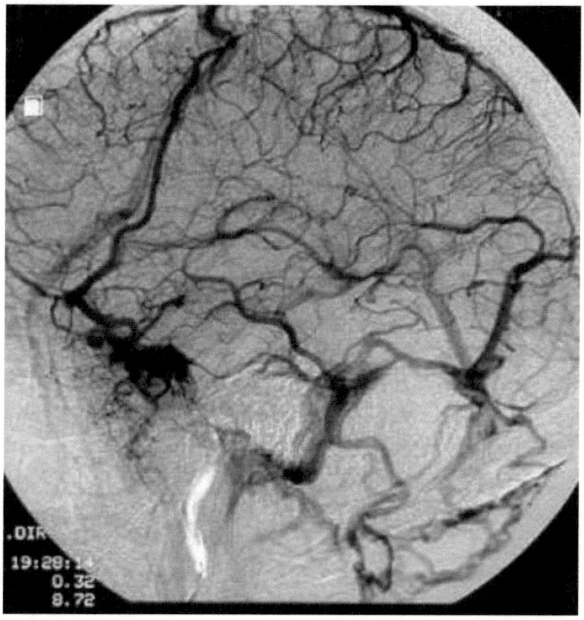

Fig. 4. CVST diagnosis: CT, MRI and venography. MR venography with limited spatial resolution, saturation of flow signal; CT venography; IA venography with hypoplasia vs. occlusion; high anatomical variability. *Reproduced with the written permission from the presentation by Ferro (2010).*

In patients with persistent or progressive symptoms despite medical treatment, repeated neuroimaging (including a CTV or MRV) may help identify the development of a new ischemic lesion, ICH, edema, propagation of the thrombus, or other brain parenchymal lesions. The deep venous system is readily seen on CT and MRI and may be less impacted by artifact because of the separation from bony structures. A potential pitfall at the junction of the straight sinus and vein of Galen on TOF MRI is the appearance of absence of flow if image acquisition is in an axial plane to the skull. This pitfall may be overcome with contrast-enhanced MRI and DWI.

Invasive diagnostic angiographic procedures. The *cerebral angiographic procedures* are less commonly needed to establish the diagnosis of CVST given the availability of MRV and CTV. These techniques are reserved for situations in which the MRV or CTV results are inconclusive or if an endovascular procedure is being considered. Cerebral angiography (arteriographic) findings include the failure of sinus appearance due to the occlusion; venous congestion with dilated cortical, scalp, or facial veins; enlargement of typically diminutive veins from collateral drainage; and reversal of venous flow. The venous phase of cerebral angiography will show a filling defect in the thrombosed cerebral vein/sinus. Because of the highly variable cerebral venous structures and inadequate resolution, CT or MRI may not provide adequate visualization of selected veins, especially cortical veins and in some situations the deep venous structures. Hypoplasia or atresia of cerebral veins or dural sinuses may lead to inconclusive results on MRV or CTV and can be clarified on the venous phase of cerebral angiography. Acute dural sinus and cortical vein thrombosis typically causes a delay in cerebral venous circulation, and cerebral angiography will demonstrate delayed and slow visualization of cerebral venous structures. Normally, the early veins begin to opacify at 4 to 5 seconds after injection of contrast material into the carotid artery, and the complete cerebral venous system is opacified in 7 to 8 seconds. If cerebral veins or dural sinuses are not visualized in the normal sequences of cerebral angiography, the possibility of acute thrombosis is suspected. This finding accounts for the observed delayed cerebral perfusion seen with perfusion/weighted MRI with prolonged transit time. The *direct cerebral venography* (DCV) is performed by direct injection of contrast material into a dural sinus or cerebral vein from microcatheter insertion via the internal jugular vein. DCV is usually performed during endovascular therapeutic procedures. In direct cerebral venography, intraluminal thrombus is seen either as a filling defect within the lumen in the setting of nonocclusive thrombosis or as complete nonfilling in occlusive thrombosis. Complete thrombosis may also demonstrate a "cupping appearance" within the sinus. Venous pressure measurements may be performed during direct cerebral venography to identify venous hypertension. Normal venous sinus pressure is <10 mm H_2O. The extent of parenchymal change correlates with increased venous pressure and with the stage of thrombosis, with changes being maximal in acute thrombosis. *Transfontanellar ultrasound* may be used to evaluate pediatric patients, including newborn or young infants with open anterior or posterior fontanels. Ultrasound, along with transcranial Doppler, may be useful to support the diagnosis of CVST and for ongoing monitoring. Evidence on *perfusion imaging methods* (PIM) using positron emission tomography, although scarce, showed a reduction of the cerebral blood flow after ligation of the superior sagittal sinus with a concomitant venous infarction. An increased regional cerebral blood volume was also observed in a young adult with sagittal sinus thrombosis. A prolonged mean transit time and increased cerebral blood volume have been suggested as venous congestion, contrary to the pattern observed in patients with an ischemic arterial stroke (prolonged mean transit time with reduction in cerebral blood volume).

Of note, some common pitfalls in the diagnostic imaging should be also mentioned. The positive findings of intraluminal thrombus are the most important feature to a confident diagnosis of CVST by CT or MRI. Unfortunately, these findings are not always evident, and the diagnosis rests on nonfilling of a venous sinus or cortical vein. Given the variation in venous anatomy, it is sometimes impossible to exclude CVST on noninvasive imaging studies. Anatomic variants of normal venous anatomy may mimic sinus thrombosis, including sinus atresia/hypoplasia, asymmetrical sinus drainage, and normal sinus filling defects related to prominent arachnoid granulations or intrasinus septa. Angiographic examination of 100 patients with no venous pathology showed a high prevalence of asymmetrical lateral (transverse) sinuses (49%) and partial or complete absence of one lateral sinus (20%). Flow gaps are commonly seen on TOF MRV images, which sometimes affects their interpretation. The hypoplastic dural sinus may have a more tapering appearance than an abrupt defect in contrast-enhanced images of the sinus. The lack of identification of a thrombus within the venous sinus on MRI or contrast-enhanced MRV or CTV is helpful to clarify the diagnosis. As mentioned, sinus signal-intensity variations may also affect the interpretation of imaging in the diagnosis of CVST. The direct cerebral venography may be difficult to interpret owing to retrograde flow of contrast from the point of injection, and the venous pressure may not be accurate because of relative compartmentalization within the system.

The following specific recommendations for diagnostic imaging in CVST may be summarised (Saposnik et al, 2011):

- Plain CT or MRI is useful in the initial evaluation of patients with suspected CVST, however, a negative plain CT or MRI does not rule out CVST. A venographic study (either CTV or MRV) should be performed in suspected CVST if the plain CT or MRI is negative or to define the extent of CVST if the plain CT or MRI suggests CVST;
- Early follow-up CTV or MRV is recommended in CVST patients with persistent or evolving symptoms despite medical treatment or with symptoms suggestive of propagation of thrombus;
- For patients who present with recurrent symptoms suggestive of CVST and had had a previous CVST, a repeat CTV or MRV is recommended;
- Gradient echo T2 susceptibility-weighted images combined with magnetic resonance can be useful to improve the accuracy of CVST diagnosis;
- Catheter cerebral angiography can be useful in patients with inconclusive CTV or MRV in whom a clinical suspicion for CVST remains high;
- A follow-up CTV or MRV at 3 to 6 months after diagnosis is reasonable to assess for recanalization of the occluded cortical vein/sinuses in stable patients.

3.2 Management of CVST - Technological advances and treatment options

Acute management and treatment of CVST. A summary algorithm for the diagnosis and management of patients with CVST is provided (**Figure 5**). The initial anticoagulation therapy (AT) has 3 aims in CVST: a) to prevent thrombus growth, b) to facilitate recanalization, and c) to prevent DVT or pulmonary embolism (PE). There is a controversy in the consideration for recommendations regarding AT, because a cerebral infarction with hemorrhagic transformation or ICH is commonly present at the time of diagnosis of CVST,

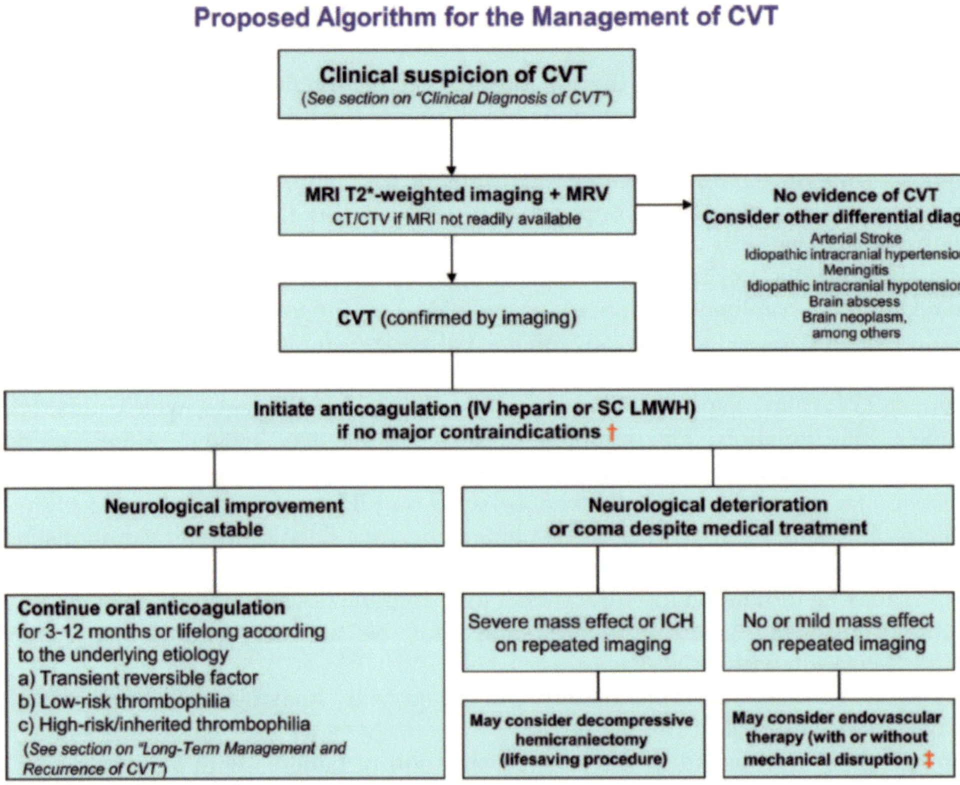

Fig. 5. Algorithm for initial management of CVST. *Symbols and abbreviations:* CVST indicates cerebral venous and sinus thrombosis; LMWH, low molecular weight heparin; Tx, therapy; ICH, intracerebral hemorrhage; CTV, CT venogram; MRV, MR venogram. †Intracranial hemorrhage that occurred as the consequence of CVST is not a contraindication for anticoagulation. ‡Endovascular therapy may be considered in patients with absolute contraindications for anticoagulation therapy or failure of initial therapeutic doses of anticoagulant therapy. *Note:* Anticoagulation remains the principal therapy and is aimed at preventing thrombus propagation and increasing recanalization. This algorithm is not comprehensive, nor applicable to all clinical scenarios and patient management must be individualized. Limited evidence is available on the benefits of decompressive hemicraniectomy and endovascular therapy for the management of CVST as reflected by the low grade and level of recommendations. Anticipated future advances in imaging techniques, new pharmacological agents and endovascular procedures may provide other therapeutic alternatives to be considered in patients with CVST. *Reproduced with the written permission from the paper by Saposnik et al (2011).*

and it may also complicate treatment. A number of observational studies, both prospective and retrospective, are available, primarily from single centers. Not all studies reported specifically on outcomes of anticoagulation treatment, because the majority of patients in most studies were treated with intravenous UFH or low-molecular-weight heparin (LMWH) at the time of diagnosis, with eventual use of vitamin K antagonists. Mortality rates were low, typically less than 10%, often due to the underlying disease (eg, cancer, etc (Knopp, 1995)) rather than CVST and rarely due to ICH. The majority of patients fully recovered neurological function, and few became disabled. In a retrospective study of 102 patients with CVST, 43 had an ICH. Among 27 (63%) who were treated with doseadjusted intravenous heparin after the ICH, 4 died (15%), and 14 patients (52%) recovered completely. Of the 13 patients who did not receive heparin, mortality was higher (69%) with lower improvement in functional outcomes (only 3 patients completely recovered). The largest study by far was the ISCVST, which included 624 patients at 89 centers in 21 countries. Nearly all patients were treated with anticoagulation initially, and mortality was 8.3% over 16 months; 79% had complete recovery (modified Rankin scale [mRS] score of 0 to 1), 10.4% had mild to moderate disability (mRS score 2-3) and 2.2% remained severely disabled (mRS score 4-5).10 Few studies had sufficient numbers of patients not treated with anticoagulation to adequately address the role of anticoagulation in relation to outcome. Data from observational studies suggest a range of risks for ICH after anticoagulation for CVST from zero to 5.4%.

There are two available randomized controlled trials comparing anticoagulant therapy with placebo or open control in patients with CVST confirmed by contrast imaging (cited in Saposnik et al, 2011). Taken together, these trials included only 79 patients. Meta-analysis of these 2 trials revealed a non-statistically significant relative risk of death or dependency with anticoagulation (relative risk 0.46, 95%CI 0.16 to 1.31), with a risk difference in favor of anticoagulation of -13% (95%CI -30% to 3%). The relative risk of death was 0.33 (95%CI 0.08 to 1.21), with a risk difference of -13% (95%CI -27% to 1%). A third randomized trial with 57 women (with puerperal CVST confirmed only by CT imaging) excluded those with hemorrhage on CT. Treatment was with subcutaneous heparin 5000 IU every 6 hours, dose adjusted to an activated partial thromboplastin time 1.5 times baseline for at least 30 days after delivery. Outcome assessment was not blinded. Three patients in the control group either died or had residual paresis compared with none in the heparin group. In the special situation of CVST with cerebral hemorrhage on presentation, even in the absence of anticoagulation, hemorrhage is associated with adverse outcomes. Highlighting this, in 1 trial of nadroparin, all 6 deaths in the trial overall occurred in the group of 29 patients with hemorrhage on their pretreatment CT scan. None of the deaths were attributed to new or enlarged hemorrhage. These 29 patients were equally divided between treatment groups. Thus, cerebral hemorrhage was strongly associated with mortality but not with cerebral bleeding on treatment. Other studies suggested low rates of cerebral hemorrhage after anticoagulation for CVST. In the special situation of a patient with a major contraindication for anticoagulation (such as recent major hemorrhage), the risks and benefits of anticoagulation must be balanced. In these settings, as for venous thrombosis in general, consultation with an expert in anticoagulation management may be appropriate, and low-intensity anticoagulation may be considered if possible in favor of no anticoagulation until such time as it might be safe to use full-intensity anticoagulation. *In conclusion,* limited data from randomized controlled clinical trials in combination with observational data on outcomes and bleeding complications of anticoagulation support a role for anticoagulation in treatment of CVST, regardless of the presence of pretreatment ICH. On the basis of the available data, it is unlikely that researchers will have equipoise on this question, so a new randomized trial may not be feasible. Anticoagulation appears safe and effective. There was consensus in the writing group to support anticoagulation therapy in the management of patients with CVST. If anticoagulation is given, there are no data supporting differences in outcome with the use of UFH in adjusted doses or LMWH in CVST patients. However, in the setting of DVT or PE, a recent systematic review and meta-analysis of 22 studies showed a lower risk of major hemorrhage (1.2% vs. 2.1%), thrombotic complications (3.6% vs. 5.4%), and death (4.5% vs. 6.0%) with LMWH.

Fibrinolytic therapy (FT) Although patients with CVST may recover with anticoagulation therapy, 9% to 13% have poor outcomes despite anticoagulation. Anticoagulation alone may not dissolve a large and extensive thrombus, and the clinical condition may worsen even during heparin treatment. Incomplete recanalization or persistent thrombosis may explain this phenomenon. Partial or complete recanalization rates for CVST ranged from 47% to 100% with anticoagulation alone. Unfortunately, most studies reporting partial or complete recanalization at 3 to 6 months have a small sample size. When 4 studies that included 114 CVST patients were combined, partial or complete recanalization at 3 to 6 months was observed in 94 (82.5%). Recanalization rates may be higher for patients who receive thrombolytic therapy (Stolz et al, 2004). In general, thrombolytic therapy is used if clinical deterioration continues despite anticoagulation or if a patient has elevated intracranial pressure that evolves despite other management approaches (Smith et alm 1997). Many invasive therapeutic procedures have been reported to treat CVST. These include direct catheter chemical thrombolysis and direct mechanical thrombectomy with or without thrombolysis. There are no randomized controlled trials to support these interventions compared with anticoagulation or with each other. Most evidence is based on small case series or anecdotal reports. Here, we review the studied interventions.

In direct catheter thrombolysis (DCT), a standard microcatheter and microguidewire are delivered to the thrombosed dural sinus through a sheath or guiding catheter from the jugular bulb. Mechanical manipulation of the thrombus with the guidewire increases the amount of clot that might be impacted by the thrombolytic agent, potentially reducing the amount of fibrinolytic agent used. In a retrospective multicenter study of CVST in the United States, 27 (15%) of 182 patients received endovascular thrombolysis. Ten patients were receiving concomitant anticoagulation therapy. Recanalization was achieved in 26 patients (96%), 4 developed an intracranial hemorrhage, and 1 patient (4%) died. A systematic review that included 169 patients with CVST treated with local thrombolysis showed a possible benefit for those with severe CVST, which indicates that fibrinolytics may reduce case fatality in critically ill patients. ICH occurred in 17% of patients after thrombolysis and was associated with clinical worsening in 5%.

The other available options include mechanical thrombectomy/thrombolysis (MTT) techniques. The *balloon-assisted thrombectomy and thrombolysis (BATT)* may be more efficient in cases where (despite above approaches) the sinus thrombosis may still persist the inflated balloon may reduce washout of fibrinolytic agents, potentially lessening the dose of fibrinolytic agents required, the occurrence of hemorrhage, and procedure time. The balloon may be used to perform partial thrombectomy before thrombolysis. A rheolytic *catheter thrombectomy* may be considered in patients with extensive thrombus that persists despite local administration of a fibrinolytic agent. One such device is the AngioJet (MEDRAD, Inc, Warrendale, PA), which uses hydrodynamic thrombolytic action occurring at the tip of the catheter via the Venturi effect from high-velocity saline jets. Thrombus is disrupted and directed down the second lumen of the device. A perforation of the venous sinus wall may occur rarely, at a rate that is unknown but reported in the existing small series. It may be avoided by removal of the AngioJet after partial recanalization of the thrombosis and follow-up with additional microcatheter thrombolysis. The Merci retrieval device (Concentric Medical, Mountain View, CA) has also been used to remove thrombus in the cerebral venous system. This technique also requires direct catheter access to the venous sinus. The small corkscrewshaped device is dispensed via the tip of the catheter, advanced into the thrombus, and then slowly pulled back into the catheter with the adherent thrombus. Here again, the device may be used to perform partial recanalization, followed by thrombolysis to avoid damaging the wall or trabeculae of the dural sinus. As mentioned above, the evidence available at the present time is anecdotal. The Penumbra System (Penumbra, Inc, Alameda, CA) is a new-generation neuroembolectomy device that acts to debulk and aspirate acute clots. It uses a reperfusion catheter that aspirates thrombus while passing a wire-based separator within the catheter to break up the clot and facilitate aspiration. Only anecdotal evidence for its efficacy is available. The risks associated with use of the Penumbra System for cerebral venous thrombosis are likely similar to those seen with the Merci and AngioJet systems.

As endovascular options for management of venous thrombosis have evolved, surgery has played an increasingly limited role. *Surgical thrombectomy* is needed uncommonly but may be considered if severe neurological or visual deterioration occurs despite maximal medical therapy. In a recent review, among 13 patients with severe CVST who underwent decompressive craniectomy, 11 (84.6%) achieved a favorable outcome (mRS score equal or less than 3). Decompressive craniotomy may be needed as a life-saving measure if a large venous infarction leads to a significant increase in intracranial pressure. Likewise, large hematomas rarely may need to be considered for surgical evacuation if associated with a progressive and severe neurological deficit.

It is to note that, in summary, the use of these direct intrasinus thrombolytic techniques and mechanical therapies is only supported by case reports and small case series. If clinical deterioration occurs despite use of anticoagulation, or if the patient develops mass effect from a venous infarction or ICH that causes intracranial hypertension resistant to standard therapies, then these interventional techniques may be considered. Further, conservative parallel treatment with *aspirin, steroids and antibiotics* may be also discussed. In particular, there are no controlled trials or observational studies that directly assess the role of aspirin in management of CVST. The steroids may have a role in CVST by decreasing vasogenic edema, but may enhance hypercoagulability. In a matched case-control study among the 624 patients in the ISCVST, 150 patients on steroids were compared with matched 150 patients without. Those treated with steroids thus had similar characteristics as control subjects, except they were more likely to have vasculitis. At 6 months, there was a trend toward a higher risk of death or dependence with steroid treatment (OR 1.7, 95%CI 0.9 to 3.3), and this did not differ after the exclusion of those with vasculitis, malignancy, inflammatory disease, and infection. Among those with parenchymal brain lesions on CT/MRI, results were striking, with 4.8-fold increased odds of death or dependence with steroid treatment (95%CI 1.2 to 19.8). Sensitivity analyses that used different analytic approaches yielded similar findings. Also, local (eg, otitis, mastoiditis) and systemic (meningitis, sepsis) infections can be complicated by thrombosis of the adjacent or distant venous sinuses. The management of patients with such suspected infection and CVST should include administration of the appropriate antibiotics and the surgical drainage of infectious sources (ie, subdural empyemas or purulent collections within the paranasal sinuses).

3.3 Prognosis of the main clinical outcome and complications

The understanding that CVST is a rare and severe disease with a poor prognosis had to be revised after more recent clinical studies reporting a much better outcome. Mortality rates range from 6–10% and independent survival is reported in 82–90% of patients (as cited in Masuhr et al, 2004). Besides severe underlying medical conditions (e. g. infectious and malignant causes), coma on admission, clinical worsening after admission and ICH are the most important predictors of a poor outcome. In addition, the site of thrombosis is also a relevant factor and thrombosis of the internal and cerebellar veins carry the worst prognosis. A recently published follow-up study of 40 patients with CVST suggested also a correlation between the degree of recanalization and clinical outcome. Whereas the prevalence of persisting neurological deficits did not differ between patients with complete or partial recanalization, patients with no recanalization had significantly more neurological sequelae (Masuhr et al, 2004).

3.3.1 Main outcome and prognosis

There are several studies and reviews on the outcome and prognosis of CVST. The majority of such studies are mainly retrospective. Of the few prospective studies, some did not analyze prognostic factors or performed only a bivariate analysis of such predictors or analyzed specific subgroups of patients. There are only 5 cohort studies that analyzed prognostic factors for the short-term and the long-term outcome of CVST patients (Saposnik et al, 2011).

Neurological and neuropsychiatric prognosis after the diagnosis of CVST. Neurological worsening may occur in 23% of patients, even several days after diagnosis. Neurological worsening can feature depressed consciousness, mental status disturbance, new seizure, worsening of or a new focal deficit, increase in headache intensity, or visual loss. About 30% of the patients with neurological deterioration will have new parenchymal lesions when neuroimaging is repeated. Patients with depressed consciousness on admission are more likely to deteriorate. In the view of the *neuropsychiatric sequelae*, the information on the long-term outcome in CVST survivors is limited. Despite the apparent general good recovery in most patients with CVST, approximately one half of survivors feel depressed or anxious, and minor cognitive or language deficits may be observed. Risk factors for poor long-term prognosis in the ISCVST cohort were central nervous system infection, any malignancy, thrombosis of the deep venous system, intracranial hemorrhage on admission CT/MRI, Glasgow Coma Scale score <9, mental status disturbance, age>37 years, and male sex. Brain herniation leading to early death was more frequent in young patients, whereas late deaths due to malignancies and less favorable functional outcome were more frequent in elderly patients. A Glasgow Coma Scale score of 14 to 15 on admission, a complete or partial intracranial hypertension syndrome (including isolated headache) as the only manifestation of CVST, and absence of aphasia were variables associated with a favorable outcome. Below we provide separately a more extensive and detailed encounter of the cognition, behavioural changes and functional outcomes after CVST.

Death. Approximately 3% to 15% of patients die in the acute phase of the disorder (*early death*). In the ISCVST (3.4%) of 624 patients died within 30 days from symptom onset; however, in a recent multicenter US study, the mortality (13%) was higher. The risk factors for 30-day mortality were depressed consciousness, altered mental status, and thrombosis of the deep venous system, right hemisphere hemorrhage, and posterior fossa lesions. The main cause of acute death with CVST is transtentorial herniation secondary to a large hemorrhagic lesion, followed by herniation due to multiple lesions or to diffuse brain edema. *Status epilepticus*, medical complications, and PE are among other causes of early death. The deaths after the acute phase (*late death*) are related mainly to the underlying conditions, in particular malignancies. In the ISCVST study, a complete recovery at last follow-up (median 16 months) was observed in 79% of the patients; however, the overall death rate was 8.3% and the dependency rate of 5.1% at the end of follow-up was observed.

In a systematic review that included both retrospective and prospective studies, overall mortality was 9.4%, and the proportion of dependency (mRS score ≥3 or Glasgow Outcome Scale score ≥3) was 9.7%. Two new studies were reported after this systematic review. In the Pakistan-Middle East registry,63 the dependency rate (mRS score≥3) was higher (11%), whereas in the US multicenter registry, 28% of patients were dependent at 12 months. Of note, some studies include patients transferred to tertiary care centers, whose strokes are usually more severe, with the potential for a referral bias. Among the 7 cohort studies (including the prospective part of retrospective/prospective studies in which information can be analyzed separately), the overall death and dependency rate was 15% (95%CI 13% to 18%).

3.3.2 Ealry and late complications – Management and prevention

Up to 40% of patients with CVST present with isolated *intracranial hypertension*. This is characterized by diffuse brain edema, sometimes seen as slit ventricles on CT scanning. Clinical features include progressive headache, papilledema, and third or sixth nerve palsies. Intracranial hypertension is primarily caused by venous outflow obstruction and tissue congestion compounded by CSF malabsorption. No randomized trials are available to clarify the optimal treatment; however, rational management of intracranial hypertension includes a combination of treatment approaches. First, measures to reduce the thrombotic occlusion of venous outflow, such as anticoagulation and possibly thrombolytic treatment, may result in resolution of intracranial hypertension. Second, reduction of increased intracranial pressure can be accomplished immediately by lumbar puncture with removal of CSF until a normal closing pressure is achieved. Unfortunately, lumbar puncture requires temporary cessation of anticoagulants, with an attendant risk of thrombus propagation. Despite the lack of randomized clinical trials, acetazolamide is a commonly used therapeutic alternative for the treatment of intracranial hypertension with CVST. It may have a limited role in the acute management of intracranial hypertension for patients with CVST. Acetazolamide, a carbonic anhydrase inhibitor, is a weak diuretic and decreases production of CSF. Serial lumbar punctures may be necessary when hypertension is persistent. In refractory cases, a lumboperitoneal shunt may be required. Because prolonged pressure on the optic nerves can result in permanent blindness, it is of paramount importance to closely monitor visual fields and the severity of papilledema during the period of increased pressure. Ophthalmologic consultation is helpful for this. Although rarely required, optic nerve fenestration is a treatment option to halt progressive visual loss. Decompressive craniectomy has been used in patients with malignant arterial stroke to treat elevated intracranial pressure unresponsive to conventional treatment. In a pooled analysis of randomized trials, surgical decompression within 48 hours of stroke onset reduced case fatality and improved functional outcome. Limited evidence is available on the role of decompressive craniectomy in CVST with either brain edema, venous infarction, neurological deterioration, or impending cerebral herniation. A disadvantage of craniectomy is that it precludes anticoagulation for the immediate postoperative period.

Seizures are present in 37% of adults, 48% of children, and 71% of newborns who present with CVST. No clinical trials have studied either the optimal timing or medication choice for anticonvulsants in CVST. Whether to initiate anticonvulsants in all cases of CVST or await initial seizures before treatment is controversial. Because seizures increase the risk of anoxic damage, anticonvulsant treatment after even a single seizure is reasonable. In the absence of seizures, the prophylactic use of antiepileptic drugs may be harmful (the risk of side effects may outweigh its benefits). A few studies have reported the occurrence and characteristics of patients with seizures accompanying CVST. One study reported that 32% out of 91 patients presented with seizures and 2% developed them during hospitalization; only 9.5% developed late seizures, and seizures were not a predictor of prognosis at 12 months. Early seizures were 3.7-fold more likely (95%CI 1.4 to 9.4) in those with parenchymal lesions on CT/MRI at diagnosis and 7.8-fold more likely (95%CI 0.8 to 74.8) in those with sensory defects. A more recent report from the ISCVST showed 245 (39%) of 624 patients presented with seizures and 43 (6.9%) experienced early seizure within 2 weeks after diagnosis. Besides seizures on presentation, only a supratentorial parenchymal lesion on CT/MRI at diagnosis (present in 58%) was associated with occurrence of early seizures (OR 3.1, 95%CI 1.6 to 9.6). Furthermore, among those with a supratentorial lesion and no presenting seizure, use of antiepileptic drugs was associated with a 70% lower risk of seizures within 2 weeks, although this was not statistically significant (OR 0.3, 95%CI 0.04 to 2.6). On the basis of these findings, the authors suggested the prescription of antiepileptic agents in acute CVST patients with supratentorial lesions who present with seizures. Hydrocephalus The superior sagittal and lateral dural sinuses are the principal sites for CSF absorption by the arachnoid granulations, highly vascular structures that protrude across the walls of the sinuses into the subarachnoid space and drain into the venous system. In CVST, the function of the arachnoid granulations may be impaired, potentially resulting in failure of CSF absorption and communicating hydrocephalus (6.6%).

Obstructive hydrocephalus is a less common complication of CVST and results from hemorrhage into the ventricular system. This is typically associated with thrombosis that involves the internal cerebral veins and may be associated with thalamic hemorrhage. This syndrome is well described in term neonates but occurs at all ages. Neurosurgical evacuation of CSF with ventriculostomy, or in persistent cases, ventriculoperitoneal shunt, is necessary. The brain is under increased venous pressure, and tissue perfusion is at increased risk compared with other situations with obstructive hydrocephalus. Therefore, close monitoring and neurosurgical consultation are important, because intervention may be required at lesser severities of ventricular enlargement.

Recurrence of CVST. The overall risk of recurrence of any thrombotic event (*CVST or systemic*) after a CVST is 6.5% per year. The risk of other manifestations of VTE after CVST ranges from 3.4% to 4.3% on the basis of the largest studies of this medical condition (Ferro et al, 2004; Saposnik et al, 2011). Patients with severe thrombophilia have an increased risk of VTE. The secondary Prevention of CVST and Other VTE Events DVT/PE and CVST share some similarities. The chronic and transient risk factors appear to be similar, although women are more likely to have CVST and selected thrombophilia subtypes may differ between CVST and DVT/PE. In the ISCVST cohort, the overall rate of recurrent CVST or other VTE recurrence was 4.1 per 100 person-years, with male sex and polycythemia/thrombocythemia being the only independent predictors found. The same study reported a steady increase in the cumulative risk of thrombotic recurrences not influenced by the duration of anticoagulation, which emphasizes the need for a clinical trial to assess the efficacy and safety of short versus extended anticoagulant therapy. Given that systemic VTE after CVST is more common than recurrent CVST, one may reasonably adopt the VTE guidelines for prevention of both new VTE and recurrent CVST. However, each individual patient should undergo risk assessment and the patient's risk level and preferences regarding long-term anticoagulation treatment, the risk of bleeding, and the risk of thrombosis without anticoagulation should then be considered. In particular, when considered in a more detail, the secondary prevention strategies focus on preventing recurrence of CVST or other VTE in those CVST patients at high risk of such outcomes. There are no available risk stratification schemes in CVST. There are no randomized clinical trials of long-term prevention of first or recurrent CVST. Because there are no secondary prevention trials of anticoagulation in adults with CVST, evaluation of prevention strategies can only be performed with observational studies that evaluate CVST or VTE recurrence. In a cohort of 154 patients treated at Mayo Clinic between 1978 and 2001, 56 patients initially received both heparin and warfarin, 12 received heparin only, and 21 received warfarin only. Seventy-seven (50%) were treated with warfarin for an average of 9 months, with 25 committed to lifelong therapy. During 36 months of follow-up (464 patient-years), there were 23 recurrent VTEs in 20 patients (13%), the majority in the first year. Ten patients had recurrent CVST (2.2 per 100 patient-years), and 11 had DVT or PE (2.8 per 100 patient-years). Nine of the recurrent events occurred while the patients were taking warfarin. After 8 years of follow-up, there was no impact of warfarin on survival or recurrence-free survival. In a cohort of 54 CVST patients treated consecutively at University Hospital Gasthuisberg, Leuven, Belgium, 8 (14.8%) had a recurrence of VTE (7 with DVT or PE and one with CVST and mesenteric vein thrombosis) over a median of 2.5 years of follow-up (4.5 per 100 patient-years). Median time to recurrence was 2.5 months (range 2 weeks to 4 years). Only 2 of these 8 patients were taking anticoagulants at the time of recurrence, 1 with an international normalized ratio (INR) of 1.6 and the other with an INR of 2.1. Among the 6 patients with recurrent VTE who were not taking anticoagulants, recurrence occurred between 2 weeks and 10 months after the index event. Those with recurrence more often had a thrombophilic disorder, had a history of DVT, and had not received oral anticoagulation because of perceived contraindications. In the ISCVST study, among 624 patients with CVST, there were 14 (2.2%) recurrent CVSTs and 27 (4.3%) other thrombotic events (16 DVT, 3 PE, 2 ischemic stroke, 2 transient ischemic attack, and 4 acute limb ischemia) over a mean follow-up of 16 months. Seventeen (41.5%) of the 41 patients with recurrent or other thrombotic events were receiving anticoagulants, but the type of anticoagulation and the number who were receiving therapeutic doses of anticoagulation were unknown. It was not reported whether anticoagulation was given long-term and whether recurrent events differed based on its use. The Cerebral Venous Thrombosis Portuguese Collaborative Study Group (VENOPORT) evaluated outcomes for 142 CVST patients, of whom 51 were retrospectively enrolled and 91 were prospectively enrolled. There were 2 (2%) recurrent CVSTs and 10 (8%) other arterial or venous thrombotic events (maximum 16 years of follow-up for the retrospective cases and 12 months of follow-up for prospective cases). For the prospectively followed cases, the incident risk of a thrombotic event was 4% per year (5 thrombotic events in 4 patients: 2 DVTs, 1 PE, 1 ischemic stroke, and 1 acute limb ischemia). Three of these events occurred with anticoagulation use, although the INR levels were unknown at the time of the event. In addition, all of these events occurred within 12 months of the index CVST. A cohort of 77 CVST patients diagnosed in France between 1975 and 1990 was followed up for 63 months. Nine (11.7%) had a recurrence of CVST, 8 during the first 12 months, and none were receiving anticoagulation at the time of recurrence. Eleven patients (14.3%) had other thrombotic events, including retinal vein thrombosis, PE, and arterial thromboses. Use of anticoagulation at the time of recurrent thromboses that were not CVSTs was not reported. More recently, 145 patients with a first CVST were followed up for a median of 6 years after discontinuation of anticoagulation therapy. CVST recurred in 5 patients (3%), and other manifestations of VTE (*defined as DVT of the lower limbs or PE*) were seen in 10 additional patients (7%). The recurrence rate accounted for 3.4% of all VTEs in the first 16 months (or 2.03 per 100 person-years; 95%CI 1.16 to 3.14) and 1.3% of CVSTs in the first 16 months (or 0.53 per 100 person-years; 95%CI 0.16 to 1.10). Approximately half of the recurrences occurred 20 within the first year after discontinuation of anticoagulant therapy. Mild thrombophilia abnormalities were not associated with recurrent CVST, but severe thrombophilia showed an increased risk of DVT or PE. In summary, the prevalence of CVST recurrence was similar in the Italian and ISCVST studies (1.3% and 2.2%, respectively) at the 16-month follow-up.

In patients with DVT or PE, increasing evidence suggests there is clinical utility to D-dimer measurement when used to define risk of recurrent VTE. For example, in a randomized controlled trial (n_608), patients with an abnormal D-dimer level 1 month after the discontinuation of 21 anticoagulation had a significant incidence of recurrent VTE (15% versus 2.9%), which was reduced by the resumption of anticoagulation (compared with those not receiving vitamin K antagonists). During 1.4 years of follow-up, 120 subjects with an abnormal D-dimer level were randomized to no anticoagulation and 15% in this group developed a recurrent VTE. Of 103 patients with abnormal D-dimer randomized to resume anticoagulation, only 2.9% had a recurrent VTE. Although the study was randomized, it was unblinded, and D-dimer levels were only obtained once. In addition, there were no subjects with CVST and no similar studies in CVST patients. Although the clinical utility of D-dimer for longer-term anticoagulation for VTE secondary prevention appears promising, the lack of standardization of D-dimer assays may limit their clinical applicability and reliability.

In particular, thrombophilias may be hereditary or acquired, and hereditary thrombophilias have been stratified as mild or severe on the basis of the risk of recurrence in very large family cohorts. Among VTE patients, the hereditary thrombophilias with the highest cumulative recurrence rates for VTE in the absence of ongoing anticoagulation have been deficiencies of antithrombin, protein C, and protein S, with a 19% recurrence at 2 years, 40% at 5 years, and 55% at 10 years. Homozygous prothrombin G20210A, homozygous factor V Leiden, deficiencies of protein C, protein S, or antithrombin, combined thrombophilia defects and antiphospholipid syndrome are categorized as severe. Interestingly, the more common hereditary thrombophilias, such as heterozygous factor V Leiden and prothrombin G20210A or elevated factor VIII, have a much lower risk of recurrence (7% at 2 years, 11% at 5 years, and 25% at 10 years) and could be categorized as mild. Hyperhomocysteinemia, a common hereditary or acquired risk factor for VTE, was not significantly associated with a high risk of recurrence. In addition, the annual incidence and the risk of recurrence increased markedly in those with combined thrombophilic defects, described as double heterozygous/homozygous. There are several important points regarding the hereditary thrombophilia data described above. First, the familial nature of these deficiencies of protein C, S, or antithrombin was clearly established, which distinguishes these patients from those with sporadic or acquired abnormalities. Second, testing for deficiencies of protein C, S, and antithrombin must be performed at least 6 weeks after a thrombotic event and then confirmed with repeat testing and family studies. In addition, protein C and S functional activity and antithrombin levels are difficult to interpret during treatment with warfarin. Therefore, testing for these conditions is generally indicated 2 to 4 weeks after completion of anticoagulation. Lastly, clearly established deficiencies of proteins C, S, and antithrombin are relatively uncommon. Antiphospholipid antibody syndrome (Atanassova, 2007) is an acquired thrombophilia associated with specific laboratory criteria (lupus anticoagulant, anticardiolipin antibody, and anti-_2-glycoprotein I) and a history of a venous or arterial event or fetal loss. Caution must be taken when the results of antiphospholipid antibody testing are interpreted. A normal result may occur at the time of the clinical presentation, which rules out antiphospholipid antibody syndrome. On the other hand, abnormal tests may occur transiently due to the disease process, infection, certain medications (antibiotics, cocaine, hydralazine, procainamide, quinine, and others), or unknown causes. Approximately 5% of the general population at any given time has evidence of abnormal tests, and these mainly have no clinical consequence. A diagnosis of antiphospholipid syndrome requires abnormal laboratory testing on 2 or more occasions at least 12 weeks apart. Patients diagnosed with antiphospholipid syndrome have an increased risk of recurrent thrombotic events; however, test results cannot predict the likelihood of complications, their type, or their severity in a particular patient. Although there are no prospective studies that report recurrence rates for CVST specifically, the high risk of recurrent VTE with this disorder meets the definition of severe thrombophilia. The Duration of Anticoagulation Study Group reported a 29% recurrence of VTE in patients with anticardiolipin antibodies versus 14% in those without over 4 years and the risk increased with the titer of the antibodies. In a randomized controlled trial of warfarin for 3 months versus extended treatment for 24 months after first-ever idiopathic DVT or PE, the presence of antiphospholipid antibodies was associated with a 4-fold increased risk of recurrence (hazard ratio [HR] 4.0, 95%CI 1.2 to 13), and the presence of a lupus anticoagulant was associated with a 7-fold increased risk (HR 6.8, 95%CI 1.5 to 31) in the placebo group. Further recommendations, with associated class and level of evidence, are provided in the recent guidelines by Saposnik et al (2011). In particular, a testing for prothrombotic conditions, including protein C, protein S, antithrombin deficiency, antiphospholipid syndrome, prothrombin G20210A mutation, and factor V Leiden, can be beneficial for the management of CVST patients.

Other late complications. *Headache* is common and occurs in about half of the patients during the follow-up. In general, headaches are primary and not related to CVST. In the Lille study, 53% of patients had residual headache, 29% fulfilled criteria for migraine, and 27% had headache of the tension type. In VENOPORT, 55% of patients reported headaches during the follow-up, and these were mild to moderate in 45%. At follow-up, severe headaches that required bed rest or hospital admission were reported in 14% of patients in the ISCVST and 11% in VENOPORT. In patients with persistent or severe headaches, appropriate investigations should be completed to rule out recurrent CVST. Occasionally, MRV may show stenosis of a previously occluded sinus, but the clinical significance of this is unclear. Headache during follow-up is more common among patients who present acutely as having isolated intracranial hypertension. In these patients, if headache persists and MRI is normal, lumbar puncture may be needed to exclude elevated intracranial pressure. *Focal or generalized post-CVST seizures* can be divided into early or remote (2 weeks after diagnosis) seizures. On the basis of case series, remote seizures affect 5% to 32% of patients. Most of these seizures occur in the first year of follow-up. In ISCVST, 11% of the patients experienced remote seizures (36 patients by 6 months, 55 by 1 year, and 66 by 2 years). Risk factors for remote seizures were hemorrhagic lesion on admission CT/MRI (HR 2.62, 95%CI 1.52 to 4.52), early seizure (HR 2.42, 95%CI 1.38 to 4.22), and paresis (HR 2.22, 95%CI 1.33 to 3.69). Five percent of the patients had post-CVST epilepsy. Post-CVST epilepsy was also associated with hemorrhagic lesion on admission CT/MRI (OR 6.76,

95%CI 2.26 to 20.41), early seizure (OR 3.99, 95%CI 1.16 to 11.0), and paresis (OR 2.75, 95%CI 1.33 to 6.54). Initiation of antiepileptic drugs for a defined duration is recommended to prevent further seizures in patients with CVST and parenchymal lesions who present with a single seizure. *Severe visual loss* due to CVST is rare (2% to 4%). Papilledema can cause transient visual impairment, and if prolonged, optic atrophy and blindness may ensue. Visual loss is often insidious, with progressive constriction of the visual fields and relative sparing of central visual acuity. Visual deficits are more common in patients with papilledema and those who present with increased intracranial pressure. Delayed diagnosis is associated with an increased risk of later visual deficit. Patients with papilledema or visual complaints should have a complete neuroophthalmological study, including visual acuity and formal visual field testing. Further, a thrombosis of the cavernous, lateral, or sagittal sinus can later induce a *dural arteriovenous fistula*. A pial fistula can also follow a cortical vein thrombosis. The relationship between the 2 entities is rather complex, because (1) dural fistulas can be a late complication of persistent dural sinus occlusion with increased venous pressure, (2) the fistula can close and cure if the sinus recanalizes, and (3) a preexisting fistula can be the underlying cause of CVST. The exact frequency of dural fistula after CVST is not known because there are no cohort studies with 22 long-term angiographic investigation. The incidence of dural arteriovenous fistula was low in cohort studies without systematic angiographic follow-up (1% to 3%). A cerebral angiogram may help identify the presence of a dural arteriovenous fistula.

Specific recommendations for management of CVST and its complications can be summarised as follows (Saposnik et al, 2011):

- Patients with CVST and a suspected bacterial infection should receive appropriate antibiotics and surgical drainage of purulent collections of infectious sources associated with CVST when appropriate;
- In patients with CVST and increased intracranial pressure, monitoring for progressive visual loss is recommended, and when this is observed, increased intracranial pressure should be treated urgently;
- In patients with CVST and a single seizure with parenchymal lesions, early initiation of antiepileptic drugs for a defined duration is recommended to prevent further seizures;
- In patients with CVST and a single seizure without parenchymal lesions, early initiation of antiepileptic drugs for a defined duration is probably recommended to prevent further seizures;
- In the absence of seizures, the routine use of antiepileptic drugs in patients with CVST is not recommended;
- For patients with CVST, initial anticoagulation with adjusted-dose UFH or weight-based LMWH in full anticoagulant doses is reasonable, followed by vitamin K antagonists, regardless of the presence of ICH;
- Admission to a stroke unit is reasonable for treatment and prevention of complications of patients with CVST;
- In CVST patients with increased intracranial pressure, it is reasonable to initiate treatment with acetazolamide. Other therapies (lumbar puncture, optic nerve decompression, or shunts) can be effective if there is progressive visual loss;
- Endovascular intervention may be considered if deterioration occurs despite intensive anticoagulation treatment;

- In patients with neurological deterioration due to severe mass effect or intracranial hemorrhage causing intractable intracranial hypertension, decompressive hemicraniectomy may be considered;
- For patients with CVST, steroid medications are not recommended, even in the presence of parenchymal brain lesions on CT/MRI, unless needed for another underlying disease;
- The current recommendations for VTE patients call for indefinite anticoagulation (adjusted-dose warfarin INR 2.0 to 3.0 or heparin) for patients with antiphospholipid syndrome;
- In patients with a history of CVST who complain of new, persisting, or severe headache, evaluation for CVST recurrence and intracranial hypertension should be considered.

3.3.3 Clinical prediction rules (CPRs) or risk score models in CVST

Although the overall outcome of CVST is favourable, about 15% of the patients become dependent or die. Clinical prediction rules (CPRs) or risk stratification models and scores (McGinn et al, 2000; McNally et al, 2010) might improve the ability to inform doctors about the individual prognosis of different disease conditions, including CVST. There are specific methodological standards that are applied to CPRs before their use in the clinical practice can be recommended. Ideally, a rule or scale undergoes three steps: derivation, narrow and broad validation, and impact analysis (randomised controlled trial assessing its effectiveness and cost-effectiveness) (McGinn et al, 2000). In this way, if a rule is applied, it is possible to further identify those CVST patients who could benefit from more intensive monitoring and/or invasive interventions at most. For instance, Barinagarrementeria et al (1992) proposed a prognostic scale based on clinical, CT and cerebrospinal fluid (CSF) analysis. The presence of coma or bilateral pyramidal signs was rated at 3, that of generalized seizures at 2 and that of meningeal signs, bilateral lesions on CT scan and haemorrhagic CSF all at 2 points. The prognosis was found to be 100% good when total score was <3, usually good (85%) with a score of 4-5, usually bad (90%) with a score of 6-8 and 100% bad with a score of >9. This scale, however, has not been consistently validated further in other CVST datasets. Another risk score model to predict a poor outcome has also been derived and validated. The score ranged from 0 (lowest risk) to 9 (highest risk), and a cut-off value equal or higher than 3 indicated a higher risk of death or dependency at 6 months. One point was assigned for male sex, presence of decreased level of consciousness, or ICH while 2 points indicated the presence of malignancy, coma, or thrombosis of the deep venous system. The discrimination performance, or area under the receiver operating characteristics (ROC) curve (AUC or c-statistics) in the derivation cohort was 85.4%, 84.4%, and 90.1% in the validation cohorts samples (Ferro et al, 2004; Dentali et al, 2006). Another study incorporated the age above 37 years and central nervous system infection as additional risk factors into the latter model. The authors validated the score in 90 patients and obtained AUC_{ROC}=81% to predict mortality (with sensitivity of 88% and specificity of 70% at a cut-off value equal or above 14) (Koopman et al, 2009). Notably, further validation studies are needed to better quantify and estimate the discrimination and calibration performance and overall generalisability of the above clinical prediction rule in other populations and settings.

3.4 Cognition, behavioural changes and functional outcomes after CVST

For many years CVST has been considered rare and lethal disease, diagnosed postmortem. The use of neuroimaging techniques as computer tomography, the magnetic resonance imaging and the cerebral angiography has made possible the early diagnoses and has changed the knowledge about this condition (Bousser et al., 2007; Breteau et al.,2003; Preter et al., 1996). The increase of the data about it in the scientific literature enlarges the aspects studied and poses new questions. One of these questions is related to the functional outcome after CVST and the impact of cognitive impairments and behavioural changes on it. Due to the heterogeneity of study methodology and design, it is very difficult to compare the obtained results. Another important obstacle is due to the differences in the diagnostic process, in the extent of control for the underlying causes for CVST, for the clinical presentations and the treatment strategy.

Most of the authors reported good functional outcome after CVST (Cakmak et al.,2003; de Bruijn et al., 2001; Ferro et al., 2001; Ferro et al., 2002; Hameed et al.,2006; Kirmani et al., 2005). In a 77 months follow-up 86% of the patients recovered without neurological sequelae (Preter et al., 1996). The conclusions from the largest, for the time being, international study - ISCVST (Ferro et al., 2004) and from a large systematic review of 19 papers on CVST (Dentali et al., 2006) were for a better prognosis than reported previously. Most of the patients examined by Stolz et al. (2004) showed significant improvement on hospital discharge and 89% of them had significant functional improvement 12 months after the discharge. A review of long-term follow-up studies found that from 1943 patients examined, only 180 had poor recovery with permanent neurological deficit (Dentali et al.,2006). At the same time Bender et al. (2006) found that the severe CVST cases had not been studied in details and that cognitive impairments could influence negatively the quality of life of survived patients. De Bruijn et al. (2000) reported less favorable CVST outcome than reported previously.

CVST is a condition that requires a prompt diagnose and treatment. The mode of onset of CVST is acute in 37,2% and sub-acute in 55,5% of the participants in ISCVST. Probably this is the reason for the lack of data about the cognitive functioning of the patients. But it is difficult to explain the absence of neuropsychological techniques from the set of methods, assessing the long-term recovery of surviving patients. Most of the outcome studies of CVST do not include testing of cognition and assessment of behavioural changes (Breteau et al., 2003; Cakmak et al.,2003; de Bruijn et al., 2001; Ferro et al., 2001; Ferro et al., 2002; Stolz et al., 2004).

The assessment of the extent of functional recovery after CVST is limited. The outcome after CVST is traditionally described by modified Rankin Scale score, that gives information only about the patient motor activity and the capacity for carrying out previous activities. Some of the studies report data received by mail or by phone.

Abulia, executive deficits, and amnesia may result from thrombosis of the deep venous system, with bilateral panthalamic infarcts. Memory deficits, behavioral problems, or executive deficits may persist. The importance of more detailed examination and neuropsychological testing could be confirmed by a paper, reporting the results of functionally independent patients, having long-term symptoms with negative impact on their everyday functioning: 75% of patients, included in this 63 months follow-up, reported concentration impairments (Koopman et al.,2009).

Aphasia was a clinical feature of CVST, found in 19% of the participants from 21 countries in ISCVST study (Ferro et al., 2004). Aphasia, in general of the fluent type, results from left lateral sinus thrombosis with temporal infarct or hemorrhage. Recovery is usually favorable, but minor troubles in spontaneous speech and naming might persist. Cognitive assessment for aphasia, apraxia and working memory found aphasia in 3 patients and working memory deficit in 6 out of 34 patients in a follow-up study (Buccino et al., 2003). Preter et al. (1996)

report 1 patient with aphasia and 3 patients with memory loss and dementia in a 78 months' follow-up of 77 patients with CVST. A detailed neuropsychological testing of participants in a long-term CVST outcome study showed that 35% of patients had abnormal performance on two or more cognitive tests, 33% - had impairments in two or more cognitive functions. Prevalence was found for visuospatial, constructive and language impairments (de Bruijn et al.,2000). Another interesting finding is the presence of cognitive impairments in patients with low scores for functional health. This report warrants for more detailed long-term assessment of CVST patients, including cognitive testing, because cognition is an important factor for everyday functioning and for the level of quality of life. The data about behavioural changes and the quality of life are even scarcer than these, related to cognitive domains. Psychiatric symptoms are rarely described during the diagnostic phase (Bousser et al., 2007). Behavioural changes are mentioned in the study of Preter et al., (1996). Data exist about depression and fatigue as long-term sequelae after CVST (Koopman et al.,2009; Buccino et al., 2003). Assessment with questionnaires for quality of life and for well-being after CVST is very rare as well (Bender et al.,2007).

4. Conclusions

The main findings of this review were that all age groups can be affected by CVST and the large sinuses such as the superior sagittal sinus are most frequently involved. Extensive collateral circulation within the cerebral venous system allows for a significant degree of compensation in the early stages of thrombus formation. Systemic inflammatory diseases and inherited as well as acquired coagulation disorders are frequent causes, although in up to 30% of cases no underlying cause can be identified. The diagnosis is usually made by venographic studies with computer tomography (CT or CTV) or magnetic resonance imaging (MRI or MRIV) to demonstrate obstruction of the venous sinuses or cerebral veins by a thrombus. The MRI with venography (MRIV) is the investigation of choice; computed tomography alone will miss a significant number of cases. Additionally, the use of such precise neuro-imaging techniques gives the possibility for early diagnosis and treatment of emerging neuropsychological impairments in the set of the clinical symptoms in CVST; for instance, a cognitive deficit as part of the long-term outcome; a range of psychiatric complications and, last but not least, to collect data and explore the various aspects of the health-related quality of life or HRQOL) in such patients. It should be noted that the neuropsychological impairments that could be present during CVST are not well known, including various aspects of the assessment of the eventually impaired mental status. For instance, various data exist about disorientation, lack of coordination, incapacity to follow commands, neglect, apraxia, recent memory impairments and language impairments, among others. In the same time, very little is known about the long term outcome of CVST - for instance, it has been observed that many patients experience some persistent neurologic and cognitive deficits, but data are scarce and difficult to collect and summarise. The management of CVST includes treatment of the underlying condition; symptomatic treatment; the prevention or treatment of complications of increased intracranial pressure, ICH, or venous infarction; and typically, anticoagulation therapy. It has now been conclusively shown that intravenous heparin is the first-line treatment for cerebral venous sinus thrombosis because of its efficacy, safety and feasibility. Local thrombolysis may be indicated in cases of deterioration, despite adequate heparinisation. This should be followed by oral anticoagulation for 3-6 months. The prognosis of cerebral venous sinus thrombosis is generally favourable. A high index of clinical suspicion is needed to diagnose this uncommon condition so that appropriate treatment can be initiated. Complications, in a short- and a long-term, include but are not limited to cognition and behavioural changes.

5. References

Atanassova, P. A. (2007). Antiphospholipid syndrome and vascular ischemic (occlusive) diseases: an overview. *Yonsei Medical Journal* 48(6): 901-926.

Atanassova PA, et al. (2006). Abnormal ECG patterns during the acute phase of subarachnoid hemorrhage in patients without previous heart disease. *Central European Journal of Medicine* 1(2): 148-157.

Barinagarrementeria, F, Cantu, C, Arredondo, H. (1992). Aseptic cerebral venous thrombosis: proposed prognostic scale. *Journal of Stroke and Cerebrovascular Disease* 2: 34-39.

Bender A, Schulte-Altedorneburg G, Mayer T et al. (2007) Functional outcome after cerebral venous thrombosis. *J Neurol*; 254:465-470.

Bousser MG, Ferro JM. (2007). Cerebral venous thrombosis: an update. *Lancet* 6: 162-170.

Breteau G, Mounier-Vehier F, Godefroy O *et al.* (2003). Cerebral venous thrombosis: 3-year clinical outcome in 55 consecutive patients. *J Neurol* 250: 29-35.

Brown, W. R. and C. R. Thore (2011). Review: cerebral microvascular pathology in ageing and neurodegeneration. *Neuropathol Appl Neurobiol* 37(1): 56-74.

Buccino G, Scoditti U, Patteri I et al. (2003) Neurological and cognitive long-term outcome in patients with cerebral venous sinus thrombosis. *Acta Neurologica Scandinavica* 107(5): 330-335.

Cakmak S, Derex L, Berruyer M et al. (2003). Cerebral venous thrombosis: Clinical outcome and systematic screening of prothrombothic factors. *Neurology* 60: 1175-1178.

Chang, Y. J., et al. (1995). Isolated cortical venous thrombosis--discrepancy between clinical features and neuroradiologic findings. A case report. *Angiology* 46(12): 1133-1138.

Ciccone A, Canhão P, Falcão F, Ferro JM, Sterzi R. (2004). Thrombolysis for cerebral vein and dural sinus thrombosis. *Cochrane Database of Systematic Reviews* Issue 1. Art. No.: CD003693.

De Bruijn SF, Budde M, Teunisse S *et al.* for the Cerebral Venous Sinus Thrombosis Study Group. (2000). Long-term outcome of cognition and functional health after cerebral venous sinus thrombosis. *Neurology* 54(8): 1687-1689.

De Bruijn SF, Haan RJ, Stam J. (2001). Clinical features and prognostic factors of cerebral venous thrombosis in a prospective series of 59 patients. *J Neurol Neurosurg Psychiatry*: 70: 105-108.

Dentali, F., Gianni, M., Crowther, M.A., Ageno, W. (2006). Natural history of cerebral vein thrombosis: a systematic review. *Blood* 108: 1129–1134.

Ferro, J. M. (2010). Cerebral venous thrombosis. Presentation at 14th ESO Stroke Summer School, Warsaw, Poland, 27 June – 3 July 2010 (last accessed on 13 July 2011 at http://www.skolamed.pl/img/panel/files/eso2010/pdf/FerroJ_Cerebral_venous_thrombosis.pdf)

Ferro JM, Correia M, Pontes C *et al.* for the Cerebral Venous Thrombosis Portuguese Collaborative Study Group (VENOPORT). (2001). Cerebral Vein and Dural Sinus Thrombosis in Portugal 1980–98. *Cerebrovasc Dis* 11: 177-182.

Ferro JM, Lopes MG, Rosas MJ *et al.* (2002). Long-term prognosis of cerebral vein and dural sinus thrombosis. Results of the VENOPORT Study. *Cerebrovasc Dis; 13* (4) : 272-278.

Ferro, J. M., Canhao, P. (2011). Etiology, clinical features, and diagnosis of cerebral venous thrombosis. UpToDate. Ver.19.2 (last updated on June 6, 2011, last accessed on July 12, 2011 at http://www.uptodate.com/contents/etiology-clinical-features-and-diagnosis-of-cerebral-venous-thrombosis#H1)

Ferro, J. M., Canhao, P., Stam, J., Bousser, M.G., Barinagarrementeria, F.; ISCVST Investigators. (2004). Prognosis of cerebral vein and dural sinus thrombosis: results of the International Study on Cerebral Vein and Dural Sinus Thrombosis (ISCVST). *Stroke* 35: 664–670.

Hameed B, Syed NA. (2006). Prognostic indicators in cerebral venous sinus thrombosis. *J Pak Med Assoc* 56(11): 551-553.

Kirmani J , Janhua N, Kawi A et al. (2005). Therapeutic advances in interventional neurology. *NeuroRx* 2(2): 304–323.

Knopp, E. A. (1995). Venous disease and tumors. *Magn Reson Imaging Clin N Am* 3(3): 509-528.

Koopman K, Uyttenboogaart M, Vroomen PC et al. (2009). Long-term sequelae after cerebral venous thrombosis in functionally independent patients. *J Stroke* 18(3): 198-202.

Koopman, K., Uyttenboogaart, M., Vroomen, P. C., van der Meer, J., De Keyser, J., Luijckx, G. J. (2009) Development and validation of a predictive outcome score of cerebral venous thrombosis. *J Neurol Sci* 276: 66–68.

Kwan J, Günther A. (2006). Antiepileptic drugs for the primary and secondary prevention of seizures after intracranial venous thrombosis. *Cochrane Database of Systematic Reviews* Issue 3. Art.No.: CD005501.

Leach, J. L., K. Meyer, et al. (2008). Large arachnoid granulations involving the dorsal superior sagittal sinus: findings on MR imaging and MR venography. *AJNR Am J Neuroradiol* 29(7): 1335-1339.

Manolidis, S., Kutz, J.W. Jr. (2005). Diagnosis and management of lateral sinus thrombosis. *Otol Neurotol* 26:1045–1051.

Masuhr, F., Mehraein, S., Einhäupl, K. (2004). Cerebral venous and sinus thrombosis. *J Neurol* 251 : 11–23

McGinn TG, Guyatt GH,Wyer PC, et al. (2000). Users' guides to the medical literature: XXII: how to use articles about clinical decision rules. Evidence-Based MedicineWorking Group. *JAMA* 284(1): 79–84.

McNally M, et al. (2010). Validity of British Thoracic Society guidance (the CRB-65 rule) for predicting the severity of pneumonia in general practice: systematic review and meta-analysis. *Br J Gen Pract* 60(579): e423-433.

Plata R, Cornejo A, Arratia C, Perna A, Dimitrov BD, Remuzzi G, Ruggenenti P. (2002). Effects of ACE inhibition therapy in altitude polycytemia. *Lancet* 359: 663-666.

Preter M, Tzourio C, Ameri A et al. (1996). Long-term prognosis in cerebral venous thrombosis. Follow-up of 77 patients. *Stroke* 27: 243–246.

Saposnik G, Barinagarrementeria F, Brown RD Jr, et al.; and the American Heart Association Stroke Council and the Council on Epidemiology and Prevention. (2011). Diagnosis and management of cerebral venous thrombosis: a statement for healthcare professionals from the American Heart Association/American Stroke Association. *Stroke* 42(4): 1158-1192.

Schmidek, H. H., L. M. Auer, et al. (1985). The cerebral venous system. *Neurosurgery* 17(4): 663-678.

Siddiqui, F. M., Kamal, A. K. (2006). Incidence and epidemiology of cerebral venous thrombosis. *J Pak Med Assoc* 56(11): 485-487.

Smith, A. G., W. T. Cornblath, et al. (1997). Local thrombolytic therapy in deep cerebral venous thrombosis. *Neurology* 48(6): 1613-1619.

Stam J (2005). Thrombosis of the cerebral veins and sinuses. *New England Journal of Medicine* 352 (17): 1791–8

Stolz E, Trittmacher S, Rahimi A et al. (2004) Influence of recanalization on outcome in dural sinus thrombosis: A Prospective Study. *Stroke; 35* : 544-547.

van den Bergh, W. M., I. van der Schaaf, et al. (2005). The spectrum of presentations of venous infarction caused by deep cerebral vein thrombosis. *Neurology* 65(2): 192-196.

9

Venous Thrombosis and the Eye

Bob Z. Wang and Celia S. Chen
Flinders Medical Centre and Flinders University
Australia

1. Introduction

Venous thrombosis is associated with Virchow's triad. This involves the combination of hypercoagulability, damage to the vessel endothelium and haemodynamic changes in the form of stasis or turbulence. These features ultimately contribute to thrombosis formation (Heit 2008).

Venous thrombosis can affect the eyes, resulting in serious ocular symptoms and is a significant cause of vision loss worldwide (Rogers, McIntosh et al. 2010). In the eye, venous thrombosis can result in a branch or a central retinal vein occlusion. The eye can also be affected by systemic venous thrombosis such as that which occurs in cerebral venous sinus thrombosis presenting with papilloedema, or in anti-phospholipid syndrome resulting in retinal arteriole occlusion, ischemic optic or cranial neuropathies.

In this chapter, we will discuss the ocular features of venous thrombosis, the presentation of retinal vein occlusion, and its ocular and systemic management. We will then examine the ophthalmic manifestations of systemic venous thrombosis.

2. Retinal vein occlusion

2.1 Pathogenesis

Retinal venous obstruction occurs as a result of Virchow's triad in the retinal vessels with stasis, hypercoagulability and endothelial change. In the retina, disruption of venous return results in elevated intravascular pressure and culminates in retinal haemorrhage and oedema. Retinal ischaemia then follows, leading to non-perfusion of the capillary beds.

Retinal vein occlusion RVO can be classified as either a branch retinal vein occlusion (BRVO) (Figure 1) or a central retinal vein occlusion (CRVO) (Figure 2) depending upon the location of the obstruction (Hayreh 2005). Each of BRVO and CRVO can be further sub-classified into ischaemic and non-ischaemic categories.

Ischaemic RVO is characterised by retinal capillary non-perfusion and results in more severe signs and symptoms including significant decrease in visual acuity, cotton wool spots (indicating retinal ischaemia) and a relative afferent pupil defect. An ischemic RVO is usually associated with ocular complications such as intraocular neovascularisation.

In non-ischaemic RVO stasis of the retinal veins occurs. There is leakage from the capillary bed but capillary perfusion is still present. A non-ischaemic RVO is associated with decreased visual acuity as a result of leaking retinal capillaries that cause macular oedema.

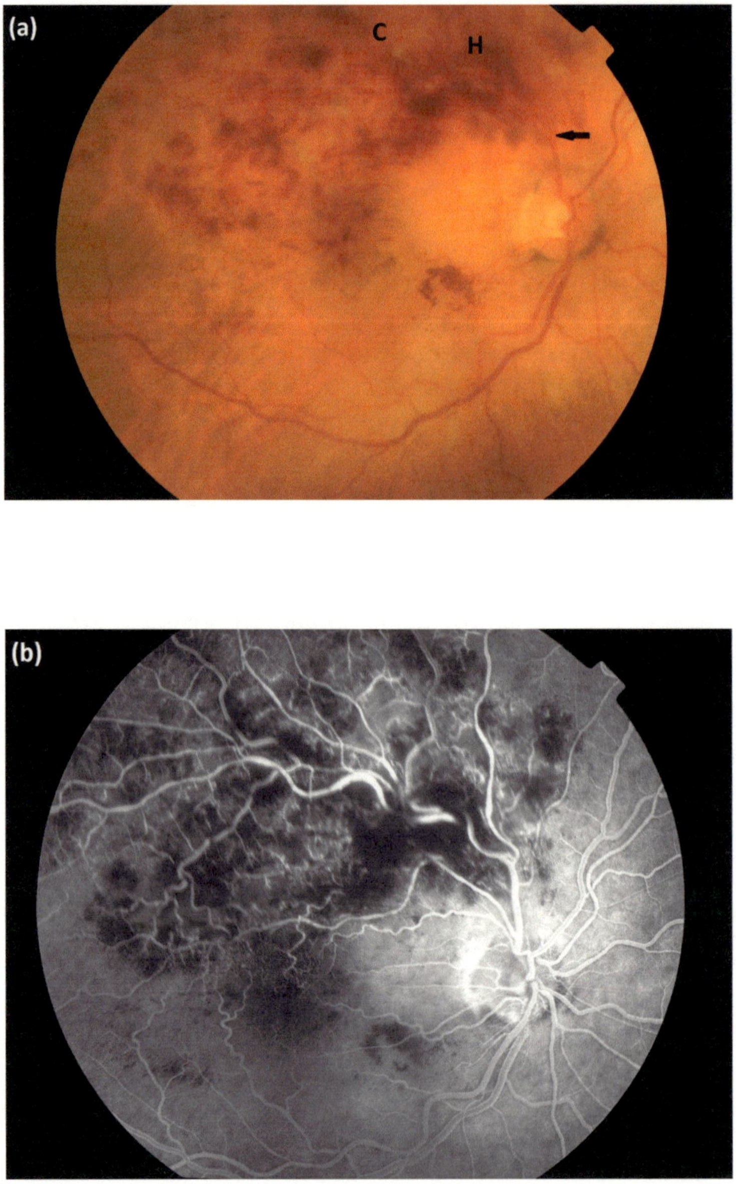

Fig. 1. Fundus photograph of a superior-temporal branch retinal vein occlusion in the right eye (a) with the corresponding fluorescein angiogram (b). The retina shows a sectoral area of retinal haemorrhages (H) and cotton wool spots (C) in the area distal to the vein occlusion (black arrow).

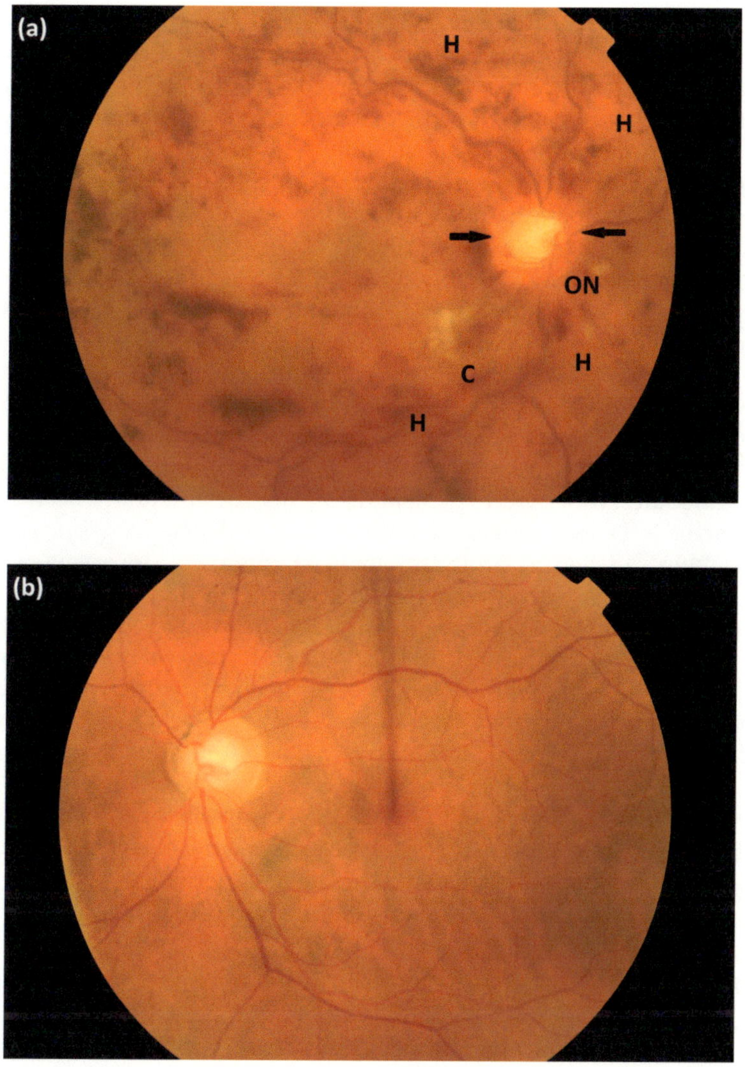

Fig. 2. Fundus photograph of a central retinal vein occlusion in the right eye (a) with normal left eye (b) of the same patient. In central retinal vein occlusion, there are scattered haemorrhages (H) in all four quadrants of the retina, cotton wool spots (C), and optic nerve swelling (ON), which is characterised by indistinct disc margins (black arrows).

2.2 Prevalence

The prevalence of RVO is approximately 1 in 200 people, with an estimated 16.4 million people being affected worldwide (Rogers, McIntosh et al. 2010). Prevalence appears to increase with age (Rogers, McIntosh et al. 2010), whereas gender or ethnicity does not appear to affect prevalence (Rogers, McIntosh et al. 2010). Retinal vein occlusion is usually unilateral and very rarely bilateral. A BRVO is four times more common than a CRVO (Rogers, McIntosh et al. 2010), with its prevalence ranging from 0.3% (Wong, Larsen et al. 2005) to 1.1% (Mitchell, Smith et al. 1996).

2.3 Risk factors

The risk factors for RVO include systemic or local conditions which result in vascular stasis or endothelial damage. Systemic risk factors for RVO are often associated with atherosclerotic vessel changes, and these risk factors include age (Hayreh, Zimmerman et al. 1994), hypertension (Mitchell, Smith et al. 1996; Hayreh, Zimmerman et al. 2001) and hyperlipidaemia (1993; 1996). Diabetes mellitus (Dodson, Kritzinger et al. 1992; Hayreh, Zimmerman et al. 2001), peripheral vascular disease and cerebrovascular disease also contribute to a higher likelihood of developing RVO.

Less common systemic risk factors for RVO include those associated with hypercoagulability. These include myeloproliferative disorders (Fegan 2002) such as polycythaemia, myeloma and Waldenstrom macroglobulinaemia. These account for 1% of RVO cases. Acquired and inherited hypercoagulable states (Fegan 2002) may also predispose a patient to RVO. Acquired diseases that have been shown to contribute to RVO include hyperhomocysteinaemia (Chua, Kifley et al. 2005; Janssen, den Heijer et al. 2005), anti-cardiolipin antibodies (Janssen, den Heijer et al. 2005), lupus anticoagulant and anti-phospholipid antibodies. Inherited hypercoagulable diseases that have been associated with RVO include factor V Leiden mutation, protein C or S deficiency (Greiner, Hafner et al. 1999), anti-thrombin deficiency, prothrombin gene mutation (Incorvaia, Lamberti et al. 1999)and factor XII deficiency (Incorvaia, Lamberti et al. 1999). Inflammatory diseases such as Behçet's disease, sarcoidosis, Wegener's granulomatosis and Goodpasture syndrome and chronic renal failure have also been proven to be risk factors for RVO. Oestrogen therapy may be a cause of RVO, although the evidence is inconclusive (Kirwan, Tsaloumas et al. 1997). Hormone replacement therapy has not been shown to be a major risk factor for RVO, whereas the contraceptive pill does increase the risk of RVO and is contraindicated in those with RVO.

A local risk factor for the development of a CRVO is primary open angle glaucoma (1996; Mitchell, Smith et al. 1996). This is due to stasis caused by the elevated intraocular pressure in glaucoma reducing arterial perfusion. The mean arterial perfusion pressure is the difference between the mean arterial pressure and the intraocular pressure.

2.4 Investigations

All investigations should be directed towards examining the systemic risk factors of RVO and assessing the ocular complications of neovascularization.

Systemic investigations include screening for atherosclerotic disease and hypercoagulability. This involves measuring blood pressure, electrocardiogram, a full blood count, measuring erythrocyte sedimentation rate, fasting glucose and lipids, a vasculitic screen and a thrombophilia screen. A vasculitic screen involves measuring antinuclear antibodies, rheumatoid factor, anti-neutrophil cytoplasmic antibody, serum protein electrophoresis, complement 3 and 4. Whereas a thrombophilia screen would include measuring serum homocysteine, protein C and S, Factor V Leiden, antithrombin, anticardiolipin antibodies and lupus anticoagulant.

It is important to remember that in patients with BRVO, cardiovascular risk factors are the predominant cause. In contrast, in patients with CRVO, especially when the patient's age is less than 65, there should be a more extensive search for other risk factors such as oral contraceptive use, thrombophilia or inflammatory diseases.

Ocular investigation with a fundus fluorescein angiography allows for visualisation of large retinal vessels and retinal capillary beds. This helps to differentiate between the ischemic and non-ischemic types of RVO (Figure 3). Optical coherence tomography (OCT) is another investigation that is becoming increasingly important in assessing the changes in retinal architecture and measuring the thickness of the retinal layers. OCT can assist in detecting and quantifying intraretinal cysts and the associated macular oedema (Figure 4).

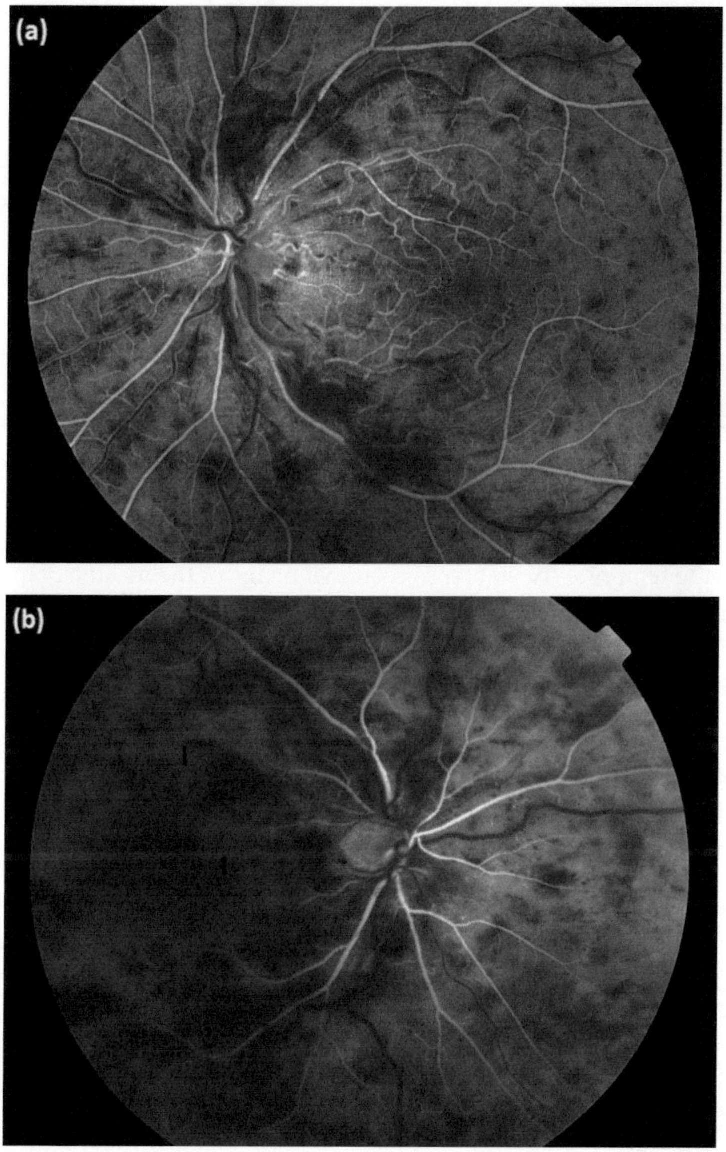

Fig. 3. Fluorescein angiogram of a non-ischaemic central retinal vein occlusion (a) compared to an ischaemic central retinal vein occlusion (b). In non-ischaemic central retinal vein occlusion, there is effective capillary perfusion and this is seen as white due to the fluorescein filling the vessels. In ischaemic central retinal vein occlusion, there are areas of capillary non-perfusion (I) and seen as black due to the absence of fluorescein filling the vessels.

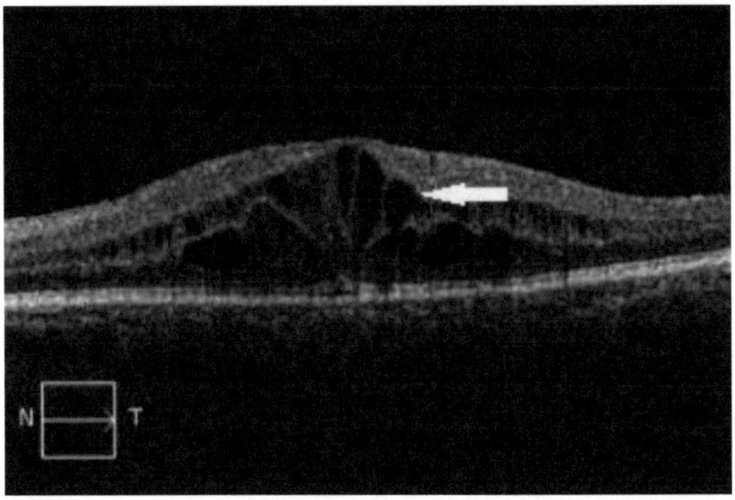

Fig. 4. Optical coherence tomography scan of the macular in an eye with retinal vein occlusion. Nasal to temporal (N→T) cross-sectional image of the macula demonstrates the presence of significant macula oedema and associated intra-retinal cysts (white arrow).

2.5 Clinical presentations

2.5.1 Branch retinal artery occlusion

In BRVO, only a branch of the retinal venous system is affected. Risk factors for BRVO are listed above. The occlusion in BRVO occurs most commonly at an arteriovenous junction, where the artery and vein share a common adventitial sheath. Venous thrombosis results from arterial wall thickening, which compresses the adjacent vein.

Vision loss is the most common presentation in patients with BRVO. The vision loss is usually sudden, unilateral and painless. This loss can be variable and is dependent upon the amount of macular and retinal involvement. If there is macular involvement, vision is usually affected. Alternatively, if the BRVO is small or located in the peripheral retina, the patient may still have 6/6 vision. Metamorphopsia or distorted vision and a visual field defect may also occur.

Ocular fundus examination often reveals a wedge shaped area of retinal abnormality. The superior temporal retinal arcade is affected in 60% of all cases of BRVO due to the higher number of arteriovenous crossings in this area. The veins distal to the occlusion may demonstrate dilatation and tortuosity, while there may be some venous attenuation proximal to the occlusion. Retinal haemorrhages are a notable feature of BRVO. Superficial retinal haemorrhages appear flame shaped, while deep haemorrhages are characteristically referred to as dot-blot haemorrhages (Figure 5). Very rarely, there may be subhyaloid or vitreous haemorrhages. Other ocular fundus features of BRVO include retinal oedema and cotton-wool spots, which is also a sign of retinal ischaemia.

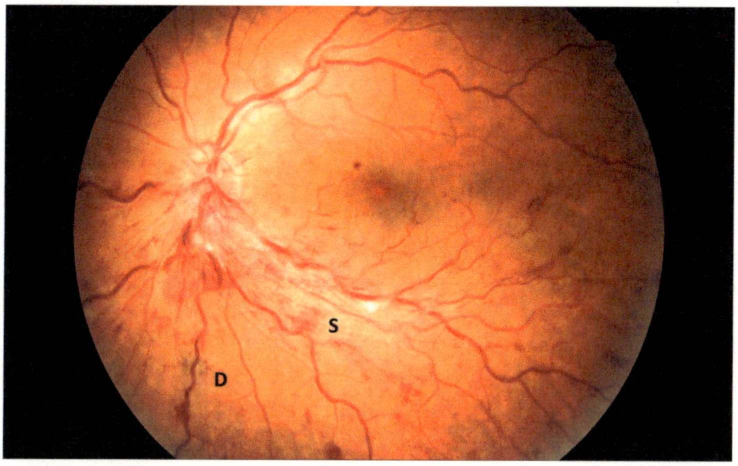

Fig. 5. Fundus photograph of an inferior branch retinal vein occlusion in the left eye showing different types of retinal haemorrhages. Superficial retinal haemorrhages (S) are flame shaped; deep retinal haemorrhages (D) are dot-blot.

2.5.2 Central retinal vein occlusion

Similar to BRVO, the most common presentation in patients with CRVO is vision loss. The vision loss is sudden, unilateral, painless and usually profound, in the range of counting fingers.

Examination reveals a relative afferent Pupillary defect. While fundus examination demonstrates tortuosity and dilatation of all the branches of the central retinal vein as well as superficial (flame-shaped) and deep (dot-blot) intraretinal haemorrhages. Cotton wool spots and oedema of the optic disc or macular may be present.

Fluorescein angiography is the ocular investigation of choice in patients with suspected CRVO. The general features of CRVO using fluorescein angiography include delayed arteriovenous transit time and blockage by retinal haemorrhages. Fluorescein angiography is vital in distinguishing between non-ischaemic and ischaemic CRVO (Figure 3). There is effective capillary perfusion in non-ischaemic CRVO and capillary non-perfusion in ischaemic CRVO.

2.6 Treatment

Treatment involves management of the systemic risk factors and local treatment for complications of RVO, such as macular oedema and neovascularisation.

With regard to systemic treatment of RVO, there is no strong evidence in current literature for the use of anticoagulant, fibrinolytic agents or antiplatelet agents. Best practice management involves treating the atherosclerotic risk factors, such as hypertension and hyperlipidaemia.

Local treatment for BRVO differs from the treatment of CRVO. For BRVO, the Branch Vein Occlusion Study (BVOS) suggested that retinal haemorrhages and any macular oedema should be observed for 3 months to allow for spontaneous resolution. After 3 months, if the macular oedema is still present, treatment may be warranted. The BVOS recommends grid laser photocoagulation for the treatment of macular oedema (1984). Use of intravitreal anti-VEGF agents, such as ranibizumab, has been shown to be beneficial (Campochiaro, Heier et al. 2010). There has been some conflicting evidence regarding the use of triamcinolone acetonide in the treatment of macular oedema in BRVO. Jonas et al. found it to beneficial in the treatment of macular oedema (Jonas, Akkoyun et al. 2005), however Scott et al found intravitreal triamcinolone to be no more effective than grid laser photocoagulation and was even associated with a higher risk of adverse events (Scott, Ip et al. 2009). Dexamethasone has been shown to be beneficial, but there is also a risk that dexamethasone can increase intraocular pressure (Haller, Bandello et al. 2010). Optic disc or retinal neovascularisation requires treatment with pan-retinal (scatter) laser photocoagulation in the distribution of occluded vein (1986; Hayreh, Rubenstein et al. 1993). Prophylactic PRP is not indicated to prevent neovascularisation, as the harmful effects of PRP outweigh the benefits in prophylaxis (1984).

Treatment of CRVO should initially involve determining the type of CRVO present. In patients with non-ischaemic CRVO, the macular oedema can be treated with intravitreal steroids such as triamcinolone acetonide (Ip, Scott et al. 2009) or dexamethasone (Haller, Bandello et al. 2010). Treatment with intravitreal anti-VEGF agents, such as Ranibizumab has been shown to be useful in a double-blinded randomized controlled trial (Brown, Campochiaro et al. 2010). Laser photocoagulation for the treatment of macular oedema in CRVO has not been found to be beneficial (1995). In ischaemic CRVO, the presence of anterior chamber angle neovascularisation or rubeosis iridis should immediately be treated with laser pan-retinal photocoagulation (1995). Prophylactic PRP is not warranted and PRP is only indicated once anterior segment neovascularisation becomes apparent. Unproven treatments include the use of Ticlopidine, Troxerutin and Epoprostenol.

2.7 Prognosis

Prognosis is dependent upon the type of RVO.

BRVO tends to have a better prognosis, but it may take 6 to 12 months to resolve. The affected area is commonly replaced by hard exudates and venous sheathing. Collateral vessels can form between the affected and unaffected retina. If there are improvements in visual acuity and the development of efficient collaterals, the prognosis is often good. The prognosis is poor if there are complications associated with the BRVO such as the development of chronic macular oedema, which occurs in 57% of temporal branch occlusions. Another serious complication is neovascularisation, which can lead to recurrent vitreous and pre-retinal haemorrhages as well as retinal detachments and ultimately adversely affects the visual outcome.

Similarly, the acute stage of CRVO takes approximately 6 to 12 months to resolve. Disc collaterals between the retinal and choroidal vascular network usually form during this time. The final visual acuity is dependent upon the initial visual acuity following RVO (1997), with better visual outcomes in those with good initial visual acuity. The complications and prognoses are different for the different types of CRVO. The complications of non-ischaemic CRVO include chronic macular oedema and conversion to ischaemic CRVO. The prognosis of non-ischaemic CRVO is often good, unless a conversion to ischaemic CRVO occurs. One-third of non-ischaemic CRVO convert to become ischemic by 3 years, with half of these conversions occurring within the first 4 months following the CRVO (1997). Ischaemic CRVO may be complicated by neovascularization, which occurs in 5% of eyes. When rubeosis iridis develops, it results in neovascular glaucoma, due to the neovascular membrane occluding the trabecular meshwork where the aqueous fluid drains out of the eye. Neovascular glaucoma commonly occurs within 3 months of the onset of the

CRVO and is characterised by a sudden increase in pain due to a rise in intraocular pressure. The risk factors for its development include poor visual acuity, extensive retinal haemorrhage and significant retinal non-perfusion on fluorescein angiography (1997). In patients with less than 10 optic disc areas of retinal non-perfusion, less than 10% of eyes will develop rubeosis iridis. However, if there are more than 30 optic disc areas of retinal non-perfusion, the risk of rubeosis iridis increases significantly. The prognosis of ischaemic CRVO is usually poor due to the development of macular ischaemia or neovascularization.

RVO in one eye increases the risk for the development of a RVO in the contralateral eye. This occurs in 9-15% of patients within 5 years of the initial diagnosis of RVO (Hayreh, Zimmerman et al. 1994). Unfortunately, at present there is no treatment available to prevent the development of RVO in the contralateral eye or a recurrence of RVO in the same eye.

RVO is also associated with an increased likelihood of death from cerebral vascular and cardiovascular causes (Tsaloumas, Kirwan et al. 2000; Cugati, Wang et al. 2007).

3. Ophthalmic manifestations of systemic thrombosis

Systemic venous thrombosis can cause significant ocular symptoms and signs. Evidence suggests that ocular manifestation in systemic thrombosis increases the risk of cerebral events (Asherson, Khamashta et al. 1989) and ultimately, this impacts the prognosis of the patient.

It is, therefore, important to consider ocular features of systemic venous thrombosis, but, it is also equally important that clinicians are aware of the ophthalmic features of systemic conditions that predispose to a venous thrombosis, such as thrombophilias.

It is clearly impossible to consider all systemic conditions that cause a predisposition to venous thrombosis in this chapter. Therefore, here we will consider two systemic conditions that have important ocular manifestations. Firstly, we will discuss cerebral venous sinus thrombosis and to highlight the ocular features of systemic thrombosis. Then we will examine anti-phospholipid syndrome to review the ocular features of a condition that is a risk factor for venous thrombosis.

3.1 Ophthalmic manifestations of cerebral venous sinus thrombosis

Cerebral venous sinus thrombosis (CVT) is a condition that results from thrombosis and occlusion of the cerebral veins or dural sinus. This thrombosis causes increased venous pressure and subsequently results in impairment of cerebrospinal fluid (CSF) absorption and increased intracranial pressure (ICP). Regardless of the site, all CVT can cause raised ICP. The common sites for CVT include the cavernous sinus, sigmoid sinus, transverse sinus and sagittal sinus. Rarer sites of thrombosis include the lateral sinus, jugular vein, posterior fossa vein and the deep cerebral venous system (straight sinus).

Impaired CSF absorption is associated with increased intracranial pressure, while increased capillary pressure disrupts the blood-brain barrier, decreases capillary perfusion and results in capillary damage. This increased capillary pressure ultimately causes vasogenic and cytotoxic oedema as well as cerebral parenchyma lesions (Gotoh, Ohmoto et al. 1993; Yoshikawa, Abe et al. 2002).

3.1.1 Prevalence

CVT is a rare thrombotic occurrence with an incidence of 3-4 per million (Stam 2005). It is more common in females compared to males with a ratio of 3:1 (Ferro, Canhao et al. 2004), and is also more common in children compared to adults (Agnelli and Verso 2008).

3.1.2 Clinical presentation

The ophthalmic presentation of CVT can be quite variable and it may have an acute or chronic onset. The most common ocular feature is papilloedema due to raised intracranial pressure. Acute papilloedema appears as flame shaped haemorrhages and cotton wool spots, which are an indication of nerve fibre layer infarction (Figure 6); whereas chronic papilloedema may have a 'champagne cork' like appearance (Figure 7). Despite the presence of papilloedema, visual acuity is often initially unaffected and the first ocular symptom to occur is usually visual field constriction (Figure 7). Patients can also present with visual obscuration with bending or coughing; and there may be diplopia due to cranial nerve VI palsy (Figure 8).

In cases of cavernous sinus thrombosis, ocular features are the predominant feature and can include ocular pain, chemosis, proptosis and cranial nerve palsies affecting the extraocular muscles. This is due to the close association between the oculomotor (cranial nerve III), trochlear (cranial nerve IV) and abducens (cranial nerve VI) nerve and the cavernous sinus.

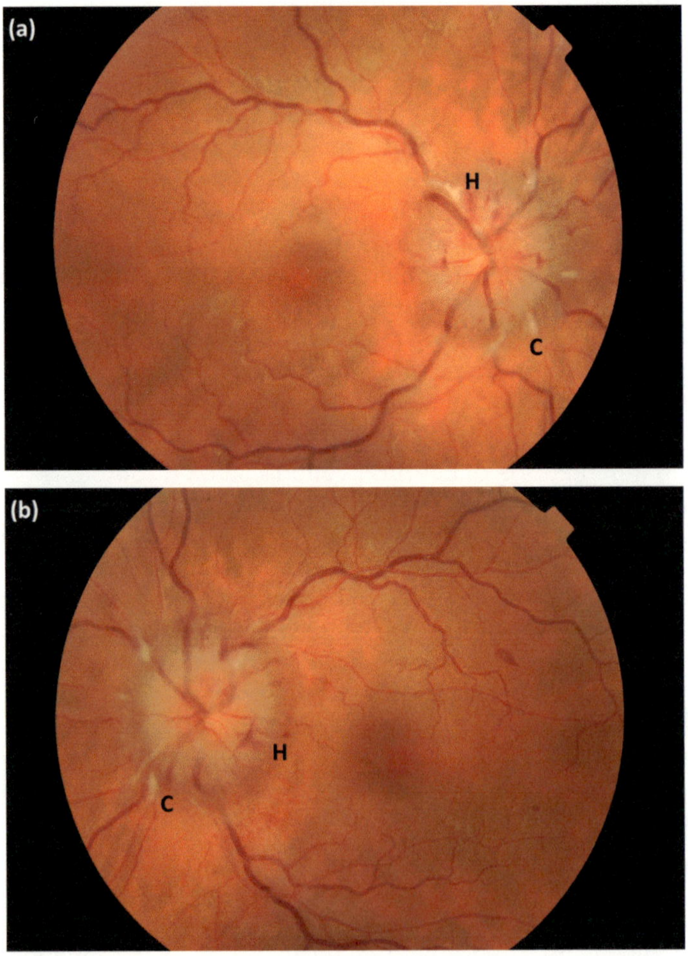

Fig. 6. Fundus photograph showing acute papilloedema with haemorrhages (H) and cotton wool spots (C) in the right eye (a) and the left eye (b) of the same patient.

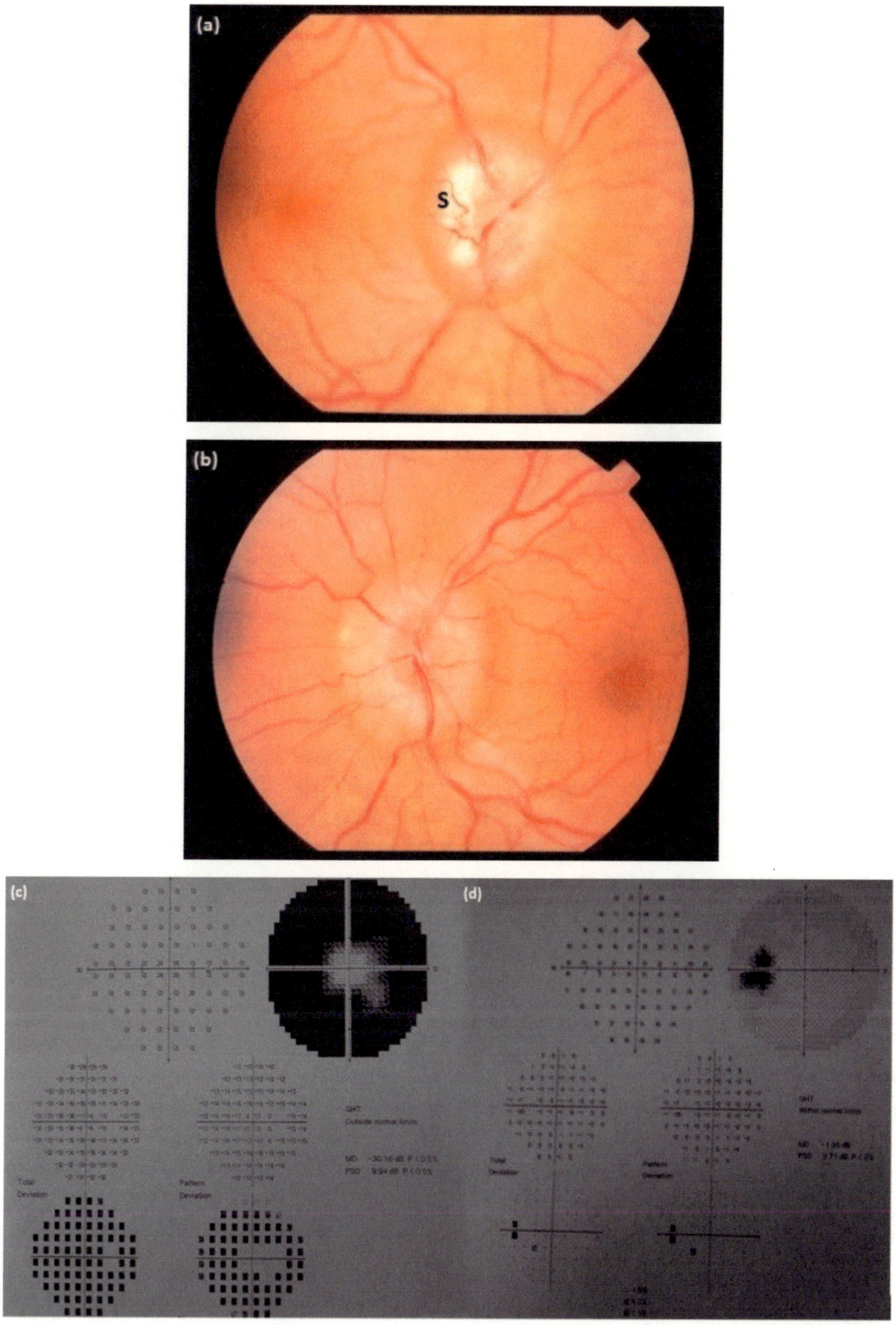

Fig. 7. Fundus photograph showing a 'champagne cork' like appearance in chronic papilloedema in the right eye (a) and left eye (b) of the same patient. In the right eye, there is a Y shaped retinochoroidal shunt (S) due to the retinal vessels diverting towards the choroidal vessels and is another fundus feature of chronic papilloedema. Corresponding visual fields images shows significant field constriction in the right eye (c) and an enlarged blind spot in the left eye (d).

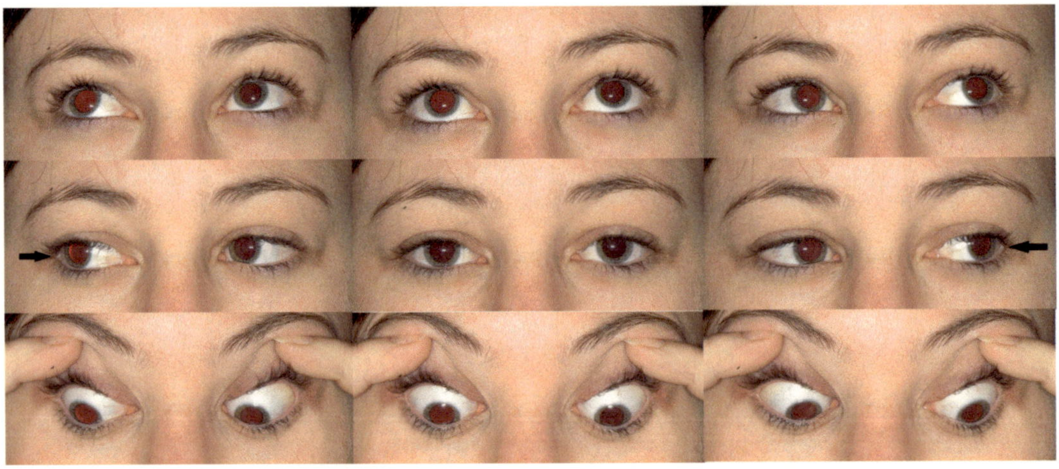

Fig. 8. Clinical photograph of all nine positions of gaze in a patient with a cranial nerve VI palsy associated with raised intracranial pressure. The patient complains of diplopia and there is weakness in the lateral rectus as indicated by the visibility of the sclera on lateral gaze (arrows).

3.1.3 Investigations

Magnetic resonance imaging (MRI) with magnetic resonance venography is the most sensitive method for diagnosing CVT and visualising brain parenchymal lesions. However, this sensitivity depends upon the location of the thrombosis (Ferro, Morgado et al. 2007).

Given its wide availability, computed tomography (CT) is often used for investigation of CVT. The radiological findings of CVT on CT are often non-specific and the scan may be normal in 30% of cases with CVT. Signs that assist in the diagnosis of CVT include the dense triangle sign on non-contrast CT (hyperdensity in the posterior part of the superior sagittal sinus caused by venous thrombosis), the cord sign on contrast CT (linear hyperdensity over cerebral cortex caused by venous thrombosis) and the empty delta sign on contrast CT (area where there is absence of contrast enhancement in the posterior part of the superior sagittal sinus) (Boukobza, Crassard et al. 2007). These signs occur in one-third of patients with CVT.

Ocular assessment in patients with CVT should involve serial visual acuity, visual field measurements and imaging of the optic nerve head with stereophotographs or other imaging modalities such as OCT in order to monitor progression.

Once diagnosed, an investigation for the possible causes of CVT may be warranted. This involves blood tests to screen for thrombophilias, as well as a search for a malignancy.

3.1.4 Treatment

Treatment aims to recanalise the occlusion, prevent thrombus propagation, address the underlying cause, and then control the symptoms of the condition such as vision loss.

The most important principle of treatment of CVT is anticoagulation (Coutinho and Stam 2010) in patients who have no contraindications to anticoagulation. Treatment with either unfractionated heparin or low molecular weight heparin has been shown to reduce the risk of death and dependency (Stam, De Bruijn et al. 2002). Anticoagulation appears to be safe in CVT patients with intracranial haemorrhages (Einhaupl, Stam et al. 2010), as the haemorrhages in CVT are the result of venous occlusion.

Although controversial, failure in improvement with anticoagulation may require the use of direct endovascular thrombolysis (Einhaupl, Stam et al. 2010) which involves either mechanically (Scarrow, Williams et al. 1999) or chemically (Wasay, Bakshi et al. 2001) dissolving the clot. This is generally reserved for patients with poorer prognoses (Stam 2005), as there is the potential that thrombolysis may cause death or dependency in up to 40% of patients with CVT (Stam, Majoie et al. 2008). However, in critically ill patients, thrombolysis may reduce death compared to other treatments or no treatment at all (Canhao, Falcao et al. 2003).

Aside from treatment of the CVT, it is important to manage any associated symptoms. In particular, control of elevated intracranial pressure is vital in patients with headaches, as well as preserving visual function. In cases of decreasing visual acuity associated with CVT, optic nerve sheath fenestrations may help to reduce pressure, thereby preventing optic nerve atrophy. Equally important in CVT treatment is the control of seizures.

3.1.5 Prognosis

The prognosis of CVT is generally good. At 16 months, approximately 57% of patients with CVT have no signs or symptoms, and a further 22% of patients with CVT have only minor residual symptoms (Ferro, Canhao et al. 2004). Characteristics that are associated with a poorer prognosis include age over 37, male , previously having a coma or mental status abnormality; haemorrhage noted on imaging; deep venous system thrombosis; central nervous system infection and CVT associated with malignancy (Ferro, Canhao et al. 2004).

Approximately 3% of patients die in the acute phase of CVT and 8% of patients die within the first 30 days following initial symptoms of CVT (Canhao, Ferro et al. 2005). Death is often due to transtentorial herniation or due to diffuse oedema and multiple parenchymal lesions (Canhao, Ferro et al. 2005).

Significant visual loss in CVT is rare (Purvin, Trobe et al. 1995), and if present, is often associated with prolonged elevated intracranial pressure. Visual prognosis depends upon the duration and severity of elevation in pressure.

There is often recanalisation after CVT and this commonly occurs within the first four months. The likelihood of recanalisation occurring depends on the location of the CVT (Baumgartner, Studer et al. 2003). Following a CVT, approximately 3% develop a recurrent CVT and 6% develop another form of venous thromboembolism at 6 years (Martinelli, Bucciarelli et al. 2010).

3.2 Ophthalmic manifestations of antiphospholipid syndrome

Antiphospholipid syndrome (APS) is an autoimmune disease associated with both arterial and venous thrombosis. It is characterised by lupus anticoagulant, anticardiolipin antibody and anti-β2 glycoprotein-I antibody (Miyakis, Lockshin et al. 2006).

3.2.1 Prevalence

The prevalence of ocular involvement in APS is variable, with studies suggesting that ocular features can occur in 8% to 88% of patients with APS (Utz and Tang 2011).

3.2.2 Clinical presentation

Ocular manifestations of APS include occlusive vascular disease (Miserocchi, Baltatzis et al. 2001; Suvajac, Stojanovich et al. 2007), vasculitis (Miserocchi, Baltatzis et al. 2001) and neuro-ophthalmic manifestations. Occlusive vascular disease may occur in the form of central and branch retinal artery or vein occlusion, and choroidal infarction (Ang, Yap et al. 2000) (Figure 9). Vasculitis may manifest as anterior uveitis, episcleritis (Figure 10), scleritis (Figure 11) or retinal vasculitis causing retinal artery occlusion (Figure 12). APS may also be associated with cranial nerve III (Genevay, Hayem et al. 2002) (Figure 13), cranial nerve IV (Shin and Lee 2006) and cranial nerve VI (Shin and Lee 2006) palsies, in addition to ischaemic optic neuropathy (Giorgi and Balacco Gabrieli 1999), and optic neuritis (Giorgi and Balacco Gabrieli 1999).

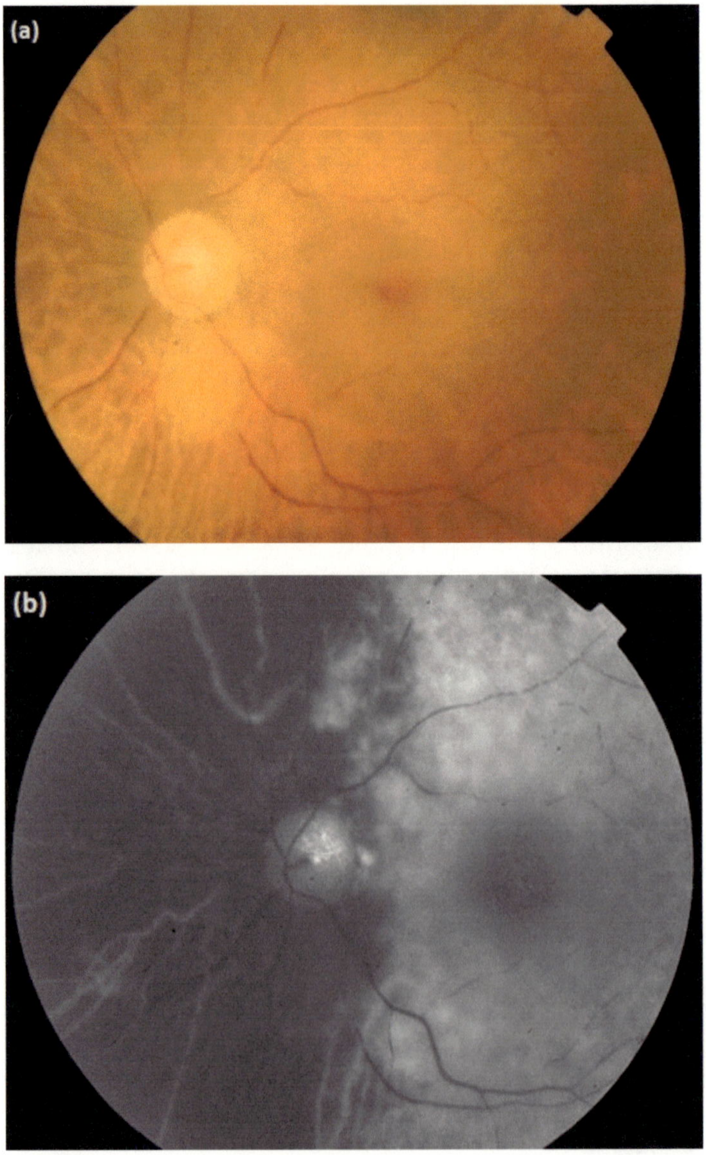

Fig. 9. Fundus photograph showing central retinal artery occlusion with associated choroidal infarction in the left eye (a) and the corresponding fluorescein angiogram (b).

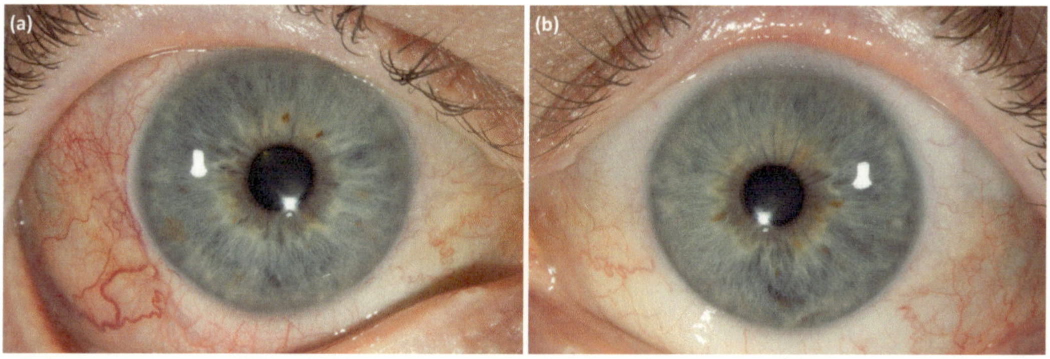

Fig. 10. External photograph showing episcleritis of both eyes of the same patient with antiphospholipid syndrome. The right eye (a) is clinically more severe than the left eye (b).

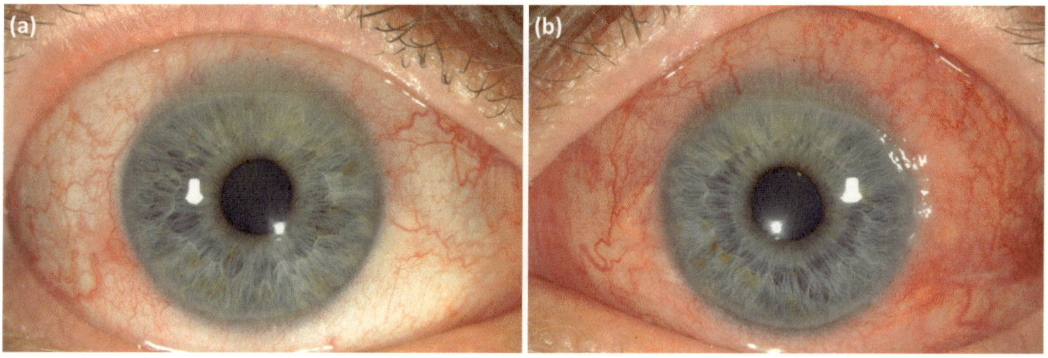

Fig. 11. External photograph showing scleritis of both eyes with the right eye (a) less severe than the left eye (b). The scleritis associated with antiphospholipid syndrome is often a necrotising scleritis.

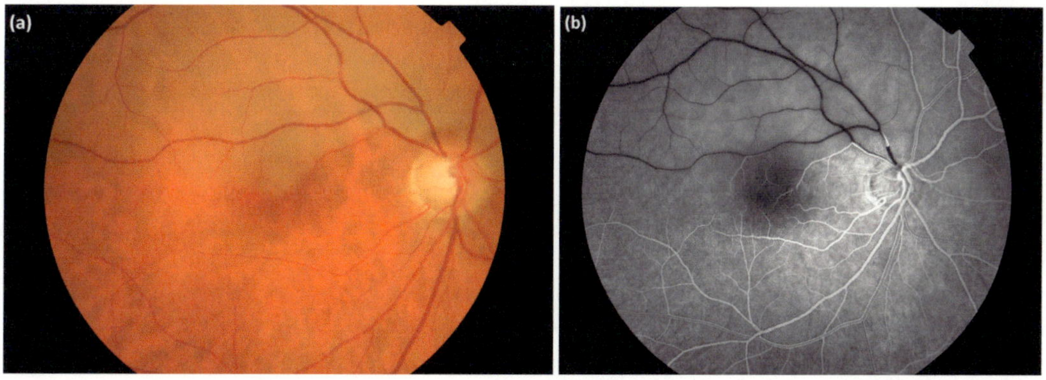

Fig. 12. Fundus photograph of a branch retinal artery occlusion in the right eye due to vasculitis (a). The superior retina is pale due to infarction and the occluded artery is clearly visible on the corresponding fluorescein angiogram (b).

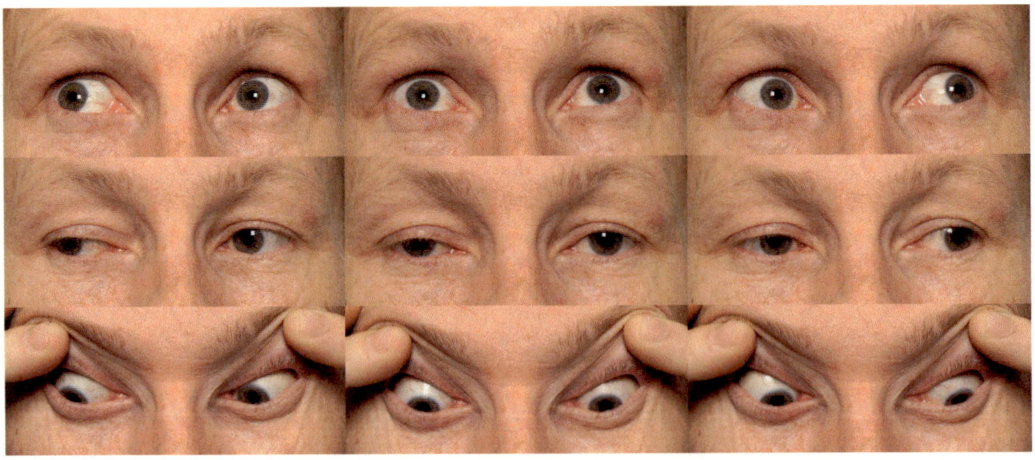

Fig. 13. Clinical photograph of all nine positions of gaze in a patient with a right pupil involving cranial nerve III palsy with right ptosis and exotropia on primary gaze.

Patients with retinal vaso-occlusion usually present with pain, unilateral or bilateral decreased visual acuity, visual field defect or amaurosis fugax. Bilateral amaurosis fugax is a very serious condition, and may indicate the presence of central nervous system ischaemia. Those with cranial neuropathy present with acute binocular diplopia.

On examination, patients with APS may have dry eyes, conjunctival telangiectasia (Miserocchi, Baltatzis et al. 2001) and corneal infiltrates or keratitis. Ocular fundus examination may reveal tortuous and dilated retinal veins, intra-retinal haemorrhages, cotton-wool spots, optic disc and macular oedema or neovascularisation.

3.2.3 Investigations

Ocular imaging with fluorescein angiography directly visualizes the retinal vessels and occlusion. An MRI scan may be important if there is visual loss without ocular fundus changes, as it is important to investigate the possibility of CNS ischaemia.

In addition to imaging, a full thrombophilia work-up may be necessary in the absence of traditional thrombophilia risk factors. This would include searching for antiphospholipid antibodies, including lupus anticoagulant, anticardiolipin antibody and anti-β2 glycoprotein-I antibody. Other screening tests should include homocysteine, protein C and S, plasminogen, anti-thrombin levels, activated protein C resistance and factor V Leiden mutation.

3.2.4 Treatment

Early detection of ocular manifestations of APS is important as it allows treatment and prevention of further systemic disease. This first involves determining the patient's thrombotic risk.

The treatment of the systemic disease is vital as it may reverse the retinal ischaemia (Srinivasan, Fern et al. 2001). This should include reducing modifiable risk factors such as hypertension, hyperlipidaemia, diabetes mellitus, oral contraceptive use, hormone replacement therapy and smoking.

Treatment should also target the cause of the thrombosis. APS with venous thrombosis requires anticoagulation with warfarin while APS with arterial thrombosis requires anti-platelet agents (Ruiz-Irastorza, Hunt et al. 2007).

3.2.5 Prognosis

Ocular prognosis depends upon the presence of complications such as neovascularisation and therefore, regular ocular monitoring is required.

In patients with antiphospholipid syndrome, the risk of further thromboembolic complications ranges from 22% to 29% (Ruiz-Irastorza, Hunt et al. 2007)

4. Conclusion

Similar to systemic venous thrombosis, venous thrombosis in the eye is a manifestation of Virchow's triad. Ocular venous thrombosis presents as retinal vein occlusion. The eye can also be affected by systemic venous thrombosis. Accurate diagnosis of venous thrombosis is vital and early treatment should be implemented in order to preserve existing vision and to prevent serious visual, and life threatening complications.

5. References

Agnelli, G. and M. Verso (2008). "Epidemiology of cerebral vein and sinus thrombosis." Front Neurol Neurosci 23: 16-22.

Ang, L. P., E. Y. Yap, et al. (2000). "Bilateral choroidal infarction in a patient with antiphospholipid syndrome: a case report." Clin Experiment Ophthalmol 28(4): 326-328.

Anonymous (1984). "Argon laser photocoagulation for macular edema in branch vein occlusion. The Branch Vein Occlusion Study Group." Am J Ophthalmol 98(3): 271-282.

Anonymous (1986). "Argon laser scatter photocoagulation for prevention of neovascularization and vitreous hemorrhage in branch vein occlusion. A randomized clinical trial. Branch Vein Occlusion Study Group." Arch Ophthalmol 104(1): 34-41.

Anonymous (1993). "Risk factors for branch retinal vein occlusion. The Eye Disease Case-control Study Group." Am J Ophthalmol 116(3): 286-296.

Anonymous (1995). "Evaluation of grid pattern photocoagulation for macular edema in central vein occlusion. The Central Vein Occlusion Study Group M report." Ophthalmology 102(10): 1425-1433.

Anonymous (1995). "A randomized clinical trial of early panretinal photocoagulation for ischemic central vein occlusion. The Central Vein Occlusion Study Group N report." Ophthalmology 102(10): 1434-1444.

Anonymous (1996). "Risk factors for central retinal vein occlusion. The Eye Disease Case-Control Study Group." Arch Ophthalmol 114(5): 545-554.

Anonymous (1997). "Natural history and clinical management of central retinal vein occlusion. The Central Vein Occlusion Study Group." Arch Ophthalmol 115(4): 486-491.

Asherson, R. A., M. A. Khamashta, et al. (1989). "Cerebrovascular disease and antiphospholipid antibodies in systemic lupus erythematosus, lupus-like disease, and the primary antiphospholipid syndrome." Am J Med 86(4): 391-399.

Baumgartner, R. W., A. Studer, et al. (2003). "Recanalisation of cerebral venous thrombosis." J Neurol Neurosurg Psychiatry 74(4): 459-461.

Boukobza, M., I. Crassard, et al. (2007). "When the "dense triangle" in dural sinus thrombosis is round." Neurology 69(8): 808.

Brown, D. M., P. A. Campochiaro, et al. (2010). "Ranibizumab for macular edema following central retinal vein occlusion: six-month primary end point results of a phase III study." Ophthalmology 117(6): 1124-1133 e1121.

Campochiaro, P. A., J. S. Heier, et al. (2010). "Ranibizumab for macular edema following branch retinal vein occlusion: six-month primary end point results of a phase III study." Ophthalmology 117(6): 1102-1112 e1101.

Canhao, P., F. Falcao, et al. (2003). "Thrombolytics for cerebral sinus thrombosis: a systematic review." Cerebrovasc Dis 15(3): 159-166.

Canhao, P., J. M. Ferro, et al. (2005). "Causes and predictors of death in cerebral venous thrombosis." Stroke 36(8): 1720-1725.

Chua, B., A. Kifley, et al. (2005). "Homocysteine and retinal vein occlusion: a population-based study." Am J Ophthalmol 139(1): 181-182.

Coutinho, J. M. and J. Stam (2010). "How to treat cerebral venous and sinus thrombosis." J Thromb Haemost 8(5): 877-883.

Cugati, S., J. J. Wang, et al. (2007). "Retinal vein occlusion and vascular mortality: pooled data analysis of 2 population-based cohorts." Ophthalmology 114(3): 520-524.

Dodson, P. M., E. E. Kritzinger, et al. (1992). "Diabetes mellitus and retinal vein occlusion in patients of Asian, west Indian and white European origin." Eye (Lond) 6 (Pt 1): 66-68.

Einhaupl, K., J. Stam, et al. (2010). "EFNS guideline on the treatment of cerebral venous and sinus thrombosis in adult patients." Eur J Neurol 17(10): 1229-1235.

Fegan, C. D. (2002). "Central retinal vein occlusion and thrombophilia." Eye (Lond) 16(1): 98-106.

Ferro, J. M., P. Canhao, et al. (2004). "Prognosis of cerebral vein and dural sinus thrombosis: results of the International Study on Cerebral Vein and Dural Sinus Thrombosis (ISCVT)." Stroke 35(3): 664-670.

Ferro, J. M., C. Morgado, et al. (2007). "Interobserver agreement in the magnetic resonance location of cerebral vein and dural sinus thrombosis." Eur J Neurol 14(3): 353-356.

Genevay, S., G. Hayem, et al. (2002). "Oculomotor palsy in six patients with systemic lupus erythematosus. A possible role of antiphospholipid syndrome." Lupus 11(5): 313-316.

Giorgi, D. and C. Balacco Gabrieli (1999). "Optic neuropathy in systemic lupus erythematosus and antiphospholipid syndrome (APS): clinical features, pathogenesis, review of the literature and proposed ophthalmological criteria for APS diagnosis." Clin Rheumatol 18(2): 124-131.

Gotoh, M., T. Ohmoto, et al. (1993). "Experimental study of venous circulatory disturbance by dural sinus occlusion." Acta Neurochir (Wien) 124(2-4): 120-126.

Greiner, K., G. Hafner, et al. (1999). "Retinal vascular occlusion and deficiencies in the protein C pathway." Am J Ophthalmol 128(1): 69-74.

Haller, J. A., F. Bandello, et al. (2010). "Randomized, sham-controlled trial of dexamethasone intravitreal implant in patients with macular edema due to retinal vein occlusion." Ophthalmology 117(6): 1134-1146 e1133.

Hayreh, S. S. (2005). "Prevalent misconceptions about acute retinal vascular occlusive disorders." Prog Retin Eye Res 24(4): 493-519.

Hayreh, S. S., L. Rubenstein, et al. (1993). "Argon laser scatter photocoagulation in treatment of branch retinal vein occlusion. A prospective clinical trial." Ophthalmologica 206(1): 1-14.

Hayreh, S. S., B. Zimmerman, et al. (2001). "Systemic diseases associated with various types of retinal vein occlusion." Am J Ophthalmol 131(1): 61-77.

Hayreh, S. S., M. B. Zimmerman, et al. (1994). "Incidence of various types of retinal vein occlusion and their recurrence and demographic characteristics." Am J Ophthalmol 117(4): 429-441.

Heit, J. A. (2008). "The epidemiology of venous thromboembolism in the community." Arterioscler Thromb Vasc Biol 28(3): 370-372.

Incorvaia, C., G. Lamberti, et al. (1999). "Idiopathic central retinal vein occlusion in a thrombophilic patient with the heterozygous 20210 G/A prothrombin genotype." Am J Ophthalmol 128(2): 247-248.

Ip, M. S., I. U. Scott, et al. (2009). "A randomized trial comparing the efficacy and safety of intravitreal triamcinolone with observation to treat vision loss associated with macular edema secondary to central retinal vein occlusion: the Standard Care vs Corticosteroid for Retinal Vein Occlusion (SCORE) study report 5." Arch Ophthalmol 127(9): 1101-1114.

Janssen, M. C., M. den Heijer, et al. (2005). "Retinal vein occlusion: a form of venous thrombosis or a complication of atherosclerosis? A meta-analysis of thrombophilic factors." Thromb Haemost 93(6): 1021-1026.

Kirwan, J. F., M. D. Tsaloumas, et al. (1997). "Sex hormone preparations and retinal vein occlusion." Eye (Lond) 11 (Pt 1): 53-56.

Martinelli, I., P. Bucciarelli, et al. (2010). "Long-term evaluation of the risk of recurrence after cerebral sinus-venous thrombosis." Circulation 121(25): 2740-2746.

Miserocchi, E., S. Baltatzis, et al. (2001). "Ocular features associated with anticardiolipin antibodies: a descriptive study." Am J Ophthalmol 131(4): 451-456.

Mitchell, P., W. Smith, et al. (1996). "Prevalence and associations of retinal vein occlusion in Australia. The Blue Mountains Eye Study." Arch Ophthalmol 114(10): 1243-1247.

Miyakis, S., M. D. Lockshin, et al. (2006). "International consensus statement on an update of the classification criteria for definite antiphospholipid syndrome (APS)." J Thromb Haemost 4(2): 295-306.

Purvin, V. A., J. D. Trobe, et al. (1995). "Neuro-ophthalmic features of cerebral venous obstruction." Arch Neurol 52(9): 880-885.

Rogers, S., R. L. McIntosh, et al. (2010). "The prevalence of retinal vein occlusion: pooled data from population studies from the United States, Europe, Asia, and Australia." Ophthalmology 117(2): 313-319 e311.

Ruiz-Irastorza, G., B. J. Hunt, et al. (2007). "A systematic review of secondary thromboprophylaxis in patients with antiphospholipid antibodies." Arthritis Rheum 57(8): 1487-1495.

Scarrow, A. M., R. L. Williams, et al. (1999). "Removal of a thrombus from the sigmoid and transverse sinuses with a rheolytic thrombectomy catheter." AJNR Am J Neuroradiol 20(8): 1467-1469.

Scott, I. U., M. S. Ip, et al. (2009). "A randomized trial comparing the efficacy and safety of intravitreal triamcinolone with standard care to treat vision loss associated with macular Edema secondary to branch retinal vein occlusion: the Standard Care vs

Corticosteroid for Retinal Vein Occlusion (SCORE) study report 6." Arch Ophthalmol 127(9): 1115-1128.

Shin, S. Y. and J. M. Lee (2006). "A case of multiple cranial nerve palsies as the initial ophthalmic presentation of antiphospholipid syndrome." Korean J Ophthalmol 20(1): 76-78.

Srinivasan, S., A. Fern, et al. (2001). "Reversal of nonarteritic anterior ischemic optic neuropathy associated with coexisting primary antiphospholipid syndrome and Factor V Leiden mutation." Am J Ophthalmol 131(5): 671-673.

Stam, J. (2005). "Thrombosis of the cerebral veins and sinuses." N Engl J Med 352(17): 1791-1798.

Stam, J., S. F. De Bruijn, et al. (2002). "Anticoagulation for cerebral sinus thrombosis." Cochrane Database Syst Rev(4): CD002005.

Stam, J., C. B. Majoie, et al. (2008). "Endovascular thrombectomy and thrombolysis for severe cerebral sinus thrombosis: a prospective study." Stroke 39(5): 1487-1490.

Suvajac, G., L. Stojanovich, et al. (2007). "Ocular manifestations in antiphospholipid syndrome." Autoimmun Rev 6(6): 409-414.

Tsaloumas, M. D., J. Kirwan, et al. (2000). "Nine year follow-up study of morbidity and mortality in retinal vein occlusion." Eye (Lond) 14(Pt 6): 821-827.

Utz, V. M. and J. Tang (2011). "Ocular manifestations of the antiphospholipid syndrome." Br J Ophthalmol 95(4): 454-459.

Wasay, M., R. Bakshi, et al. (2001). "Nonrandomized comparison of local urokinase thrombolysis versus systemic heparin anticoagulation for superior sagittal sinus thrombosis." Stroke 32(10): 2310-2317.

Wong, T. Y., E. K. Larsen, et al. (2005). "Cardiovascular risk factors for retinal vein occlusion and arteriolar emboli: the Atherosclerosis Risk in Communities & Cardiovascular Health studies." Ophthalmology 112(4): 540-547.

Yoshikawa, T., O. Abe, et al. (2002). "Diffusion-weighted magnetic resonance imaging of dural sinus thrombosis." Neuroradiology 44(6): 481-488.

Part 4

Venous Thrombosis in Special Patient Populations

10

Approaching Venous Thrombosis in General Surgery Patients

Gulcin Hepgul[1], Fatih Yanar[2] and Meltem Küçükyılmaz[1]
[1]Bagcilar, Training and Research Hospital, General Surgery Clinic
[2]Bakirkoy Dr Sadi Konuk Training and Research Hospital, General Surgery Clinic
Turkey

1. Introduction

Venous thromboembolism (VTE) manifesting as deep vein thrombosis(DVT) or pulmonary embolism (PE), is one of the most common complications of hospitalization and is associated with short and long-term morbidity, mortality and resource expenditure. Routine use of thromboprophylaxis reduces adverse patient outcomes while at the same time decreasing overall costs. Almost all hospitalized patients have at least one associated risk factor for VTE, and approximately 40% have three or more risk factors **(Table 1)**(1).

Surgery
Trauma (major trauma or lower-extremity injury)
Immobility, lower-extremity paresis
Cancer (active or occult)
Cancer therapy (hormonal, chemotherapy, angiogenesis inhibitors, radiotherapy)
Venous compression (tumor, hematoma, arterial abnormality)
Previous VTE
Increasing age
Pregnancy and the postpartum period
Estrogen -containing oral contraceptives or hormone replacement therapy
Selective estrogen receptor modulators
Erythropoiesis-stimulating agents
Acute medical illness
Inflammatory bowel disease
Nephrotic syndrome
Myeloproliferative disorder
Paroxysmal nocturnal hemoglobinuria
Obesity
Central venous catheterization
Inherited or acquired thrombophilia

Table 1. Risk Factors for VTE

Without thromboprophylaxis, the incidence of objectively confirmed, hospital-acquired DVT is approximately 10 to 40% among medical or general surgical patients and 40 to 60% following major orthopedic surgery **(Table 2)**(1-2).

Patient Group	DVT Prevalence, %
Medical patients	10-20
General, surgery	15-40
Major gynecologic surgery	15-40
Major Urologic surgery	15-40
Neurosurgery	15-40
Stroke	20-50
Flip or knee arthroplasty, HFS	40-60
Major trauma	60-80
SCI	60-80
Critical care patients	10-80

* Rates based on objective diagnostic: screening for asymptomatic DVT in patients not receiving thromboprophylaxis.

Table 2. Approximate Risk of DVT in Hospitalized Patients

Several hundred clinical trials of thromboprophylaxis, conducted over the past 50 years, have shown that the use of prophylaxis reduces the rates of deep vein thrombosis (DVT), proximal DVT, pulmonary embolism (PE), and fatal PE by more than 60% in a broad spectrum of hospitalized patients with a very low risk of adverse effects. Although effective strategies for the prevention of venous thromboembolism (VTE) are widely available and existence of several guidelines for individual risk assessments to determine thrombosis risk and prophylaxis, a significant number of patients still develop VTE because appropriate thromboprophylaxis is not correctly prescribed. Adapting evidence-based practice guidelines into existing local policies and protocols has been shown to significantly increase the proportion of at-risk patients receiving appropriate thromboprophylaxis.

The American College of Chest Physicians (ACCP) sponsor and publish what are generally considered to be the most comprehensive and most commonly utilized of these guidelines(3). A summary of the 2008 ACCP Guidelines on the Prevention of VTE is presented in **Table 3**, (4).

The type and duration of surgery clearly influence the risk of DVT. Numerous efforts have been made to identify the patients most at risk for DVT and PE. The studies of this problem categorize risk levels as low, medium, high, and very high.

Patients at *low risk* are under 40 years of age contemplating minor surgery and with no associated risk factors. The incidence of DVT is less than 2%, proximal DVT 0.4%, PE at 0.2%, and fatal PE 0.02%. This group requires no special prophylaxis other than early ambulation.

Patients at *moderate risk* are those aged 40–50 who are undergoing major surgery, have no associated risk factors, and expect a prompt recovery. The frequency of DVT is 10%–20% proximal DVT, 2%–4%, clinical PE 1%–2%, and fatal PE 0%– 1.4%. This group will benefit from prophylactic treatment with LMWH, or LDUH and ES.

Patient groups	**Recommended thromboprophylaxis options***	**Optimal duration of prophylaxis**
Low VTE Risk: •Medical - fully mobile, brief admission, no additional risk factors • Surgical - procedure < 30 minutes, patient mobile, no additional risk factors	No prophylaxis Early and frequent ambulation	Not applicable.
Moderate VTE Risk: •Acute medical illness •Major general surgery •Major gynecologic surgery " Major urologic surgery •Thoracic surgery •Bariatric surgery	Low-molecular-weight heparin Low-dose heparin Fondaparinux Combinations of a mechanical method and an anticoagulant	Continue until discharge for the majority of patients. Selected patients may benefit from post-discharge prophylaxis.
High VTE Risk: •Hip or knee arthroplasty •Hip fracture surgery	Low-molecular-weight heparin Fondaparinux Rivaroxaban or dabigatran Warfarin (target INR 2-3)	Minimum of 10 days and up to 35 days.
High VTE Risk: •Major trauma, (including spinal cord injury)	Low-molecular-weight heparin Combinations of a mechanical method and an anticoagulant	Continue until discharge for the majority of patients. Prophylaxis should be continued for the inpatient rehabilitation period.
High bleeding risk	Mechanical method of prophylaxis (GCS, PCD, VFP) Consider anticoagulant prophylaxis when bleeding risk decreases	Duration appropriate for the specific patient risk group.

GCS indicates graduated compression stocking; PCD, pneumatic compression device, VFP, venous foot pump.

Table 3. Risk stratification, recommended thromboprophylaxis and optimal duration of prophylaxis by patient group.

The *high-risk* group are patients over 60, candidates for major surgery, with associated risk factors. The prevalence of DVT is 20%-40%; proximal DVT 4%-8%, clinical PE 2%-4% and fatal PE 0.4%-1%. Higher doses of LMWH or LDUH should be used, together with 1 PC devices and ES.

In the *very-high-risk* group of patients with major trauma (multiorgan, spinal, pelvic, long bone fractures), intermittent compression devices and ES should be started as early as possible, and LMWH or LDUH initiated as soon as it is safe. In cases of major trauma, with absolute contraindications for anticoagulants, the prophylactic indication of an inferior vena cava (IVC) filter should be considered, especially in cases with duplex ultrasonography demonstration of DVT.

2. Mechanical methods of thromboprophylaxis and the role of combined thromboprophylaxis modalities

Early and frequent mobilizitation of hospitalized patients at risk for VTE is an important part of patient care. However, many patients cannot be fully ambulatory early after surgery. Furthermore, the majority of hospital-associated, symptomatic thromboembolic events occur after patients have started to ambulate, and mobilization alone does not provide adequate thromboprophylaxis for hospital patients. Specific mechanical methods of thromboprophylaxis, which include graduated compression stockings (GCS), intermittent pneumatic compression (IPC) devices, and the venous foot pump (VFP), increase venous outflow and/or reduce stasis within the leg veins. Use of mechanical thromboprophylaxis is the preferred option for patients at high risk for bleeding. If the high bleeding risk is temporary, consideration should be given to starting pharmacologic thromboprophylaxis once this risk has decreased. Mechanical thromboprophylaxis may also be considered in combination with anticoagulant thromboprophylaxis to improve efficacy in patient groups for which this additive effect has been demonstrated(3,5,6). However, since they are not associated with bleeding, and some methods have demonstrated efficacy as DVT prevention in clinical trials, the use of mechanical prophylaxis in combination with pharmacological prophylaxis may be helpful in certain situations. For example, in major trauma patients who have a high risk of bleeding at presentation (as after head injury), we use mechanical prophylaxis initially followed by anticoagulant prophylaxis with LMWH when safe (5,6). This strategy could be adopted in any postoperative situation in which the initial risk of bleeding is high.

3. VTE in cancer patients

The association of cancer with thrombosis has been known for more than 100 years. Since the beginning it was regarded as a 2-way association, first cancer increases the risk of thrombosis(as first observed by Armand Trousseau in 1865), and secondy clotting activation increases the progression of cancer(as postulated by Billroth in 1878). Patients with cancer have at least a sixfold-increased risk of VTE compared to those without cancer and active cancer accounts for almost 20% of all new VTE events occurring in the community. Furthermore, VTE is one of the most common and costly complications seen in cancer patients. Although the association between cancer and thrombosis has been known for years, there is now an increasing recognition among cancer providers of the impact of thrombotic complications on patients with cancer (7,8). Several factors have contributed to this heightened awareness. Firstly, cancer-associated VTE is increasingly prevalent. In a recent analysis of more than 1 million hospitalized patients with cancer, the rate of VTE increased by 28% from 1995 to 2003 ($P < .0001$)(9). Secondly, the consequences of VTE are better understood. Thrombosis is the second-leading cause of death in patients with cancer and is associated with worsened mortality (10-12). In addition, patients with cancer who suffer VTE have an increased risk of recurrent VTE, bleeding complications, morbidity, and utilization of health care resources(13,14). Finally, newer anticancer agents particularly antiangiogenic drugs, appear to be more thrombogenic than conventional chemotherapy (15,16). Selected cancer patients with established VTE will need extended treatment to prevent its recurrence. In addition, a number of new cancer therapies have been associated with a further increase in the risk of VTE, warranting primary prophylaxis. Given the high mortality rate for VTE in cancer patients, it is imperative to ensure that all health-care professionals become familiar with and utilize the latest guidelines and tools for timely and evidence-based risk assessment, prevention, and treatment of VTE(17,18).

A hypercoagulable state or low-grade DIC is common in patients with cancer. The results of laboratory tests indicate that a process of fibrin formation and removal is ongoing during the development of malignancy. Reported rates of venous thromboembolism (VTE) in patients with cancer range from 4% to 31%(19,23). Cancer alone elevates the risk of thrombosis 4-fold; chemotherapy increases the risk 6.5-fold(24,25). Patients who undergo cancer surgery have a higher risk of postoperative VTE than those who have surgery for a nonmalignant disease (26). VTE is the second leading cause of death in cancer patients, and the presence of VTE in patients with cancer has been reported to increase the likelihood of death by 2- to 8-fold (27-32).

Results of the FRONTLINE (Fundamental Research in Oncology and Thrombosis) survey underscored the need for development of clinical guidelines focusing on VTE in cancer patients: surgeons and medical oncologists reported that they used VTE prophylaxis in only about 50% and 5% of their patients, respectively(33). Two sets of guidelines devoted specifically to oncology patients are available to help guide clinicians: recommendations by the American Society of Clinical Oncology (ASCO) and by the National Comprehensive Cancer Network (NCCN) (34-35). Both sets of recommendations direct that all adults hospitalized with cancer receive prophylactic anticoagulation therapy in the absence of contraindications. However, a recent review of more than 70,000 hospitalized patients with cancer in whom an indication for thromboprophylaxis had been identified showed that the rate of appropriate prophylaxis was only 27%(36).

Alcalay et al. was found VTE as a significant predictor of death within 1 year of colorectal cancer diagnosis, among the patients with local or regional stage disease, but not among the patients with metastatic disease(37).

Thromboembolic events are a major cause of morbidity and mortality in patients undergoing surgery. Cancer patients requiring curative abdominal surgery are considered to be at a particularly high risk for VTE, and thromboprophylaxis is strongly recommended (38). Studies of Western populations have shown that DVT rates range from 15% to 30% for cancer patients not receiving thromboembolic prophylaxis, and a meta-analysis by Colditz et al. estimated fatal PE rates of 0.1%-0.8% (39,40). Colorectal surgery is associated with a specific high risk of postoperative thromboembolic complications relative to other general surgery (41-43). The incidences of DVT and PE in colorectal cancer surgery patients who do not receive thromboembolic prophylaxis are approximately 40% and 5%, respectively (42-43). Moreover, late VTE rates of 10%- 20% have been reported in patients who received LMWH thromboprophylaxis in the first postoperative week (44).

The randomized double-blind ENOXACAN II study, and the multicenter randomized Denmark/Norway study found that thromboprophylaxis for 4 weeks after abdominal or pelvic cancer surgery reduced the incidence of venographically demonstrated asymptomatic thrombosis (45-46). In those studies, the rate of asymptomatic thrombosis was 5%–7% after prolonged prophylaxis. Although the majority of asymptomatic DVT is not clinically significant, there is an association between asymptomatic DVT and the subsequent development of symptomatic VTE (47). In most studies, the ratio of asymptomatic DVT to symptomatic VTE ranges from 5:1 to 10:1. If a ratio of 10:1 is applied, the incidence of symptomatic DVT is approximately 0.5%–0.7% after prolonged thromboprophylaxis (4 weeks), similar to that found in the present study (0.63%). It shows the comparable incidence with that of Western countries, although in the present study thromboprophylaxis was administered only to high-risk patients and the treatment was of much shorter duration (median 3 days) and at a lower dose than that reported in those other studies.

Venous thromboembolism is a common complication in cancer patients due to the hypercoagulable state induced by changes in the coagulation system (48). A prothrombotic state is present in many cancer patients as a result of an increase in procoagulants, such as tissue factor, cancer procoagulant, and factor VIIa, and hypercoaguability increases as the cancer progresses (49,50). Patients with metastatic cancers are at an increased risk of VTE. Several studies have shown a direct association between cancer stage and thrombosis risk. Recent studies showed that a higher initial cancer stage was a strong independent risk factor for developing VTE within the first year after diagnosis of cancer (51). In the Korean study, multivariate analysis showed metastatic colorectal cancer (stage IV) was found a predictor of VTE. Moreover, advanced colorectal cancer (stage III, IV) was also a predictor of VTE, and patients with advanced cancer were twice as likely to be diagnosed with VTE as patients with less-advanced cancer (52).

4. Anticoagulant use in renal insufficiency

Renal clearance is the primary mode of elimination for several anticoagulants, including LMWH, fondaparinux, and the new oral factor Xa and Ha inhibitors. Therefore, with reduced renal function, these drugs may accumulate and may increase the risk of bleeding, particularly in elderly patients and those at high risk for bleeding (53). The relationship between renal impairment and drug accumulation for the various LMWHs appears to be variable and may be related to the chain length distribution of the different LMWH preparations (54). Two recent studies in hospitalized patients, the majority of whom were critically ill and had creatinine clearances less than 30 mL/min, have shown no bioaccumulation of dalteparin 5000 U once daily based on serial anti-factor Xa levels (55,56). Therefore, we do not reduce the prophylaxis dose of dalteparin in patients with renal insufficiency. In patients receiving intermittent hemodialy-sis, we suggest that the LMWH be administered after the dialysis session. With enoxaparin thromboprophylaxis, we suggest that 30 mg once daily be used. We also suggest that fondaparinux, rivaroxaban and dabigatran be avoided unless future evidence demonstrates that these agents can be used safely in patients with severe renal insufficiency.

5. Concomitant use of regional anesthesia techniques and anticoagulant prophylaxis

Neuraxial blockade (spinal or epidural anesthesia and continuous epidural analgesia) results in a significant reduction in cardiopulmonary morbidity compared with general anesthesia and narcotic-based systemic analgesia, as well as better pain control and patient satisfaction (57). However, concerns have been raised about a possible increased risk of epidural or spinal hematoma and spinal cord ischemia or paraplegia with use of concomitant anticoagulant prophylaxis (58,59).We believe that anticoagulant thromboprophylaxis with LMWH or LDH can safely be given along with neuraxial blockade with proper patient selection and timing of doses. Further details can be found in Section 1.5 of the 8th ACCP Prevention of VTE guidelines(3). In summary:

1. Neuraxial blockade should be avoided in patients with systemic bleeding disorders and if hemostasis is impaired by an anticoagulant. The spinal needle or epidural catheter should be inserted at a time when there is minimal or no anticoagulant effect present.
2. Anticoagulant prophylaxis should be delayed if a hemorrhagic aspirate ("bloody tap") is encountered during initial needle or catheter placement.
3. Removal of an epidural catheter should be done when the anticoagulant effect is at a minimum (usually just before the next scheduled injection) and anticoagulant prophylaxis should be delayed for at least 2 hours after spinal needle or epidural catheter removal.
4. In patients with an indwelling epidural catheter, we suggest that warfarin be avoided altogether or that the catheter be removed less than 48 hours after starting warfarin because of its unpredictable anticoagulant effect.
5. The safety of continuous epidural analgesia with concomitant administration of fondaparinux or one of the new oral anticoagulants is not known and this combination is best avoided at this time.
6. Patients with epidural catheters who are given anticoagulant thromboprophylaxis should be carefully monitored for symptoms and signs of spinal cord compression. If spinal hematoma is suspected, diagnostic imaging and surgical decompression should be performed rapidly to reduce the risk of permanent spinal cord damage.
7. Every hospital using neuraxial blockade along with anticoagulant prophylaxis should develop a written protocol.
8. For patients receiving deep peripheral nerve blocks along with anticoagulant prophylaxis, it is reasonable to use the same cautions described above.

6. Trauma

Deep venous thrombosis DVT and pulmonary embolism are among the most common preventable sources of mortality and morbidity in trauma patients treated in intensive care units. In various studies, DVT and PE have been demonstrated to range from 6%to 40% and from2%to 22%, respectively, in patients with serious spinal/head trauma (5, 6, 60-62). Knudson et al. and Geerts et al. reported that in trauma patients other than the ones with head trauma LMWH was better than unfractionated heparin for DVT prophylaxis (61,62). Vanek, with a metaanalysis, showed that intermittent pneumatic compression (IPC) decreased the relative risk of DVT by 62%, 47%, and 48% compared to placebo, high-pressure stockings, and LMWH, respectively (63). Norwood et al. reported that enoxaparin for DVT prophylaxis in patients with acute brain injury having an Abbreviated Injury Score of > 3 did not increase the morbidity (64). Early use of LMWH for DVT prophylaxis in the presence of intraabdominal solid organ injury (liver, spleen, kidney) may also be safe (6, 61). A properly placed and managed intermittent pneumatic compression device could provide thromboprophylaxis of comparable efficacy to that of LMWH, in patients with moderate and severe injury (65).

7. Laparoscopic surgery

The expanding use of laparoscopy last 3 decades has profoundly changed surgical diagnosis and therapy. However there is still some controversy over the best practice for prevention of deep vein thrombosis (DVT) during laparoscopic surgery. There is considerable uncertainty related to the thromboembolic risk after laparoscopic procedures, and the use of thromboprophylaxis is controversial. Surgical trauma is generally less with laparoscopic than with open abdominal surgery, but activation of the coagulation system is similar to or only slightly less with laparoscopic procedures. Laparoscopic operations may be associated with longer surgical times than comparable open procedures. Both pneumoperitoneum and the reverse Trendelenburg position reduce venous return from the legs, creating venous stasis. Patients undergoing laparoscopic procedures may have shorter hospital stays, but they may not mobilize more rapidly at home than those who have had open procedures.

Despite the paucity of evidence, the European Association for Endoscopic Surgery has recom mended that intraoperative IPC be used for all prolonged laparoscopic procedures (66). In 2006, the Society of American Gastrointestinal Endoscopic Surgeons recommended the use of similar thromboprophylaxis options for laparoscopic procedures as for the equivalent open surgical procedures (67). However, available evidence does not support a recommendation for the routine use of thromboprophylaxis in these patients (68,69,70). Furthermore, with anticoagulant thromboprophylaxis, the risk of major bleeding may exceed the rate of thrombotic complications(71). Patients who are at particularly high thromboembolic risk can be considered for thromboprophylaxis with any of the modalities currently recommended for surgical patients (3,72).

8. Treatment of VTE

Treatment for VTE has been widely studied, and treatment guidelines have been published and frequently updated by the American College of Chest Physicians (ACCP), American College of Emergency Physicians, Eastern Association for the Surgery of Trauma, and Institute for Clinical Systems Improvement(1,3). Generally, acute treatment consists of low-molecular-weight heparin (LMWH) or unfractionated heparin (UFH) for 4 to 5 days, with overlapping therapy to warfarin until an international normalized ratio (INR) of >2 for two consecutive days is achieved. Anticoagulation should be continued for at least 3 to 12 months, depending on the site of thrombosis and risk factors. Failure to provide adequate VTE treatment can result in patient morbidity and mortality, with a substantial economic burden(73). Although the evidence and consensus strongly favor LMWH treatment for up to 6 months in patients with cancer with established VTE, evidence is lacking to support continuing treatment beyond 6 months. It is likely that anticoagulation can be safely discontinued in certain patients (eg, patients who developed a VTE while on adjuvant chemotherapy and are in complete remission withnoplans for further treatment). Conversely, certain patients will continue to be at risk for recurrent VTE (eg, a patient with cancer with metastatic disease with plans for indefinite chemotherapy). Data from well-designed randomized clinical trials are essential for clinicians to make evidencebased recommendations in these varied settings.

Activation of the hemostatic system promotes tumor growth, angiogenesis, and metastasis. Antithrombotic agents could therefore potentially influence tumor biology and outcomes in patients with cancer. Multiple recent studies have evaluated the effect of anticoagulants on survival, with encouraging but inconclusive results (74). Given that anticoagulant prophylaxis could have dual benefits for patients with cancer reducing VTE and prolonging survival it is vital to pursue well-designed clinical trials of thromboprophylaxis focusing on survival(75).

9. Appendix

An informative summary from American College of Chest Physicians Evidence-Based Clinical Practice Prevention of Venous Thromboembolism Guidelines (8th Edition)(3).

10. Guyatt grading(76)

Grade 1 recommendations are strong and indicate that the benefits do or do not outweigh risks, burden, and costs.
Grade 2 suggestions imply that individual patient values may lead to different choices

11. General surgery

- For low-risk general surgery patients who are undergoing minor procedures and have no additional thromboembolic risk factors, ACCP recommend against the use of specific thromboprophylaxis other than early and frequent ambulation (Grade 1A).
- For moderate-risk general surgery patients who are undergoing a major procedure for benign disease, patients should receive thromboprophylaxis with LMWH, LDUH, or fondaparinux (each Grade 1A).
- For higher-risk general surgery patients who are undergoing a major procedure for cancer, patient should receive thromboprophylaxis with LMWH, LDUH three times daily, or fondaparinux (each Grade 1A).
- For general surgery patients with multiple risk factors for VTE who are thought to be at particularly high risk, AACP recommend that a pharmacologic method *(ie,* LMWH, LDUH three times daily, or fondaparinux) be combined with the optimal use of a mechanical method (te, graduated compression stockings [GCS] and/or IPC) [Grade 1C].
- For general surgery patients with a high risk of bleeding, optimal use of mechanical thromboprophylaxis with properly fitted GCS or IPC is best method (Grade 1A). When the high bleeding risk decreases, we recommend that pharmacologic thromboprophylaxis be substituted for or added to the mechanical thromboprophylaxis (Grade 1C).
- For patients undergoing major general surgical procedures, we recommend that thromboprophylaxis continue until discharge from hospital (Grade 1A). For selected high-risk general surgery patients, including some of those who have undergone major cancer surgery or have previously had VTE, ACCP suggest that continuing thromboprophylaxis after hospital discharge with LMWH for up to 28 days be considered (Grade 2A).

12. Cancer patients

- For cancer patients undergoing surgical procedures, ACCP recommend routine thromboprophylaxis that is appropriate for the type of surgery (Grade 1A). Refer to the recommendations in the relevant surgical subsections. 7.0.2. For cancer patients who are bedridden with an acute medical illness, ACCP recommend routine thromboprophylaxis as for other high-risk medical patients (Grade 1A). Refer to the recommendations in Section 6.0. 7.0.3. For cancer patients with indwelling central venous catheters, ACCP recommend that clinicians not use either prophylactic doses of LMWH (Grade IB), or minidose warfarin (Grade IB) to try to prevent catheter-related thrombosis.

- For cancer patients receiving chemotherapy or hormonal therapy, ACCP recommend against the routine use of thromboprophylaxis for the primary prevention of VTE (Grade 1C). 7.0.5. For cancer patients, ACCP recommend against the routine use of primary thromboprophylaxis to try to improve survival (Grade IB).

13. Laparoscopic surgery

- For patients undergoing entirely laparoscopic procedures who do not have additional thromboembolic risk factors, routine use of thromboprophylaxis is unneccessary. Early and frequent ambulation should be forced (Grade 1B).
- For patients undergoing laparoscopic procedures in whom additional VTE risk factors are present, ACCP recommend the use of thromboprophylaxis with one or more of LMWH, LDUH, fondaparinux, IPC, or GCS (all Grade 1C).

14. Trauma

- For all major trauma patients, ACCP recommend routine thromboprophylaxis if possible (Grade 1A).
- For major trauma patients, in the absence of a major contraindication, ACCP recommend that clinicians use LMWH thromboprophylaxis starting as soon as it is considered safe to do so (Grade 1A). An acceptable alternative is the combination of LMWH and the optimal use of a mechanical method of thromboprophylaxis (Grade IB).
- For major trauma patients, if LMWH thromboprophylaxis is contraindicated due to active bleeding or high risk for clinically important bleeding, we recommend that mechanical thromboprophylaxis with IPC or possibly with GCS alone be used (Grade IB). When the high bleeding risk decreases, we recommend that pharmacologic thromboprophylaxis be substituted for or added to the mechanical thromboprophylaxis (Grade 1C).
- In trauma patients, ACCP recommend against routine DUS screening for asymptomatic deep vein thrombosis (DVT) (Grade IB). We do recommend DUS screening in patients who are at high risk for VTE (eg, in the presence of a spinal cord injury [SCI], lower-extremity or pelvic fracture, or major head injury), and who have received suboptimal thromboprophylaxis or no thromboprophylaxis (Grade 1C).
- For trauma patients, ACCP recommend against the use of an inferior vena cava (IVC) filter as thromboprophylaxis (Grade 1C).
- For major trauma patients, ACCP recommend the continuation of thromboprophylaxis until hospital discharge (Grade 1C). For trauma patients with impaired mobility who

undergo inpatient rehabilitation, ACCP suggest continuing thromboprophylaxis with LMWH or a VKA (target INK, 2.5; range, 2.0 to 3.0) (Grade 2C).

15. References

[1] Geerts WH, Pineo GF, Heit JA, et al. Prevention of venous thromboembolism: the Seventh ACCP Conference on Antithrombotic and Thrombolytic Therapy. Chest 2004; 126: 338S–400S

[2] National Institute for Health and Clinical Excellence. Reducing the risk of venous thromboembolism (deep vein thrombosis and pulmonary embolism) in inpatients undergoing surgery. NICE clinical guideline No. 46:1–160. Available at: http://www.nice.org.uk/CG046.

[3] Geerts WH, Bergqvist D, Pineo GF, Heit JA, Samama CM, Lassen MR, Colwell CW. Prevention of venous thromboembolism: American College of Chest Physicians Evidence-Based Clinical Practice Guidelines (8th Edition). Chest. 2008 Jun;133(6 Suppl):381S-453S.

[4] Selby R, Geerts W. Prevention of venous thromboembolism: consensus, controversies, and challenges. Hematology Am Soc Hematol Educ Program. 2009:286-92. Review.

[5] Serin K, Yanar H, Ozdenkaya Y, Tuğrul S, Kurtoğlu M. Venous thromboembolism prophylaxis methods in trauma and emergency surgery intensive care unit patients: low molecular weight heparin versus elastic stockings + intermittent pneumatic compression]. Ulus Travma Acil Cerrahi Derg 2010;16 (2):130-134

[6] Kurtoglu M, Yanar H, Bilsel Y, Guloglu R, Kizilirmak S, Buyukkurt D, Granit V, Ulus Travma Acil Cerrahi Derg. 2010 Mar;16(2):130-4. Venous thromboembolism prophylaxis after head and spinal trauma: intermittent pneumatic compression devices versus low molecular weight heparin. World J Surg. 2004 Aug;28(8):807-11.

[7] Khorana AA: Malignancy, thrombosis and Trousseau: The case for an eponym. J Thromb Haemost 1:2463-2465, 2003

[8] Falanga A: The incidence and risk of venous thromboembolism associated with cancer and nonsurgical cancer treatment. Cancer Invest 27:105-115, 2009

[9] Khorana AA, Francis CW, Culakova E, et al: Frequency, risk factors, and trends for venous thromboembolism among hospitalized cancer patients. Cancer 110:2339-2346, 2007

[10] Khorana AA, Francis CW, Culakova E, et al: Thromboembolism is a leading cause of death in cancer patients receiving outpatient chemotherapy. J Thromb Haemost 5:632-634, 2007

[11] Sorensen HT, Mellemkjaer L, Olsen JH, et al: Prognosis of cancers associated with venous thromboembolism. N Engl J Med 343:1846-1850, 2000

[12] Chew HK, Wun T, Harvey D, et al: Incidence of venous thromboembolism and its effect on survival among patients with common cancers. Arch Intern Med 166:458-464, 2006

[13] Prandoni P, Lensing AW, Piccioli A, et al: Recurrent venous thromboembolism and bleeding complications during anticoagulant treatment in patients with cancer and venous thrombosis. Blood 100:3484-3488, 2002

[14] Elting LS, Escalante CP, Cooksley C, et al: Outcomes and cost of deep venous thrombosis among patients with cancer. Arch Intern Med 164: 1653-1661, 2004

[15] Zangari M, Barlogie B, Anaissie E, et al: Deep vein thrombosis in patients with multiple myeloma treated with thalidomide and chemotherapy: Effects of prophylactic and therapeutic anticoagulation. Br J Haematol 126: 715-721, 2004

[16] Nalluri SR, Chu D, Keresztes R, et al: Risk of venous thromboembolism with the angiogenesis inhibitor bevacizumab in cancer patients: A metaanalysis. JAMA 300:2277-2285, 2008

[17] Sousou T, Khorana A. Identifying cancer patients at risk for venous thromboembolism. *Hamostaseologie.* 2009:29:121-124.

[18] Aki EA, Rohilla S, Barba M, et al. Anticoagulation for the initial treatment of venous thromboembolism in patients with cancer. *Cochrane Database SystRev.* 2008 Jan 23;(1):CD006649.

[19] Lee A, Levine M. The thrombophilic state induced by therapeutic agents in the cancer patient. *Semin Thromb Hemost.* 1999;25:137-145.

[20] Deitcher SR. Cancer and thrombosis: mechanisms and treatment. *J Thromb Thrombolysis.* 2003:16:21-31.

[21] Sorensen H, Mellemkjaer L, Steffensen F, et al. The risk of a diagnosis of cancer after primary deep venous thrombosis or pulmonary embolism. *N EnglJMed.* 1998:338:1169-1173.

[22] Prandoni P, Lensing A, Buller HR, et al. Deep-vein thrombosis and the incidence of subsequent symptomatic cancer. *N EnglJMed.* 1992:327:1128-1133.

[23] Levitan N, Dowlati A, Remick S, et al. Rates of initial and recurrent thromboembolic disease among patients with malignancy versus those without malignancy. *Medicine.* 1999:78:285-291.

[24] Heit JA, Silverstein MD, Mohr DN, et al. Risk factors for deep vein thrombosis and pulmonary embolism: a population-based case-control study. *Arch Intern Med.* 2000:160:809-815.

[25] Huerta C, Johansson S, Wallander MA, Garcia Rodriguez LA. Risk factors and short-term mortality of venous thromboembolism diagnosed in the primary-care setting in the United Kingdom. *Arch Intern Med.* 2007:167:935-943.

[26] Clagett GP, Reisch JS. Prevention of venous thromboembolism in general surgical patients. Results of meta-analysis. *AnnSurg.* 1988:208:227-240.

[27] Mousa SA. Low-molecular-weight heparins in thrombosis and cancer: emerging links. *Cardiovasc Drug Rev.* 2004:22:121-134.

[28] Prandoni P, Lensing AW, Cogo A, et al. The long-term clinical course of acute deep venous thrombosis. *Ann Intern Med.* 1996:125:1-7.

[29] Heit JA, Silverstein MD, Mohr DN, et al. Predictors of survival after deep vein thrombosis and pulmonary embolism: a population-based, cohort study. *Arch Intern Med.* 1999:159:445-453.

[30] Sorensen HT, Mellemkjaer L, Olsen JH, Baron JA. Prognosis of cancers associated with venous thromboembolism. *N EnglJMed.* 2000:343:1846-1850.

[31] Martino MA, Williamson E, Siegfried S, et al. Diagnosing pulmonary embolism: experience with spiral CT pulmonary angiography in gynecologic oncology. *Gynecol Oncol.* 2005:98:289-293.

[32] Lee AY, Levine MN. Venous thromboembolism and cancer: risks and outcomes. *Circulation.* 2003:107(23 suppl 1):I17-I21.

[33] Kakkar AK, Levine M, Pinedo HM, et al. Venous thrombosis in cancer patients: insights from the FRONTLINE survey. *Oncologist.* 2003:8:381-388.

[34] Lyman GH, Khorana AA, Falanga A, et al. American Society of Clinical Oncology Guideline: recommendations for venous thromboembolism prophylaxis and treatment in patients with cancer. *J Clin Oncol.* 2007:25:5490-5505.

[35] *NCCN Clinical Practice Guidelines in Oncology™ Venous Thromboembolic Disease.* V2.2008. Copyright 2008 by the National Comprehensive Cancer Network. Available at: http://www.nccn.org/professionals/physician_gls/PDF/vte.pdf.

[36] Amin A, Stemkowski S, Lin J, Yang G. Appropriate thromboprophylaxis in hospitalized cancer patients. *Clin Adv Hematol Oncol.* 2008;6(12):910-920.

[37] Alcalay A, Wun T, Khatri V, Chew HK, Harvey D, Zhou H, White RH. Venous thromboembolism in patients with colorectal cancer: incidence and effect on survival. J Clin Oncol. 2006;24(7):1112-8.

[38] Geerts WH, Bergqvist D, Pineo GF et al (2008) Prevention of venous thromboembolism: American College of Chest Physicians Evidence-Based Clinical Practice Guidelines (8th Edition). Chest 133:381S–453S

[39] Colditz GA, Tuden RL, Oster G (1986) Rates of venous thrombosis after general surgery: combined results of randomised clinical trials. Lancet 2:143–146

[40] Denstman F, Lowry A, Vernava A et al (2000) Practice parameters for the prevention of venous thromboembolism. The Standards Task Force of the American Society of Colon and Rectal Surgeons. Dis Colon Rectum 43:1037–1047

[41] Torngren S, Rieger A (1982) Prophylaxis of deep venous thrombosis in colorectal surgery. Dis Colon Rectum 25:563–566

[42] Huber O, Bounameaux H, Borst F et al (1992) Postoperative pulmonary embolism after hospital discharge. An underestimated risk. Arch Surg 127:310–313

[43] McLeod RS (1996) The risk of thromboembolism in patients undergoing colorectal surgery. Drugs 52(Suppl 7):38–41

[44] Rasmussen MS (2002) Preventing thromboembolic complications in cancer patients after surgery: a role for prolonged thromboprophylaxis. Cancer Treat Rev 28:141–144

[45] Rasmussen MS, Jorgensen LN, Wille-Jorgensen P et al (2006) Prolonged prophylaxis with dalteparin to prevent late thromboembolic complications in patients undergoing major abdominal surgery: a multicenter randomized open-label study. J Thromb Haemost 4:2384–2390

[46] Bergqvist D, Agnelli G, Cohen AT et al (2002) Duration of prophylaxis against venous thromboembolism with enoxaparin after surgery for cancer. N Engl J Med 346:975–980

[47] Mismetti P, Laporte S, Darmon JY et al (2001) Meta-analysis of low molecular weight heparin in the prevention of venous thromboembolism in general surgery. Br J Surg 88:913–930

[48] Anderson FA Jr, Spencer FA (2003) Risk factors for venous thromboembolism. Circulation 107:I-9–I-16

[49] Johnson MJ, Walker ID, Sproule MW et al (1999) Abnormal coagulation and deep venous thrombosis in patients with advanced cancer. Clin Lab Haematol 21: 51–54

[50] Sampson MT, Kakkar AK (2002) Coagulation proteases and human cancer. Biochem Soc Trans 30:201–207

[51] Alcalay A, Wun T, Khatri V et al (2006) Venous thromboembolism in patients with colorectal cancer: incidence and effect on survival. J Clin Oncol 24:1112–1118

[52] Yang SS, Yu CS, Yoon YS, Yoon SN, Lim SB, Kim JC.Symptomatic venous thromboembolism in Asian colorectal cancer surgery patients. World J Surg. 2011 Apr;35(4):881-7.

[53] Lim W, Dentali F, Eikelboom JW, Crowther MA. Metaanalysis: low-molecular-weight heparin and bleeding in patients with severe renal insufficiency. Ann Intern Med. 2006;144:673-684.

[54] Mahé I, Aghassarian M, Drouet L, et al. Tinzaparin and enoxaparin given at prophylactic dose for eight days in medical elderly patients with impaired renal function: a comparative pharmacokinetic study. Thromb Haemost. 2007;97:581-586.

[55] Douketis J, Cook D, Meade M, et al. Prophylaxis against deep vein thrombosis in critically ill patients with severe renal insufficiency with the low-molecularweight heparin dalteparin: an assessment of safety and pharmacodynamics: the DIRECT study. Arch Intern Med. 2008;168:1805-1812.

[56] Schmid P, Brodmann D, Fischer AG, Wuillemin WA. Study of bioaccumulation of dalteparin at a prophylactic dose in patients with various degrees of impaired renal function. J Thromb Haemost. 2009;7:552-558.

[57] Wu CL, Cohen SR, Richman JM, et al. Efficacy of postoperative patient-controlled and continuous infusion epidural analgesia versus intravenous patientcontrolled analgesia with opioids: a meta-analysis. Anesthesiology. 2005;103:1079-1088.

[58] Horlocker TT, Wedel DJ, Benzon H, et al. Regional anesthesia in the anticoagulated patient: defining the risks (the second ASRA Consensus Conference on Neuraxial Anesthesia and Anticoagulation). Reg Anesth Pain Med. 2003;28:172-197.

[59] Moen V, Dahlgren N, Irestedt L. Severe neurological complications after central neuraxial blockades in Sweden 1990-1999. Anesthesiology. 2004; 101: 950-959.

[60] Kurtoglu M, Buyukkurt CD, Kurtoglu M, et al. Venous thromboembolism prophylaxis with low molecular weight heparin in polytraumatized patients in intensive care unit (extended series). Ulus Travma Derg. 2003;9:37–44

[61] Knudson MM, Lewis FR, Clinton A, et al. Prevention of thromboembolism in trauma patients. J Trauma 1994;37:480–487

[62] Geerts WH, Jay RM, Code KI, et al.Acomparison of low-dose heparin with low molecular weight heparin as prophylaxis against venous thromboembolism after major trauma. N Engl J Med. 1996;335:701- 707

[63] Vanek VW. Meta-analysis of effectiveness of intermittent pneumatic compression devices with a comparison of thigh-high to knee-high sleeves. Am. Surg. 1998;64:1050–1058

[64] Norwood SH, McAuley CE, Berne JD, et al. Prospective evaluation of the safety of enoxaparin prophylaxis for venous thromboembolism in patients with intracranial hemorrhagic injuries. Arch. Surg. 2002;137: 696–702

[65] Ginzburg E, Cohn SM, Lopez J, Jackowski J, Brown M, Hameed SM; Miami Deep Vein Thrombosis Study Group. Randomized clinical trial of intermittent pneumatic compression and low molecular weight heparin in trauma. Br J Surg. 2003 Nov;90(11):1338-44.

[66] Neudecker J, Sauerland S, Neugebauer E, et al. The European Association for Endoscopic Surgery clinical practice guideline on the pneumoperitoneum for laparoscopic surgery. Surg Endosc 2002; 16:1121-1143

[67] Dabrowiecki S, Rose D, Jurkowski P. The influence of laparoscopic cholecystectomy on perioperative blood clotting and fibrinolysis. Blood Coagul Fibrinol 1997; 8:1-5

[68] Ljungstrom KG. Is there a need for antithromboembolic prophylaxis during laparoscopic surgery? Not always. J Thromb Haemost 2005; 3:212-213

[69] Blake AM, Toker SI, Dunn E. Deep venous thrombosis prophylaxis is not indicated for laparoscopic cholecystec-tomy. J Soc Laparosc Surg 2001; 5:215-219

[70] Bergqvist D, Lowe G. Venous thromboembolism in patients undergoing laparoscopic and arthroscopic surgery and in leg casts. Arch Intern Med 2002; 162:2173-2176

[71] Montgomery JS, Wolf JS. Venous thrombosis prophylaxis for urological laparoscopy: fractionated heparin versus sequential compression devices. J Urol 2005; 173:1623-1626

[72] Caprini JA, Arcelus JI, Laubach M, et al. Postoperative hypercoagulability and deep-vein thrombosis after laparoscopic cholecystectomy. Surg Endosc 1995; 9:304-309

[73] Caprini JA, Botteman MF, Stephens JM, Nadipelli V, Ewing MM, Brandt S, et al. Economic burden of long-term complications of deep vein thrombosis after total hip replacement surgery in the United States. Value Health 2003; 6:59-74.

[74] Kuderer NM, Khorana AA, Lyman GH, et al: Ameta-analysis and systematic review of the efficacyand safety of anticoagulants as cancer treatment:Impact on survival and bleeding complications. Cancer 110:1149-1161, 2007

[75] Khorana AA, Streiff MB, Farge D, Mandala M, Debourdeau P, Cajfinger F, Marty M, Falanga A, Lyman GH. Venous Thromboembolism Prophylaxis and Treatment in Cancer: A Consensus Statement of Major Guidelines Panels and Call to Action. J Clin Oncol. 2009;27(29): 4919–4926.

[76] Guyatt G, Schünemann HJ, Cook D, Jaeschke R, Pauker S. Applying the grades of recommendation for antithrombotic and thrombolytic therapy: the Seventh ACCP Conference on Antithrombotic and Thrombolytic Therapy. Chest. 2004 Sep;126(3 Suppl):179S-187S.

Part 5

Special Issues

11

Heparin-Induced Thrombocytopenia

Kelly L. Cervellione and Craig A. Thurm
Jamaica Hospital Medical Center, Jamaica, New York, USA

1. Introduction

Heparin-induced thrombocytopenia (HIT) is an immune-mediated response to heparin administration that causes thrombocytopenia and a prothrombotic state. Heparin is the most commonly used anticoagulant drug for the prevention and treatment of thromboembolic diseases in hospitalized patients. Heparin exists in two main forms, pure unfractionated heparin (UFH) and low molecular weight heparin (LMWH), which is derived from UFH. Though HIT is relatively rare, occurring in less than 5% of patients receiving UFH and less than 1% of patients receiving LMWH, it has the potential to cause significant morbidity and mortality. The main complication of HIT is thrombosis, most commonly deep vein thrombosis (DVT) or pulmonary embolism (PE). More rarely HIT can manifest as occlusion of a limb artery, acute myocardial infarct, stroke, a systemic reaction or skin necrosis. In the current chapter the topic of HIT will be reviewed in terms of its pathophysiology, diagnosis, and treatment.

1.1 *Clinical Vignette: Patient S-B*

S-B is a 48-year-old male who was admitted to the orthopedics service for surgical repair of a right acetabular fracture resulting from a fall. He had no significant past medical history. His course was complicated by an ileus. He was given enoxaparin for thromboprophylaxis starting on day 2 of admission. During his hospital stay, he developed a pulmonary embolus and atrial fibrillation and the dose of enoxaparin was increased. An IVC filter was also placed. His platelet count dropped from 278K/uL on admission to a low of 88K/uL on hospital day 10. HIT antibody was positive. Enoxaparin was discontinued and lepirudin was started. Platelet count began improving by the next day and was 190K/uL two days after starting lepirudin. He was transitioned to warfarin. A PICC line was placed for parenteral nutrition as his ileus had not resolved.

Several days later, the patient suddenly developed shortness of breath, chest pain, nausea and fever of 102°F. His heart rate increased to 130; he was normotensive. An arterial blood gas revealed metabolic acidosis and hypoxemia; his lactate level was elevated. Chest x-ray showed no infiltrates and a CT pulmonary angiogram (CTPA) was negative for infiltrates, pulmonary emboli and other pathology. EKG showed sinus tachycardia. Antibiotics were begun for possible sepsis. Platelet count was found to be 114K/uL compared to 231K/uL the previous day. Review of his chart revealed that the patient had received heparin flushes of his PICC line as part of a standing protocol. Heparin flushes were discontinued and lepirudin was restarted. Over the next several hours his fever, tachycardia, and hypoxemia improved. His lactate level normalized and platelets rose to 160K/uL by the following morning. All cultures were negative and antibiotics were discontinued.

2. Pathophysiology

Heparin is a negatively-charged, highly sulfated glycosaminoglycan that occurs naturally in the body. It was discovered nearly one century ago (Howell & Holt, 1918) and shortly thereafter was used in the medical profession for thromboprophylaxis in post-operative patients (Crafoord, 1936). Amongst the qualities that made it an attractive option for physicians were its immediate onset of action and its short half-life. During the first three decades of its use in the medical field, case reports and series of patients developing thrombosis while on heparin began to emerge in the literature, a phenomenon known as HIT (e.g. Weismann & Tobin, 1958; Roberts et al., 1963). Over the last several decades much has been learned about heparin and the mechanisms that are responsible for this disorder.

Physiologically, two types of thrombocytopenia due to heparin exposure have been described. Non-immune heparin-associated thrombocytopenia, historically referred to as HIT type I, describes a response that is self-limiting and rarely causes major complications. Non-immune HIT occurs in 10% to 30% of patients who receive heparin and typically emerges within 4 days of exposure (Jang & Hursting, 2005). Platelet counts do not normally fall below 100K/uL. Heparin use does not need to be discontinued and no treatment is needed (Chong, 2003).

Currently the term HIT is used to denote what has been historically called HIT type 2. HIT occurs when, following heparin administration, platelet factor 4 (PF4) binds to heparin to form heparin/PF4 complexes. The body identifies these complexes as abnormal and, in response, develops antibodies. Specifically immunoglobulin G (IgG), M (IgM) and/or A (IgA) antibodies are formed. IgG is pathogenic, and binding of the IgG antibodies to the heparin/PF4 complexes results in platelet activation and aggregation. This causes thrombin generation, resulting in thrombotic events. Activated platelet aggregates are removed prematurely from circulation, which leads to development of thrombocytopenia, the main criteria for diagnosis of HIT (Warkentin et al., 1994a; Untch et al., 2002). The heparin/PF4 antibodies (also known as chemokine CXCL4) are typically activated within 5-14 days of heparin exposure, though delayed-onset cases have been reported (Warkentin & Kelton, 2001a). In patients who have a recent history of heparin use, however, significant platelet activation can occur more rapidly after reintroducing a heparin-containing product (Warkentin & Kelton, 2001b). This may be because HIT antibodies are transient and can remain in the body for up to four months after withdrawal of heparin (Lubenow et al., 2002).

Though the exact mechanisms of action are unclear, endothelial cells and monocytes also seem to play a role in the procoagulant state associated with HIT (Blank et al., 2002; Pouplard et al., 2001; Rauova et al., 2010; Arepally & Mayer, 2001). Many processes still remain unexplained in HIT, including the inability of some anti-heparin/PF4 IgG molecules to cause platelet activation (Warkentin, 2005) and the role of individual biological differences in predisposing to development of the disease. There is evidence that the length of the heparin molecule chain may positively correlate with the potential for HIT. Since LMWH's are formed from smaller molecules, this could explain why there is less immunogenic potential in these derived forms of heparin (Gruel et al., 2003). Furthermore, there may be a role of other glycosaminoglycans that are found on the surface of platelets, which may cross-react with heparin/PF4 antibodies and more directly cause thrombus formation (Rauova et al., 2006).

3. Clinical features

3.1 Epidemiology

Several factors have been identified as being associated with an increased risk of HIT. At the patient level, HIT has been more frequently reported in females (Warkentin et al., 2006) and in patients over 40 years of age (Stein et al., 2009). Patients on UFH have a higher likelihood of developing HIT than those on LMWH (Martel et al., 2005). Dosage is also an important factor; patients receiving therapeutic doses may be more likely to develop clinical manifestations of HIT than those receiving prophylactic doses (Dager & White, 2003). Patients receiving thromboprophylaxis with UFH for six or more days have a higher incidence of HIT than those receiving it for shorter periods (Martel et al., 2005; Smythe et al., 2007). Furthermore, the preparation type seems to influence risk; bovine UFH is more likely to cause HIT than porcine UFH (Green et al., 1984; Bailey et al., 1986; Francis et al., 2003).

In general, surgical patients are at a higher risk of developing HIT than medical patients (Warkentin et al., 2006), but there is variation in incidence between surgical types. Since HIT develops secondary to the formation of heparin/PF4 complexes, it would be logical to assume that patients with higher concentrations of circulating PF4 would be at greater risk, including patients undergoing cardiac surgery on cardiopulmonary bypass (Yoon & Jang, 2011). However, the incidence of HIT in these cardiac surgery patients is less than 3% (Warkentin et al,. 2000), whereas those who undergo orthopedic surgery, which is associated with less PF4 production, has incidence rates of HIT around 5% (Warkentin et al., 2003). The mechanism underlying this difference is not clearly understood, but evidence from data collected in trauma patients suggests a role of inflammatory processes in the development of heparin/PF4 complexes (Lubenow et al., 2010).

3.2 Timing

Thrombocytopenia secondary to HIT commonly occurs between 5 and 14 days after the onset of heparin therapy. Patients with recent heparin exposure (e.g. within 30 to 100 days) may develop a significant fall in platelets related to HIT more quickly, even within minutes of re-exposure (i.e. rapid-onset HIT) (Warkentin, 2004; Warkentin and Kelton, 2001b). This is likely due to the continued presence of antibodies from previous exposure (Warkentin and Kelton, 2001b; Lubenow et al., 2002). Conversely, there have been cases of HIT where symptoms do not manifest until 10-14 days or more after heparin withdrawal, a phenomenon known as delayed-onset HIT (Warkentin and Kelton, 2001a). This phenomenon is not completely understood. It is known that the anti-heparin/PF4 antibodies can remain in the system for 100 days or more following discontinuation of heparin therapy and that the antibody titers in patients who develop delayed-onset HIT are very high (Rice et al., 2002; Warkentin & Kelton, 2001a). There may be a role of cross-reactivity with other glycosaminoglycans residing on the surface of platelets, thus inducing platelet activation in the absence of heparin (Rauova et al., 2006).

3.3 Degree of thrombocytopenia

In the majority of patients with HIT the platelet count drops below 150K/uL, or falls to less than 50% of baseline. HIT may be overlooked when the platelet count remains above 100K/uL if prior values are not reviewed. The nadir platelet count in HIT typically does not fall below 20K/uL; if such an extensive drop is seen, alternate or additional diagnoses must be seriously considered (Warkentin, 1998). Generally the nadir platelet count in HIT is between 40 and 80K/uL (Greinacher et al., 2005).

3.4 Complications

Thrombosis occurs in 30% to 70% of cases of HIT, depending on the population, and can occur without the presence of significant thrombocytopenia (Warkentin, 2007). Thrombotic events may occur days prior to the onset of thrombocytopenia (Greinacher et al., 2005). In patients who develop a thrombotic event who are either on or have recently completed heparin therapy, the possibility of HIT should be considered (Levine et al., 2006). In addition, it is important to realize that small amounts of heparin, such as those used to perform heparin flushes, can also cause significant manifestations of HIT (Refaai et al., 2007).

When HIT is associated with thrombosis approximately 20-30% of cases are fatal and an additional 20-30% result in permanent disability (Greinacher, 1995). DVT (50%) and PE (25%) are the most common thrombotic events related to HIT. Arterial thrombosis, infrarenal aortic thrombosis (Karkos et al., 2011), acute myocardial infarct (Iqbal et al., 2007), cerebral ischemia (Meyer-Lindenberg et al., 1997), limb ischemia (Kreidy & Hatem, 2004), acute adrenal insufficiency (Poulain et al., 2008) and bilateral adrenal hemorrhage (Ernest & Fisher, 1991; Rosenberg et al., 2011) are less common. Skin lesions, which may or may not be necrotic, can be seen at the heparin injection site in 10% to 20% of patients who develop HIT (Jang et al., 2005). Skin lesions appear to be more common in patients with higher levels of platelet-activating IgG (Warkentin, 1996). Despite the presence of thrombocytopenia, bleeding complications related to HIT are uncommon (Selleng et al., 2007).

Systemic or anaphylactoid reactions can rapidly occur after an IV bolus of UFH. In addition to a marked decline in platelet count, patients may develop fever, chills, respiratory symptoms that may simulate a pulmonary embolus (Hartman et al., 2006; Popov et al., 1997), cardiac arrest, gastrointestinal symptoms such as nausea, vomiting and diarrhea, or even neurologic symptoms such as ischemia or transient global amnesia (Warkentin et al., 1994b; Warkentin & Greinacher, 2009). It is important to note that these reactions are due to the immune-mediated response to heparin therapy (Warkentin & Greinacher, 2009); additional cases of anaphylactic reactions due to contaminated or over-sulfated heparins also exist (Liu et al., 2009). This type of systemic reaction is illustrated in the clinical vignette at the beginning of the chapter.

In hemodialysis patients, a unique set of complications may emerge as a result of HIT. For example, there may be clotting of the extracorporeal circuit or failed arteriovenous fistulae. If an IV bolus of UFH or LMWH is given prior to hemodialysis and systemic reactions occur, it is important to consider HIT as a cause (Syed and Reilly, 2009). Increased circuit pressures, formation of a clot in the drip chambers, clotted dialyzer fibers, or an acute thrombocytopenia with at least a 20% decrease in platelet counts may also be suggestive of HIT (Yamamoto et al., 1996).

3.5 Alternative causes

Thrombocytopenia is frequently encountered in critically ill patients and can have a variety of etiologies. ICU patients often receive UFH or LMWH for either prophylaxis or treatment of venous thromboembolic disease or for treatment of a variety of other conditions, such as cardiac ischemia or atrial fibrillation. The question of HIT is therefore frequently raised (Sakr, 2011). However, HIT is actually an uncommon cause of thrombocytopenia in this patient population with an incidence of less than 1% (Crowther et al., 2010; Verma et al., 2003). Some more common causes of thrombocytopenia in critically ill patients include sepsis and infection, non-heparin drugs, disseminated intravascular coagulation (DIC), chronic liver disease, immune disorders, and pseudo-thrombocytopenia (Sakr, 2011; Rice et al., 2009). A list of drugs to consider when determining the cause of thrombocytopenia can be found in Table 1 Note that the Table does not include chemotherapeutic agents since most drugs in this class are well-known to cause thrombocytopenia. Serologic confirmation is often delayed for several days and physicians are forced to make decisions based on clinical judgment alone. Therefore, especially in very ill patients, close attention must be given to all possible causes of thrombocytopenia.

4. Diagnosis

Recent data from the CATCH (Complications After Thrombocytopenia Caused by Heparin) registry suggests that less than 10% of patients who develop thrombocytopenia receive a diagnostic evaluation for HIT (Oliveira et al., 2008). Furthermore, many do not receive diagnostic attention for possible HIT until after a thromboembolic event has occurred (Crespo et al., 2009). Given the potential for significant morbidity and mortality, timely diagnosis is of utmost importance. Diagnosis of HIT should be based on both clinical judgment and laboratory assessment. The patient's presentation and history provide the most important information for initial determination of likelihood of HIT, but verification of anti-heparin/PF4 antibodies through serum or plasma analysis is a significant step for guiding treatment and follow-up.

4.1 Clinical diagnosis

The Four T's (4T) score can be used to calculate the pre-test probability of HIT in patients experiencing signs or symptoms of the disorder (Warkentin & Heddle, 2003). The 4T score takes into account four domains and generates a score of 0–8 points depending on the patients' signs and symptoms; a total score of 0 to 3 indicates that HIT is unlikely; 4 to 5 indicates an intermediate probability; 6 to 8 indicates high likelihood of HIT. In addition to the severity of thrombocytopenia, the score also takes into account the timing of the fall in platelet count, the occurrence of thrombosis or other sequelae, and the presence of other potential causes of the thrombocytopenia. In general, studies have found that the 4T score has high sensitivity for diagnosis (>95%), but specificity is low, especially in ICU patients (Lo et al., 2006; Pouplard et al., 2007). Most authors suggest that those patients with a high likelihood of HIT based on 4T score should be immediately withdrawn from heparin therapy, be treated with an alternative, and be monitored closely while laboratory tests for HIT antibodies are performed. Withdrawal of heparin should not wait until laboratory results are obtained in any patient where HIT is being strongly considered.

Several other sets of criteria and scoring systems have been developed for determining pre-test probability of HIT in both general and specific populations (e.g. Messmore et al., 2011). The HIT Expert Probability Score has recently been developed based on a panel of expert opinions (Cuker et al., 2010), but data regarding its psychometric properties are still lacking. Scoring systems for patients on hemodialysis (Yamamoto et al., 1996) have been created owing to the unique factors associated with HIT in this population. It has also been noted that the use of some scoring systems, such as the 4T score, should be modified in the setting of a critically ill patient; in such cases more emphasis should be placed on ruling out other causes of thrombocytopenia (Hall et al., 2010).

Antibiotics	
Vancomycin	Penicillins
Cephalosporins	Ciprofloxacin
Clarithromycin	Pentamidine
Daptomycin	Meropenem
Rifampin	Linezolid
Nitrofurantoin	Ganciclovir
Fluconazole	Valganciclovir hydrochloride
Trimethoprim/sulfamethoxazole	
Glycoprotein IIb/IIIa inhibitors	
Abciximab	Eptifibatide
Tirofiban	
Thienopyridines	
Clopidogrel	Ticlopidine
Antiepileptics	
Phenytoin	Carbamazepine
Valproate	
Antiarrhythmics	
Procainamide	Amiodarone
Quinidines	
Anti-Inflammatory Drugs	
Salicylates	Acetaminophen
Nonsteroidal Anti-Inflammatory Drugs (NSAIDS)	
Diuretics	
Furosemide	Thiazides
Spironolactone	Acetazolamide
Histamine 2 Receptor Blockers	
Ranitidine	Cimetidine
Sulfonylurea Drugs	
Captopril	
Digoxin	
Morphine	
Haloperidol	

Table 1. Non-Chemotherapeutic Agents other than Heparin and Low Molecular Weight Heparin that may cause Thrombocytopenia in the Hospitalized Patient

4.2 Laboratory diagnosis

Both functional and immunologic assay tests are available for the detection of HIT antibodies. Functional tests work by detecting antibodies that induce heparin-dependant platelet activation whereas immunologic tests detect circulating anti-heparin/PF4 antibodies, regardless of their ability to activate platelets. Immunologic assays, such as polytypic ELISA, IgG-specific ELISA, and particle gel immunoassay (PGI) have a sensitivity of over 95%, but the specificity is sub-optimal and true positive diagnosis is identified in as few as half of all cases. Due to the pathogenicity of IgG, assays that are specific to this antibody are more likely to yield a true positive diagnosis than the general ELISA assays. Immunologic tests are relatively rapid, producing results within hours. Because of the high sensitivity and the fast turn-around, they are often used to rule-out HIT, but a positive test needs to be interpreted in conjunction with clinical data (Amiral, 1999; Amiral & Vissac, 1999). Mistakenly diagnosing and treating for HIT based on positive assay in the setting of a low pre-test probability score could result in serious consequences, such as venous limb gangrene or fatal hemorrhage (Smythe et al., 2011).

Functional assay tests, such as serotonin release assay (SRA), flow cytometric detection and heparin-induced platelet aggregation (HIPA) assay, have a slightly lower sensitivity (approximately 90%), but a much better specificity (>90%) than the immunologic assays. Therefore, the overall accuracy of the test for correctly identifying HIT is high (Warkentin, 2002). However, these tests are technically more demanding and are only offered at a minority of laboratories. Therefore, they are not relevant in most clinical settings.

The HemosIL AcuStar HIT-IgG (specific for IgG anti-PF4/heparin antibodies) and the HemosIL AcuStar HIT-Ab (for detecting IgG, IgA and IgM anti-PF4/heparin antibodies) are newer laboratory tests available for diagnosing HIT. These two semi-quantitative chemiluminescent immunoassays provide results in 30 minutes and can be run for single sample testing. Legnani and colleagues (2010) reported on initial data showing a 100% sensitivity and negative predictive value for these tests, making them ideal for ruling out HIT. Specificity for the HIT-IgG test was 96.5% and for the HIT-Ab test was 81.2%. These tests, especially the IgG specific test, may gain more use in the future depending on results of further studies.

A recent article advocates the use of a colorimetric test to detect HIT (Prechel et al., 2011). The test uses a tetrazolium-based indicator dye that reacts to the activity of platelets. When contact is made with inactivated or mildly activated platelets, the dye metabolizes to a dark color. When the platelets are highly activated (e.g. due to the presence of HIT antibodies) the dye is unable to metabolize and remains light in color. Preliminary analyses have shown this platelet activation assay test to have between 96% and 100% agreement with the functional assay C-SRA for HIT diagnosis.

In general, pairing the findings of a clinical diagnostic score with the results of a laboratory test significantly increases the sensitivity and specificity of the diagnostic yield (Demma et al., 2011; Ruf et al., 2011; Kim et al., 2011).

5. Treatment

When HIT is suspected or proven, all heparin and LMWH should be discontinued. A careful investigation for heparin exposure from sources such as catheter flushes and hemodialysis is necessary. Even the low doses used to flush a catheter can lead to worsening thrombocytopenia and a systemic reaction in patients with HIT, as in the case presented above. Once heparin therapy is discontinued, platelet count should begin to rise within three days, though this is dependent on the amount of antibodies present in the system (Seleng et al., 2007; Kelton, 2002).

There are several important principles in the management of HIT. The American College of Chest Physicians published evidenced-based clinical practice guidelines for the treatment and prevention of HIT in 2008 (Warkentin et al., 2008). Given the prothrombotic nature of the disorder, alternate, non-heparin anticoagulants should be administered. Just discontinuing UFH or LMWH or substituting warfarin (Coumadin®) is associated with a significant risk of thrombosis (Warkentin et al., 1998). As test results may take days to come back, treatment cannot wait until final confirmation of the diagnosis is made and should be instituted if the diagnosis is highly suspected.

For patients who develop a thrombotic event while on heparin or soon after discontinuing heparin, the platelet count should be checked and alternate non-heparin anticoagulants should be used until HIT is excluded.

Low molecular weight heparins, such as enoxaparin (Lovenox®) and dalteparin (Fragmin®) cannot be used in patients who develop HIT due to UFH as there may be cross-reactivity. The use of vitamin K antagonists such as warfarin is contraindicated during the acute phase of the illness when the patient is thrombocytopenic to avoid complications such as venous limb gangrene (Srinivasin, 2004; Warkentin et al., 1997) and multicentric skin necrosis (Warkentin et al., 1999). If the patient is on warfarin at the time HIT is diagnosed, Vitamin K should be administered. Platelet transfusions should generally be avoided, although there have been reports of their use without complication (Hopkins & Goldfinger, 2008; Refaai et al., 2010). IVC filters are not recommended during acute HIT (Warkentin et al., 2008). Ultrasound of the lower extremity can be considered as presence of DVT will affect the duration of anticoagulation (Tardy et al., 1999).

Choice of alternative, nonheparin anticoagulants include direct thrombin inhibitors (DTIs), such as argatroban and lepirudin (Refludan®), the heparinoid danaparoid (Orgaran®), and possibly the Xa inhibitor, fondaparinux (Arixtra®). Argatroban and lepirudin are approved for treatment of HIT in the United States. Danaproid has not been available in the United States since 2002. Choice of agent depends on a number of factors including availability and the presence of renal or hepatic dysfunction. An important difference between the DTIs is that argatroban is primarily hepatically eliminated, while lepirudin is primarily renally eliminated. The dose of argatroban should be reduced in the setting of liver dysfunction, congestive heart failure, anasarca, and after cardiac surgery. Lepirudin needs be adjusted for patients with renal insufficiency. Adjustments in the doses of these medications should be based on the aPTT. DTIs can elevate the INR and this can complicate the transition to warfarin when the thrombocytopenia has resolved.

Other DTI's have been utilized for the treatment of HIT. Bivalrudin is approved for patients with HIT or at risk for HIT undergoing percutaneous coronary intervention. It has also been used successfully in cardiac surgery. This agent undergoes enzymatic proteolysis and a minority is excreted renally. Desirudin, another DTI, showed promise as a more economical alternative to argatroban in a recent, small pilot study (Boyce et al., 2011). In addition, observational studies examining the role of desirudin in HIT in patients undergoing orthopedic and cardiac surgery have shown some positive results (Duncan et al., 2011; Levy & Koster, 2011). Desirudin is given subcutaneously every 12 hours as opposed to the other DTI's mentioned above, which are given as continuous intravenous infusions.

Factor Xa inhibitors make an attractive option for use in HIT. Fondaparinux can be given once a day subcutaneously. It costs less and requires less monitoring than the DTIs (monitoring of coagulation parameters to adjust dosing is not required). However, large randomized trials are lacking and it is not approved by the FDA for use in HIT. It has been used to successfully treat HIT (Lobo et al., 2008), though there have been case reports of worsening thrombocytopenia in patients with HIT or a history of HIT treated with fondaparinux (Pistulli et al., 2011; Warkentin et al., 2007; Modi et al., 2009; Rota et al., 2008). Newer Xa inhibitors such as Rivaroxiban that can be taken orally are becoming available, however their role in the treatment of HIT is not yet known.

For patients requiring longer term anticoagulation once the HIT has resolved, a transition to warfarin can be made. It should not be done until the platelet count has improved to at least 150K/uL and there should be an overlap of at least 5 days of warfarin and the non-heparin anticoagulant (Warkentin et al., 2008).

For patients who require anticoagulation with heparin and have a remote history of HIT, heparin can be used for a short duration when antibody assays are negative. Anti-heparin/PF4 antibodies are usually undetected by 100 days after discontinuation of heparin therapy (Warkentin & Kelton, 2001b). For those who are antibody positive, or those who need prolonged anticoagulation, a non-heparin alternative should be considered (Warkentin et al., 2008).

6. Conclusion

HIT is an important clinical entity to recognize as it creates a prothrombotic state that can lead to a variety of thromboembolic and systemic consequences. These most commonly include DVT and PE, though arterial thrombosis, acute myocardial infarction, stroke, acute adrenal insufficiency, and other serious complications can occur. Patients with HIT given an IV bolus of heparin may experience acute systemic reactions that can simulate pulmonary embolus or sepsis and even lead to cardiac arrest. Treatment includes discontinuation of all UFH and LMWH. A thorough search for surreptitious sources of heparin exposure should be performed. An alternative, non-heparin anticoagulant, such as a DTI should be started. HIT should be considered in patients who develop DVT or PE who are either receiving or have recently discontinued heparin. Intravenous heparin or LMWH should not be utilized to treat thrombosis in these situations. In the future, newer DTI's and possibly factor Xa inhibitors may simplify treatment and reduce cost in managing this condition.

7. References

Amiral, J. (1999). Antigens involved in heparin-induced thrombocytopenia. Seminars in Hematology, vol.36, no.1s1, (January 1999), pp.7-11.

Amiral, J., & Vissac, A.M. (1999). Generation and pathogenicity of anti=platelet factor 4 antibodies: diagnostic implications. *Clinical and Applied Thrombosis/Hemostasis*, vol.5, no.s1, (October 1999), pp.s28-s31.

Arepally, G.M., & Mayer, I.M. (2001). Antibodies from patients with heparin-induced thrombocytopenia stimulate monocytic cells to express tissue factor and secrete interleukin-8. *Blood*, vol.98, no.4, (August 2001), pp.1252-1254.

Bailey, R.T., Ursick, J.A., Heim, K.L., Hilleman, D.E., & Reich, J.W. (1986). Heparin-associated thrombocytopenia: a prospective comparison of bovine lung heparin, manufactured by a new process, and porcine intestinal heparin. *Drug Intelligence & Clinical Pharmacy* vol.20, no.5, (May 1986), pp.374-378.

Blank, M., Schoenfeld, Y., Tavor, S., Praprotnik, S., Bofia, M.C., Weksler, B., et al. (2002). Anti-platelet factor 4/heparin antibodies from patients with heparin-induced thrombocytopenia provoke direct activation of microvascular endothelial cells. *International Immunology*, vol.14, no.2 , (February 2002), pp.121-129.

Boyce, S.W., Bandyk, D., Bartholomew, J.R., Frame, J.N., & Rice, L. (2011). A randomized, open-label pilot study comparing desirudin and argatroban in patients with suspected heparin-induced thrombocytopenia with or without thrombosis: PREVENT-HIT Study. *American Journal of Therapeutics*, vol.18, pp.14-22.

Chong, B.H. Heparin-Induced Thrombocytopenia. (2003). *Journal of Thrombosis and Haemostasis*, vol.1, no.7, (July 2003), pp.1471-1478.

Crafoord, C. (1936). Preliminary report on post-operative treatment with heparin as a preventative of thrombosis. *Acta Chirurgica Scandinavica*, vol.79, (1936), pp.:407–426.

Crespo, E.M., Oliveira, G.B., Honeycutt, E.F., Becker, R.C., Berger, P.B., Moliterno, D.J., et al. (2009). Evaluation and management of thrombocytopenia and suspected heparin0induced thrombocytopenia in hospitalized patients: The Complications after Thrombocytopenia Caused by Heparin (CATCH) Registry. *American Heart Journal*, vol.157, no.4, (April 2009), pp.651-657.

Crowther, M.A., Cook, D.J., Albert, M., Williamson, D., Meade, M., Granton, J., et al. (2010). The 4Ts scoring system for heparin-induced thrombocytopenia in medical-surgical intensive care unit patients. *Journal of Critical Care*, vol.25, no.2, (June 2010), pp.287-293.

Cuker, A., Arepally, G., Crowther, M.A., Rice, L., Datko, F., Cook, K., et al. (2010). The HIT Expert Probability (HEP) Score: a novel pre-test probability model for heparin-induced thrombocytopenia. *Journal of Thrombosis and Haemostasis*, vol.8, no.12, (December 2010), pp.2642-2650.

Dager, W.E. & White, R.H. (2003). Pharmacotherapy pf heparin-induced thrombocytopenia. *Expert Opinions in Pharmacotherapy*, vol.4, no.6, (June 2003), pp.919-940.

Demma, L.J., Winkler, A.M., Levy, J.H. (2011). A diagnosis of heparin-induced thrombocytopenia with combined clinical and laboratory methods in cardiothoracic surgical intensive care unit patients. *Anasthesia and Analgesia*, vol.113, no.4, (October 2011), pp.697-702.

Duncan, L., Kurz, M., & Levy, J. (2011). Use of the subcutaneous direct thrombin inhibitor desirudin in patients with heparin-induced thrombocytopenia (HIT) requiring venous thromboembolic event (VTE) prophylaxis [abstract]. Presented at the 40th annual meeting of the Society of Critical Care Medicine. Jan 15-19 2011, San Diego, CA.

Ernest, D., & Fisher, M.M. (1991). Heparin-induced thrombocytopenia complicated by bilateral adrenal hemorrhage. *Intensive Care Medicine*, vol.17, no.4, (1991), pp.238-240.

Francis, J.L., Palmer, G.J. 3rd, Moroose, R., & Drexel, A. (2003). Comparison of bovine and porcine heparin in heparin antibody formation after cardiac surgery. *Annals of Thoracic Surgery*, vol.75, no.1, (January 2003), pp.17-22.

Green, D., Martin, G.J., Shoichet, S.H., DeBacker, N., Bomalaski, J.S., & Lind, R.N. (1984). Thrombocytopenia in a prospective, randomized, double-blond trial of bovine and porcine heparin. *American Journal of Medical Sciences*, vol.288, no.2, (September 1984), pp.60-64.

Greinacher, A., Farner, B., Kroll, H., Kohlmann, T., Warkentin, T.E., & Eichler, P. (2005). Clinical features of heparin-induced thrombocytopenia including risk factors for thrombosis. A retrospective analysis of 408 patients. *Thrombosis and Haemostasis,* vol.94, no.1 , (July 2005), pp.132-135.

Gruel, Y., Pouplard, C., Nguyen, P., Borg, J.Y., Derlon, A., Juhan-Vague, I., et al. (2003). Biological and clinical features of low-molecular-weight heparin-induced thrombocytopenia. *British Journal of Haematology,* vol.121, no.5, (June2003), pp.786-792.

Hall, A., Thachil, J., & Martlew, V. (2010). Heparin-induced thrombocytopenia in the intensive care unit. *Journal of the Intensive Care Society,* vol.11, no.1, (January 2010), pp.20-25.

Hartman, V., Malbrin, M., Daelemans, R., Meersman, P., & Zachee, P. (2006). Pseudo-pulmonary embolism as a sign of acute heparin-induced thrombocytopenia in hemodialysis patients: safety of resuming heparin after disappearance of HIT antibodies. *Nephron Clinical Practice,* vol.104, no.4, (2006), pp.c143-148.

Hopkins, C.K., & Goldfinger, D. (2008). Platelet transfusions in heparin-induced thrombocytopenia: a report of four cases and review of the literature. *Transfusion,* vol.48, no.10, (October 2008), pp.2128-2132.

Howell, W.H. & Holt, E. (1918). Two new factors in blood coagulation: heparin and pro-antithrombin. *American Journal of Physiology,* vol.47, no.3, (December 1918), pp.328–341.

Iqbal, R., Mulvihill, N.T.,Nolan,B., & Crean, P.A. (2007). Multivessel coronary thrombosis resulting from heparin-induced thrombocytopenia. *Irish Medical Journal,* vol.100, no.8, (September 2007), pp.569-571.

Jang, I.K. & Hursting, M.J. (2005). When heparins promote thrombosis: review of heparin-induced thrombocytopenia. *Circulation,* vol.111, no.20, (May 2005), pp.2671-2683.

Karkos, C.D., Mandala, E., Gerogiannis, I., Papadimitriou, D.N.,& Gerassimidis, T.S. (2011). Endovascular management of acute infrarenal aortic thrombosis caused by heparin-induced thrombocytopenia in a patient treated with low molecular weight heparin. *Journal of Vascular and Interventional Radiology,* vol.22, no.4, (April 2011), pp.581-582.

Kelton, J.G. (2002). Heparin-induced thrombocytopenia: a n overview. *Blood Reviews,* vol.16, no.1, (March 2002), pp.77-80.

Kim, S.Y., Kim, H.K., Han, K.S., Kim, I., Yoon, S.S., Park, S., et al. (2011). Utility of ELISA optical density values and clinical scores for the diagnosis of and thrombosis prediction in heparin-induced thrombocytopenia. *Korean Journal of Laboratory Medicine,* vol.31, no.1, (January 2011), pp.1-8.

Kreidy, R., & Hatem, J. (2004). Acute limb ischemia secondary to heparin-induced thrombocytopenia after cardiac surgery. *Lebanese Medical Journal,* vol.52, no.3 (July-September 2004), pp.175-181.

Legnani, C., Cini, M., Pili, C., Boggian, O., Frascaro, M., & Palareti, G. (2010). Evaluation of a new automated panel of assays for the detection of anti-PF4/heparin antibodies in patients suspected of having heparin-induced thrombocytopenia. *Thrombosis and Haemostasis,* vol.104, no.2, (August 2010), pp.402-409.

Levine, R.L., McCollum, D., & Hursting, M.J. (2006). How frequently is venous thromboembolisms in heparin-treated patients associated with heparin-induced thrombocytopenia? *Chest,* vol.130, no.3, (September 2006), pp.681-687.

Levy, J., & Koster, A. (2011). Safety of peri-operative bridging with desirudin and intraoperative bivalirudin in patients with heparin antibodies undergoing coronary artery bypass surgery (CABG) [abstract]. Presented at the 40th annual meeting of the Society of Critical Care Medicine. Jan 15-19 2011, San Diego, CA.

Liu, H., Zhang, Z., & Linhardt, R.J.(2009). Lessons learned from the contamination of heparin. *Natural Product Reports,* vol.26, no.3, (March 2009), pp.313-321.

Lo, G.K., Juhl, D., Warkentin, T.E., Sigouin, C.S., Eichler, P., & Greinacher, A. (2006). Evaluation of pre-test clinical score (4 T's) for the diagnosis of heparin-induced thrombocytopenia in two clinical settings. *Journal of Thrombosis/Haemostasis,* vol.4, no.4, (April 2006), pp.759-765.

Lobo, B., Finch, C., Howard, A., & Minhas, S. (2008). Fondaparinux for the treatment of patients with acute heparin–induced thrombocytopenia. *Thrombosis and Haemostasis,* vol.99, no.1, (January 2008), pp.208-14

Lubenow, N., Hinz, P., Thomaschewski, S., Lietz, T., Vogler, M., Ladwig, A., et al. (2010). The severity of trauma determine the immune response to PF4/heparin and the frequency of heparin-induced thrombocytopenia. *Blood,* vol.115, no.9, (March 2010), pp.1797-1803.

Lubenow, N., Kempf, R., Eichner, A., Eichler, P., Carlsson, L.E., & Greinacher, A. (2002). Heparin-induced thrombocytopenia: temporal pattern of thrombocytopenia in relation to initial use or re-exposure to heparin. *Chest,* vol.122, no.1, (July 2002), pp.37-42.

Martel, N., Lee, J., & Wells, P.S. (2005). Risk for heparin-induced thrombocytopenia with unfractionated and low-molecular weight heparin thromboprophylaxis: a meta-analysis. *Blood,* vol.106, no.8, (October 2005), pp.2710-2715.

Messmore, H.L., Fabbrini, N., Bird, M.L., Choudhury, A.M., Cerejo, M., Prechel, M., et al. (2011). Simple scoring system for early management of heparin-induced thrombocytopenia. *Clinical and Applied Thrombosis/Hemostasis,* vol.17, no.2, (April 2011), pp.197-201.

Meyer-Lindenberg, A., Quenzel, E.M., Bierhoff, E., Wolff, H., Schindler, E., & Biniek, R. (1997). Fatal cerebral venous sinus thrombosis in heparin-induced thrombocytopenia. *European Neurology,* vol. 37, no.3, (1997), pp.191-192.

Modi, C., Satani, D., Cervellione, K., Cervantes, J., Gintautas, J. (2009). *Proceedings of the Western Pharmacology Society,* vol.52, no.1, (January 2009) pp.5-7.

Oliveira, G.B., Crespo, E.M., Becker, R.C., Honeycutt, E.F., Abrams, C.S., Anstrom, K., et al. (2008). Incidence and prognostic significance of thrombocytopenia in patients treated with prolonged heparin therapy. *Archives of Internal Medicine,* vol.168, no.1, (January 2008), pp.94-102.

Pistulli, R., Oberle, V., Figulla, H.-R., Yilmaz, A., & Pfeifer, R. (2011). Fondaparinux cross-reacts with heparin antibodies in vitro in a patient with fondaparinux-related thrombocytopenia. *Blood Coagulation & Fibrinolysis,* vol.22, no.1, (January 2011), pp.76-78.

Popov, D., Zarrabi, M.H., Foda, H., & Graber, M. (1997). Pseudopulmonary embolism: acute respiratory distress in the syndrome of heparin-induced thrombocytopenia. *American Journal of Kidney Diseases,* vol.29, no.3, (March 1997), pp.449-452.

Poulain, G., Lamberto, C., Coche, E., Hainaut, P. & Lambert, M. (2008). Acute adrenal insufficiency associated with heparin-induced thrombocytopenia. *Acta Clinica Belgica,* vol.63, no.2, (March-April 2008), pp.112-115.

Pouplard, C., Gueret, P., Fouassier, M., Ternisien, C., Trossaert, M., Regina, S., et al. (2007). Prospective evaluation of the '4Ts" score and particle gel immunoassay specific to heparin/PF4 for the diagnosis of heparin-induced thrombocytopenia. *Journal of Thrombosis and Haemostasis,* vol.5, no.7, (July 2007), pp/1373-1379.

Pouplard, C., Iochmann, S., Renard, B., Herault, O., Colombat, P., Amiral, J., & Gruel, Y. (2001). Induction of monocyte tissue factor expression by antibodies to heparin-platelet factor 4 complexes developed in heparin-induced thrombocytopenia. *Blood,* vol.97, no.10, (May 2001), pp.3300-3302.

Prechel, M.M., Escalante, V., Drenth, A.F., & Walenga, J.M. (2011). A colorimetric, metabolic dye reduction assay detects highly activated platelets: application in the diagnosis of heparin-induced thrombocytopenia. *Platelets* Jul 8; e-pub ahead of print.

Rauova, L., Hirsch, J.D., Greene, T.K., Zhai, L., Hayes, V.M., Kowalska, M.A., et al. (2010). Monocyte-bound PF4 in the pathogenesis of heparin-induced thrombocytopenia. *Blood,* vol.116, no.23, (December 2010), pp.5021-5031.

Rauova, L., Zhai, L., Kowalska, M.A., Arepally, G.M., Cines, D.B., & Poncz, M. (2006). Role of platelet surface PF4 antigenic complexes in heparin-induced thrombocytopenia pathogenesis: diagnostic and therapeutic implications. *Blood,* vol.107, no.6, (March 2006), pp.2346-2353.

Refaai, M.A., Chuang, C., Menegus, M., Blumberg, N., & Francis, C.W. (2010). Outcomes after platelet transfusion in patients with heparin-induced thrombocytopenia. *Journal of Thrombosis and Haemostasis,* vol.8, no.6, (June 2010), pp.1419-1421.

Refaai, M.A., Warkentin, T.E., Axelson, M., Matevosyan, K., & Sarode, R. (2007). Delayed-onset heparin-induced thrombocytopenia, venous thromboembolisms, and cerebral venous thrombosis: a consequence of heparin "flushes". *Thrombosis and Haemostaasis,* vol.98, no.5, (November 2007), pp.1139-1140.

Rice, L., Attisha, W.K., Drexler, A., & Francis, J.L. (2002). Delayed-onset heparin-induced thrombocytopenia. *Annals of Internal Medicine,* vol.136, no.3, (February 2002), pp.210-215.

Rice, T.W., & Wheeler, A.P. (2009). Coagulopathy in critically ill patients part 1: platelet disorders. *Chest,* vol.136, no.6, (December 2009), pp.1622-1629.

Roberts, B., Rosato, F.E., & Rosato, E.F. (1963). Heparin: a cause of arterial emboli? *Surgery,* vol.55, no.6, (June 1964), pp.803–808.

Rosenberger, L.H., Smith, P.W., Sawyer R.G., Hanks J.B., Adams, R.B., & Hedrich, T.L. (2011). Bilateral adrenal hemorrhage: the unrecognized cause of hemodynamic collapse associated with heparin-induced thrombocytopenia. *Critical Care Medicine,* vol.39, no.4, (April 2011), pp.833-838.

Rota, E., Bazzan, M., & Fantino, G. (2008). Fondaparinux-related thrombocytopenia in a previous low-molecular-weight-heparin (LMWH)-induced heparin-induced thrombocytopenia (HIT). *Thrombosis and Haemostaasis,* vol.99, no.4, (April 2008), pp.1139-1140.

Ruf, K.M., Bensadoun, E.S., Davis, G.A., Flynn, J.D., & Lewis, D.A. (2011). A clinical-laboratory algorithm incorporating optical density value to predict heparin-induced thrombocytopenia. Thrombosis and Haemostasis, vol.105, no.3, (March 2011), pp.553-559.

Sakr, Y. (2011). Heparin-induced thrombocytopenia in the ICU: an overview. *Critical Care,* vol.15, no.2, (2011), pp.211-220.

Selleng, K., Warkentin, T.E., & Greinacher, A. (2007). Heparin-induced thrombocytopenia in intensive care patients. *Critical Care Medicine,* vol.35, no.4, (April 2007), pp.1165-1176.

Smythe, M.A., Koerber, J.M., & Mattson, J.C. (2007). The incidence of recognized heparin-induced thrombocytopenia in a large, tertiary care teaching hospital. *Chest,* vol.131, no.6, (June 2007), pp.1644-1649.

Smythe, M.A., arkentin, T.E., Woodhouse, A.L., & Zakalik, D. (2011). Venous limb gangrene and fatal hemorrhage: adverse consequences of HIT "overdiagnosis" in a patient with antiphospholipid syndrome. *American Journal of Hematology,* vol.86, no.2, (February 2011), pp.188-191.

Srinivasan, A.F., Rice, L., Bartholomew, J.R., Rangaswamy, C., La Perna, L., Thompson, J.E., et al. (2004). Warfarim-induced skin necrosis and venous limb gangrene in the setting of heparin-induced thrombocytopenia. *Archives of Internal Medicine,* vol.164, no.1, (January 2004), pp.66-70.

Stein, P.D., Hull, R.D., Matta, F., Yaekoub, A.Y., & Liang, J. (2009). Incidence of thrombocytopenia in hospitalized patients with venous thromboembolism. *American Journal of Medicine,* vol.122, no.10, (October 2009), pp.919-930.

Syed, S., & Reilly, R.F. (2009). Heparin-induced thrombocytopenia: a renal perspective. Nature Reviews: *Nephrology,* vol.5, no.9, (September 2009), pp.501-511.

Tardy, B., Tardy-Poncet, B., Fournel, P., Venet, C., Jospe, R., & Dacosta, A. (1999). Lower limb veins should be systematically explored in patients with isolated heparin-induced thrombocytopenia. *Thrombosis and Haemostasis,* vol.82, no.3, (September 1999), pp.1199-1200.

Untch, B., Ahmad, S., Jeske, W.P., Messmore, H.L., Hoppensteadt, D.A., Walenga, J.M., et al. (2002). Prevalence, isotype, and functionality of antiheparin-platelet factor 4 antibodies in patients treated with heparin and clinically suspected for heparin-induced thrombocytopenia: the pathogenic role of IgG. *Thrombosis Research,* vol.105, no.2, (January 2002), pp.117-123.

Verma, A.K., Levine, M., Shalansky, S.J., Carter, C.J., & Kelton, J.G. (2003). Frequency of heparin-induced thrombocytopenia in critical care patients. *Pharmacotherapy,* vol.23, no.6, (June 2003), pp.745-753.

Warkentin, T.E. (1996). Heparin-induced skin lesions. *British Journal of Haematology,* vol.92, no.2, (February 1996), pp.494-497.

Warkentin, T.E. (1998). Clinical presentation of heparin-induced thrombocytopenia. *Seminars in Hematology,* vol.35, no.4 s5, (October 1998), pp.9-16.

Warkentin, T.E. (2002). Heparin-induced thrombocytopenia. *Current Hematology Reports,* vol.1, no.1, (September 2002), pp.63-72.

Warkentin, T.E. (2004). Heparin-induced thrombocytopenia: diagnosis and management. *Circulation,* vol.110, no.18, (November 2004), pp.e454-458.

Warkentin, T.E. (2005). Heparin-induced thrombocytopenia. *Disease a Month,* vol.51, no.2-3, (February-March 2005), pp.141-149.

Warkentin, T.E. (2007). Heparin-induced thrombocytopenia. *Hematology/Oncology Clinics of North America*, vol.21, no.4, (August 2007), pp.589-607.

Warkentin, T.E., Chong, B.H., & Greinacher, A. (1998). Heparin-induced thrombocytopenia:towards consensus. *Thrombosis and Haemostasis*, vol.79, no.1, (January 1998), pp.1-7.

Warkentin, T.E., Elavathil, L.J., Hayward, C.P., Johnston, M.A., Russett, J.I., & Kelton, J.G. (1997). The pathogenesis of venous limb gangrene associated with heparin-induced thrombocytopenia. *Annals of Internal Medicine,* vol.127, no.9, (November 1997), pp.804-812.

Warkentin, T.E., Greinacher, A., Koster, A., & Lincoff, M. (2008). Treatment and Prevention of Heparin-Induced Thrombocytopenia. American College Of Chest Physicians Evidence-Based Clinical Practice Guidelines (8th Edition). *Chest,*vol.133, no.6 sup, (June 200y8), pp.340S-380S.

Warkentin, T.E., & Greinacher, A. (2009). Heparin-induced anaphylactic and anaphylactoid reactions: two distinct but overlapping syndromes. *Expert Opinions on Drug Safety,* vol.8, no.2, (March 2009), pp.129-144.

Warkentin, T.E., Hayward, C.P., Boshkov, L.K., Santos, A.V., Sheppard, J.A., Bode, A.P., & Kelton, J.G. (1994a). Sera from patients with heparin-induced thrombocytopenia generate platelet-derived microparticles with procoagulant activity: an explanation for the thrombotic complications of heparin-induced thrombocytopenia. *Blood,* vol.84, no.11, (December 1994), pp.3691-3699.

Warkentin, T.E., Hirte, H.W., Anderson, D.R., Wilson, W.E., O'Connell, G.J., & Lo, R.C. (1994b). Transient global amnesia associated with acute heparin-induced thrombocytopenia. *American Journal of Medicine,* vol.97, no.5, (November 1994), pp.489-491.

Warkentin, T.E., & Heddle, N. (2003). Laboratory diagnosis of immune heparin-induced thrombocytopenia. *Current Hematology Reports,* vol.2, no.2, (March 2003), pp.148-157.

Warkentin, T.E., & Kelton, J.G. (2001a). Delayed-onset heparin-induced thrombocytopenia and thrombosis. *Annals of Internal Medicine,* vol.135, no.7, (October 2001), pp.502-506.

Warkentin, T.E., & Kelton, J.G. (2001b).Temporal aspects of heparin-induced thrombocytopenia. *New England Journal of Medicine,* vol.334, no.17, (April 2001), pp.1286-1292.

Warkentin, T.E., Maurer, B.T., & Aster, R.H. (2007). Heparin–induced thrombocytopenia associated with fondaparinux. *New England Journal of Medicine,* vol.356, no.25, (June 2007), pp.2653-2654.

Warkentin, T.E., Roberts, R.S., Hirsh, J., & Kelton, J.G. (2003). An improved definition of immune heparin-induced thrombocytopenia in post-operative orthopedic patients. *Archives of Internal Medicine,* vol.163, no.20, (November 2003), pp.2518-2524.

Warkentin, T.E., Sheppard, J.A., Horsewood, P., Simpson, P.J., Moore, J.C., & Kelton, J.G. (2000). Impact of the patient population on the risk of heparin induced thrombocytopenia. *Blood,* vol.96, no.5, (September 2000), pp.1703-1708.

Warkentin, T.E., Sheppard, J.A., Sigouin, C.S., Kohlmann, T., Eichler, P., & Greinacher, A. (2006). Gender imbalance and risk factors interactions in heparin-induced thrombocytopenia. *Blood,* vol.108, no.9, (November 2006), pp.2937-2941.

Warkentin, T.E., Sikov, W.., & Lillicrap, D.P. (1999). Multicentric warfarin-induced skin necrosis complicating heparin-induced thrombocytopenia. *American Journal of Hematology*, vol.62, no.1, (September 1999), pp.44-48.

Weismann, R.E. & Tobin, R.W. (1958). Arterial embolism occurring during systemic heparin therapy. *AMA Archives of Surgery*, vol.76, no.2, (February 1958), pp.219–225.

Yamamoto, S., Koide, M., Matsuo, M. Suzuki, S., Ohtaka, M., Saika, S., & Matsuo, T. (1996). Heparin-induced thrombocytopenia in haemodialysis patients. *American Journal of Kidney Diseases*, vol.28, no.1, (July 1996), pp.82-85.

Yoon, J.H. & Jang, I.K. (2011). Heparin-induced thrombocytopenia in cardiovascular patients: Pathophysiology, diagnosis, and treatment. *Cardiology in Review*, vol.19, no.3, (May-June 2011), pp.143-153.

12

Cavitary Pulmonary Infarct: The Differential Diagnostic Dilemma – A Case Report

Ivanka Djordjevic and Tatjana Pejcic
Clinic for lung diseases; Clinical Center – Nis, Serbia

1. Introduction

Pulmonary infarction is localized destruction (necrosis) of lung tissue by blocking (obstruction of) the arterial blood supply. It follows an embolic event in ~10% of cases. Blockage of pulmonary artery by a clot or air bubble or other particle (called pulmonary embolism) leads to localized damage of lung tissue which results in pulmonary infarction (1, 2). The reasons for this low incidence of pulmonary infarct are the dual blood supply systems, as well as oxygenation of the lung tissues via ventilation (3).
The predisposing factors for pulmonary infarct include congestive heart failure, pleural effusion, pulmonary infection, atelectasis, hypotension, positive-pressure ventilation, chronic lung disease, central venous catheterization and an immunocompromised state. It is more common in people with chronic heart and lung diseases. Infarction condition may be mild and can be rapidly fatal (4).
Common symptoms include chest pain which may be because of difficulty in breathing, high pulse rate, mild fever, developing of fluid in the lungs, a productive cough (sputum may be blood-tinged). Blockage may also result into circulatory breakdown, like low blood pressure, presence of very little oxygen in the blood. Also, swelling of neck vein and leg, weakness, restlessness, and fainting. In the case of infection as developing complication, there is worsening of the clinical status, persistent fever, malaise, sweating, increasing pulse rate and leukocytosis (usually more than $20 \times 10^9/l$) (5).
Diseases that should be listed in the differential diagnosis include bacterial pneumonia, aspergillosis, tuberculosis, norcardia, actinomycosis, and granulomatous vasculitis. Other unusual etiologies that should be listed in the differential diagnosis include primary or metastatic angiosarcoma or leomyosarcoma and lung cancer invading the main pulmonary arteries (6,7).

2. Clinical presentation

Bacterial pneumonia and pulmonary infarction frequently mimic each other clinically, indicates that most methods for distinguishing between these illnesses are unsatisfactory. Both diseases may give rise to dyspnea, pleuritic pain, tachypnoea, fever, cyanosis, hypotension, cough, hemopthysis, jaundice, leukocytosis and similar radiographic abnormalities (8).
Shaking chills point strongly to bacterial pneumonia. Additional hints are a preceding upper respiratory tract infection followed by gradually increasing malaise and then cough, usually

productive of purulent sputum. Patients with pulmonary infarction more often become ill with dramatic suddenness, seldom have a cough and experience shaking chills only if the emboli are septic or the infarct become infected (8).
Physical signs are not specific for either diseases. Although high fever is more typical of bacterial pneumonia, it is occurs with sufficient frequency in pulmonary infarction to be unreliable as differential diagnostic sign. Patients with pulmonary infarction, as compared to those with bacterial pneumonia, generally are more dyspnoic and tachypnoic in relation to the extent of their physical and radiographic abnormalities and rarely exhibit classic signs of consolidation. They more often manifest hypotension, either transient or recurrent, and more commonly show signs suggesting pulmonary hypertension and right-sided congestive heart failure, e.g. a loud pulmonis component of the second heart sound and elevation of the jugular venous pressure (8).
A pleural friction rub helps in differentiation only when chest radiography shows no parenchymal disease. Then, infarction is more often do not cause radiographic changes early in the course of the illness (8).

3. Laboratory and other diagnostic tests

Sputum examination is one of the best ways of differentiating bacterial pneumonia from pulmonary infarction. In bacterial pneumonia the sputum classically is purulent, occasionally foul smelling and may contain bright red fleck of blood. Gram's stain typically shows many bacteria and polymorphonuclear leukocytes. In pulmonary infarction, sputum, when present, usually is frankly blood with few bacteria or inflammatory cells. If the infarct becomes infected the sputum may be indistinguishable from that in bacterial pneumonia. Blood cultures often reveal the causative microorganism in the patients with bacterial pneumonia but show no growth in cases of bland pulmonary infarction (8).
Cavitation after bland pulmonary infarcts may result from either aseptic necrosis of the infracted lung or from secondary bacterial infection with subsequent abscess formation. It is infective almost as often as it is aseptic (9).
Two types of infected pulmonary infarct have been proposed based on the mode by which infection sets in (10). One is called "primary" because the infection is from a septic embolus. The other is called "secondary" because the infection is bronchigenic origin. Some authors suggest that the development of fever and/or purulent sputum following a pulmonary infarct is highly suspicious for secondary infection. The spectrum of causative agents for infected pulmonary infarct is similar to that of nosocomial pneumonia (3).
Total leukocyte count has limited discriminatory value. It usually is normal or slightly elevated in pulmonary infarction, but there is reports of leukocytes count higher than 40 000 per mm^3 in patients with massive, bland necrosis of pulmonary tissue. Elevated serum lactic dehydrogenase (LDH) activity, normal aspartate aminotranspherase activity (AST) and increased serum bilirubin concentration forms a triad once considered a sensitive indicators of pulmonary embolism and infarction. However, subsequent studies have shown that these tests fail to differentiate pulmonary infarction from pneumonia and host of other disorders (8).
Electrocardiographic abnormalities that may appear are right ventricular conduction disturbances; right axis deviation; inverted T-waves with S-T segment deviation in the right precordial leads; peaked T-waves in leads II, III and AVF; various types of supraventricular and raraly ventricular arrhythmias and S1, Q3 or S1,S2, S3 patterns. Heart ultrasound may

reveals right ventricular dilatation, septal deviation of left ventricle, tricuspidal regurgitation or right ventricle hypokinesis with wall thinning (8, 11).
Pulmonary function test and arterial blood gas studies provide data that are too variable and nonspecific to differentiate bacterial pneumonia from pulmonary infarction (8).

4. Imaging studies

Radiographic similarities of bacterial pneumonia and pulmonary infarction are the chief source of diagnostic confusion between the two entities. Each is responsible for parenchymal infiltrates of varied size and shape, with or without pleural effusion, atelectasis or cavitation. In contrast to bacterial pneumonia, pulmonary infarcts always abut a pleural surface and predominate in lower lobes, especially the right. They also may appear in concert with dilatation of one or both main pulmonary arteries, decreased peripheral vascular markins in the affected portion of lung (oligemia) or engorged vassels in the non affected areas (pleonemia). Further radiographic clues to pulmonary infarction are infiltrates appearing first in one lung and then the other or "pneumonia" unresponsive to chemotherapy (8).
Spiral computed tomography and magnetic resonance angiography are helpful in establishing the difference between pneumonia and pulmonary infarct. Also, this imaging techniques could help tracking the resolution of the thrombo emboli, but they are expensive and unavailable in many hospitals (6,7).
Pulmonary arteriography is the most specific means of differentiating bacterial pneumonia from pulmonary infarction. In bacterial pneumonia the pulmonary arteries proximal to the subsegmental level show neither filling defect nor obstructive lesions, where in pulmonary infarction they contain filling defect, appear obstructed, or both (8).
The grater the size of infarct, more likely its centre will be hypoxic and nectrotic. Pulmonary infarct larger than 4 x 4 cm in size have a great tendency for cavitation (12).
The median time from the first detection of consolidation to cavity formation is 14 days (12).
Doppler sonography is a noninvasive and convenient tool for diagnosing pulmonary embolism and follow-up reperfusion of the lung. Dynamic changes in blood flow in consolidated areas provides information about the status of reperfusion (6).
Despite use of the aforementioned techniques, the question of infected versus infracted lung sometimes will persist. To minimize error, the physicians should think of both diseases when he considers either, particularly if the process involves the lower lobes, especially the right. Dangers of delaying treatment for pulmonary infarction rival the hazards of withholding specific chemotherapy in bacterial pneumonia. Thus, as long as the diagnosis remains in doubt, treatment for both disorders seems well advised (8).
Multiple complications have been associated with pulmonary infarct, including pneumonia, empyema, pneumothorax, lung abscess, bronchopleural fistulae and lethal haemorrhage. Large series of autopsies reveald cavitation in 4-5% of all pulmonary infarcts (5).
The mortality rate is as high as 41% and 73% for nonifected and infected cavitary pulmonary infarcts, respectively. Anticoagulants and antibiotics are the mainstay of therapy. Massive haemopthysis may persist even after discontinuation of anticoagulants. Possible explanation for this phenomenon are an overdose of anticoagulants and reperfusion of necrotic lung tissue. Anticoagulants use in cavitary pulmonary infarction, therefore, must be very carefully monitored and causation should be exercised in monitoring clinical conditions and the status of coagulation (10).

5. Case presentation

Patient was admitted to our clinic with a three week history of dyspnea, tachycardia, cough, expectoration of yellow colored sputum, fever, exhaustion and lower legs edema. Few days before admission to clinic he presented altered level of consciousness (mental confusion), caused by alcohol withdrawal. The patient suffered from congestive heart failure and chronic obstructive pulmonary disease for several years. There was no past medical history of predisposition factors for embolism or episodes of venous thrombo-embolism.

On examination he presented normal mental status, body temperature was within normal range, blood pressure 130/80 mmHg, pulse rate 90 beats/min; respiratory rate 26 breath/min; with signs of peripheral cyanosis. The chest expanded symmetrically and breathing sounds were clear. There were heart rhythm disorder (absolute arrhythmia) but no heart murmurs were detected. The liver and spleen were not palpable. Lower leg edema was noticed.

The initial laboratory blood test revealed elevated inflammatory parameters: white blood cells:15.7 x 10^9/L; with 87.6% neutrophils; 3.4% monocytes and 9.0% lymphocytes; C-reactive protein: 73 mg/L; D-dimer: 759 ηg/ml. The prothrombin time, activated partial thromboplastin time (PTT) and platelets were within normal range. There were elevated activity of aspartate aminotranspherase (160.6 U/L); alanin aminotransferase (128.0 U/L); lactic dehydrogenase (745 U/L); serum bilirubin concentration (45 µmol/L);blood urea nitrogen (16.3 mmol/L) and creatinine (120.4 µmol/L). But, all this test has limited discriminatory value.

The arterial gas blood analysis showed the following: pH 7,5; carbon dioxide tension in arterial blood (PCO_2) 31 mmHg; oxygen tension in arterial blood (PO_2) 71 mmHg; HCO3 24 mmol/L; BE 1 mmol/L and oxygen saturation (SaO_2) 95%.

Lung functional test shown severe restrictive ventilation disorder (FEV1: 8%; FVC: 44% - 1.67 L; FEV1/FVC: 72%) which is nonspecific to differentiate bacterial pneumonia from pulmonary infarction as well as the arterial gas blood analysis too.

The electrocardiography (ECG) revealed atrial fibrillation only. The initial chest radiograph was showed enlarged cardiac shadow without pulmonary opacities (**Figure 1**) because infarction is more often do not cause radiographic changes early in the course of the illness. Congestive heart failure was diagnosed and the patient was treated with diuretics and inotropes.

However, a ten days later the intensity of dyspnea, fatique, weakness and exhaustion has increased. He was febrile (38.3^0 C). A contribution to literature data, in our case, clinical condition has got worsening suddenly. Chest radiography was significant since it showed round pulmonary consolidation with central cavitation on the apical segment of the right lower lobe (**Figure 2**). The patient was placed on antibiotic therapy (intravenous ceftazidine and ertapenem) for a presumptive diagnosis of bacterial pneumonia.

However, one week later, the treatment with antibiotics was not satisfactory and there were no clinical recovery. Also, there were no microbiologic confirmation of causative microorganism which made definitive diagnosis difficult. The clinical symptoms of congestive heart failure was dominant and the patient underwent a cardiac ultrasound which revealed tricuspidal regurgitation and elevated right ventricular pressure (systolic blood pressure of right ventricule - SPRV: 46 mmHg). The increased intensity of dyspnoea, fatique, weakness and exhaustion, despite the treatment with diuretics and inotropes was due to unconfirmed hemodynamic disorder.

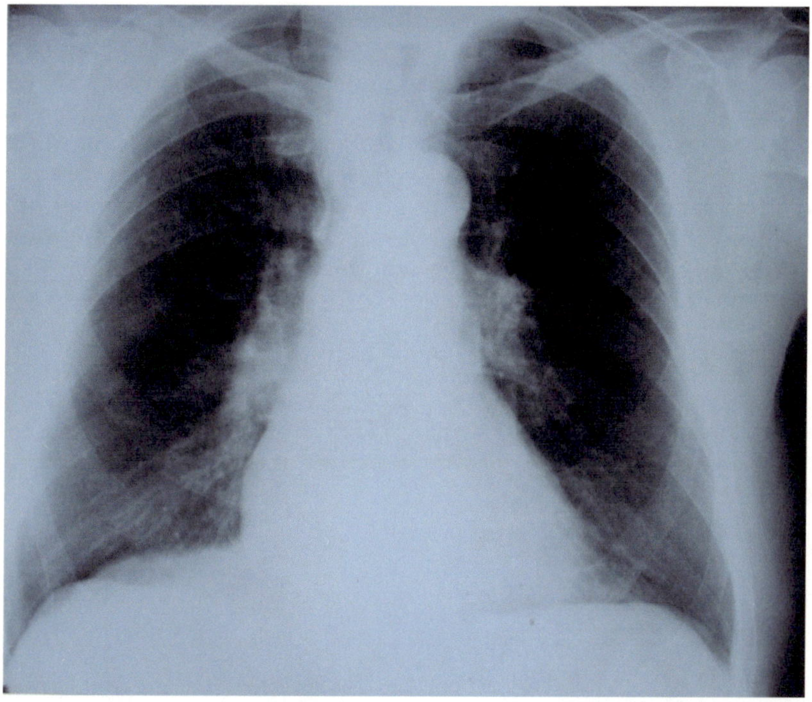

Fig. 1. Initial chest PA (postero-anterior) radiography showing enlarged cardiac shadow without pulmonary opacities

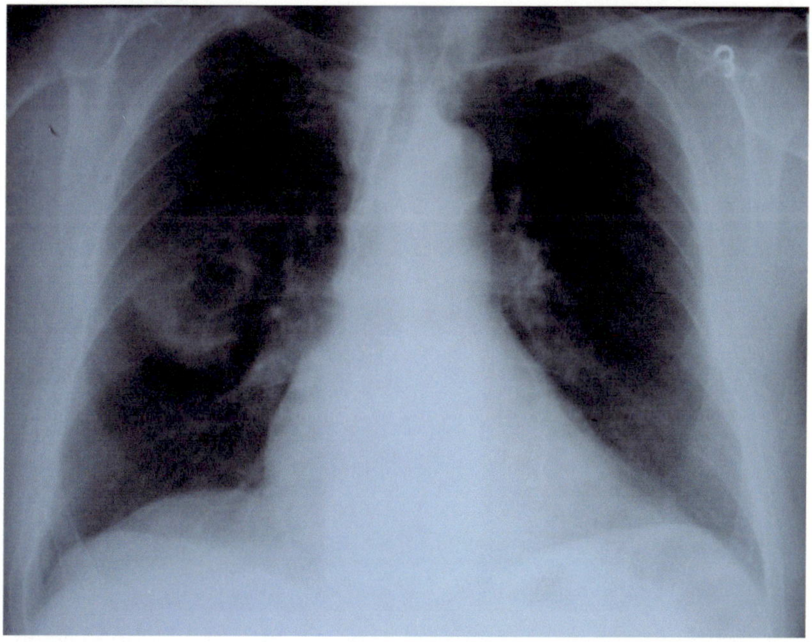

Fig. 2. PA (postero-anterior) chest radiography ten days from admission showing round pulmonary consolidation with central cavitation on the apical segment of the right lower lobe

The most striking and unexpected findings was contrast-enhanced computed tomography (CT) scan of blood vessels and identification of filling defect in the main pulmonary arteries which presumptive diagnosis of pneumonia excluded. There were pulmonary consolidation with central cavitation on the right lower and left upper lobes too. The diameter of right and left consolidation was 63 x 75 mm and 85 x 70 mm respectively (**Figure 3a and 3b**). The size of pulmonary infarct , in our case, is grater than 40 x 40 mm which explain the appearance of cavitation. Also, the velocity of cavity formation presented in our case is significantly lower than literature data pointed out. Venous duplex ultrasound of lower extremitas was negative for deep-vein thrombosis. Low-molecular heparin were administered immediately after the findings of the CT scans were obtained.

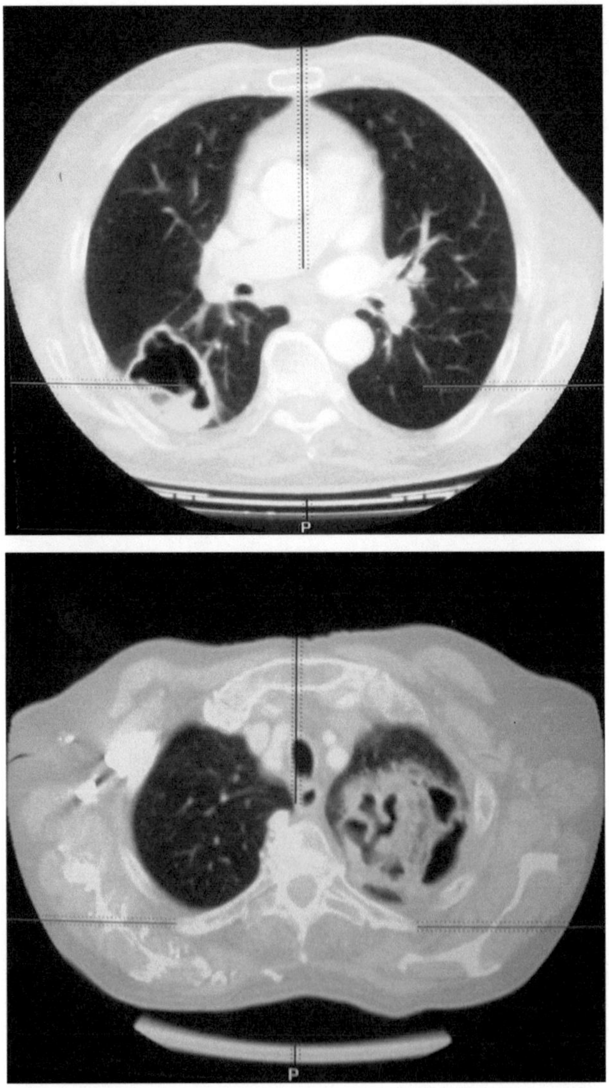

Fig. 3a. and 3b. Contrast - enhanced computed tomography scan of blood vessels showing filling defect in the main pulmonary arteries with central cavitation on the right lower and left upper lobes too

The follow-up chest radiograph (three weeks later) showed regression of mentioned pulmonary opacities (**Figure 4**). Due to anticoagulant therapy was administered immediately after the findings of the CT scans were obtained, the patient was clinicaly recovered and he was discharged with follow-up recommended.

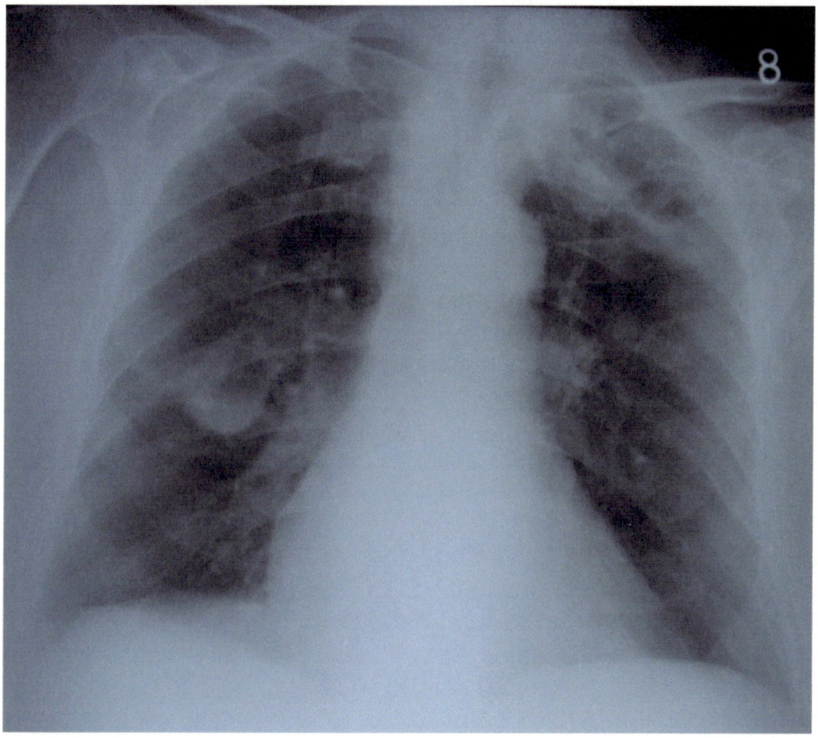

Fig. 4. Follow-up chest radiograph (three weeks later) showing regression of mentioned pulmonary opacities.

6. Conclusion

Cavitary pulmonary infarct is a rare but frequently misdiagnosed disease entity. Differentation between cavitary pulmonary infarct and multiple complications or other diseases can be a real challenge because of the similar radiographic abnormalities and clinical presentation of all this conditions. In the cases with clinical suspicion to "pneumonia" unresponsive to chemotherapy images studies are of great help. The best evidence of infarction is the angiographic demonstration of pulmonary thromboemboli. Anticoagulant and antibiotic treatment in the cases of infected cavitary pulmonary infarct must be started immediately after the diagnosis is established.

7. Acknowledgement

The authors wish to thanks all physicians from the clinic who participated in the medical care of the patient described in this report. Also, we are grateful to Marta Djordjevic for technical assistance in the computer processing of the images.

8. References

[1] Robert Baird, Pulmonary Embolism and Infarction; January 19, 2008 (www.americanchronicle.com)
[2] Libby LS, King TE, LaForce FM, Schwarz MI. Pulmonary cavitation following pulmonary infarction. Medicine (Baltimore) 1985; 64: 342-348.
[3] Urano T, Shibayama Y, Fukunchi K, Nariyama K, Ohsawa N. Interruption of pulmonary arterial flow with inadequate ventilation leads to pulmonary infarction. Virchows Arch 1996; 427: 607-612.
[4] Butler MD, Biscardi FH, Schain DC, Humphries JE, Blow O, Spontnitz WD. Pulmonary resection for treatment of cavitary pulmonary infarction. Ann Thorac Surg 1997; 63: 849-850.
[5] Lennox H Huang, MD, Pulmonary Infarction; Aug 12, 2008 (www.emedicine.com)
[6] Wang PW, Kuo PH, Chang YC, Yang PC. A patient with right upper quadrant abdominal pain, hypotension and dyspnoea. Eur Respir J 2002; 20: 238-241.
[7] Djordjevic I et all. Difficulties in establishing a timely diagnosis of pulmonary artery sarcoma misdiagnosed as chronic thrombo-emblic pulmonary disease: a case report. JMCR 2009; 3:64.
[8] Herbert L. Fred bacterial pneumonia or pulmonary infarction? Chest 1969; 55: 422-425.
[9] Morganthaler TI, Ryu JH, Utz JP. Cavitary pulmonary infarct in immunocompromised host. Mayo Clin Proc 1995; 70: 66-68.
[10] Vidal E, LeVeen HH, Yarnoz M, Piccone VA Jr. Lung abscess secondary to pulmonary infarction. Ann Thorac Surg 1971; 11: 557-564.
[11] Geibel A. et all. Prognostic value of the ECG on admission in patients with acute major pulmonary embolism. Eur Respir J 2005; 25: 843-848.
[12] Wilson AG, Joseph AEA, Butland RJA. The radiology of aseptic cavitary pulmonary infarction. Clin Radiol 1986; 37: 327-333.

13

Hypothetical Mechanism of the Formation of Dural Arteriovenous Fistula – The Role and Course of Thrombosis of Emissary Vein and Sinuses

Shigeru Miyachi
Department of Neurosurgery, Nagoya University Graduate School of Medicine, Nagoya Japan

1. Introduction

Dural ateriovenous fistula (DAVF) is the acquired and progressive arteriovenous (AV) shunt disease on or between the dura matter, and its etiology is still controversial[1-4]. This disorder occurs not in the whole dura but at very specific locations. DAVF can be divided into two types based on the intervention of the drainage route and affected sinus; sinus type and non-sinus type. The sinus type has the shunt at the sinus wall or dural vein, and includes DAVF at the cavernous sinus (CS), transverse-sigmoid sinus (TS-SS), anterior condylor confluence (ACC), and superior sagittal sinus (SSS). The non-sinus DAVF has the shunt on the dura and directly drains into the pial veins, and includes tentorial, ethmoidal, craniocervical and spinal DAVF. However, even the sinus type DAVF ultimately changes to the isolated sinus with cortical reflux due to progressive sinus occlusion, similar to the non-sinus type. Such seemingly separated and complex pathogeneses of DAVF remain elusive.

2. Previous theory about DAVF etiology

Previous recognition of the etiology of DAVF has been directed to sinus hypertension[1,4] and thrombosis[5, 8]. It is true that such abnormal situations may create the experimental AV shunt[1-4]. However, if one considers that the sinus hypertension is the initial trigger, it should be caused secondary to the thrombosis or outlet stenosis. It is unreasonable to adopt this theory into non-sinus type, because this type has no correspondence with the sinus. In other hand AV shunt formation can easily create the condition of sinus hypertension. Thus, the conventional discussion over the etiology of AV shunt formation between sinus occlusion and sinus hypertension is just a chicken-or-egg question. We consider that sinus hypertension concerning sinus wall hypertrophy may not be the cause, but rather one factor in the development of DAVF. Our theory based on inflammatory initiation affecting EV can explain both types of DAVF and subsequent development with pathological changes of the drainage route is not contradictory to the previous sinus-oriented theory.

3. Hypothesis

Etiologically, DAVF is revealed secondary to causes such as trauma, inflammation, or sinus thrombosis[5-8]. However, most causes are idiopathic and independent of the preceding hematological and immunological impairments. Therefore, comprehensive factors concerning the initiation of DAVF that covers all of the pathological features should be considered. From this perspective, we focused on the location of emissary veins (EV) and discovered that the distribution of EV definitely corresponds to those of the location of DAVF (Fig. 1). According to this previous consensus and to new information, we propose following hypothesis concerning the development of DAVF which focuses on the emissary vein.

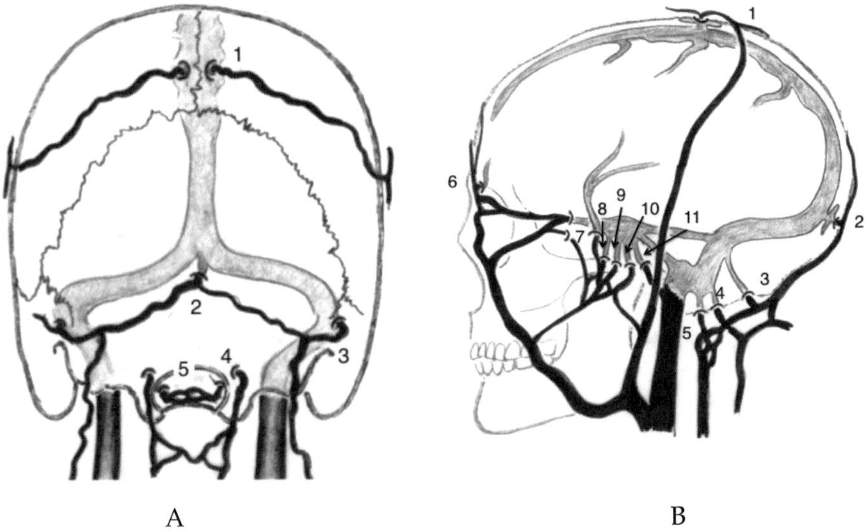

A Postero-anterior view
B Lateral view 1. parietal (parasagittal) emissary vein (EV), 2. occipital (torcular) EV, 3. mastoid EV, 4. condylar (condyloid) EV, 5. hypogroassal EV, 6. frontal (ethmoidal) emissary vein (EV), 7. petrosquamosal EV, 8. foramen ovale EV, 9. foramen spinosum EV, 10. foramen lacerum EV, 11. Basilar plexus EV and Trolard's inferior petrooccipital vein (venous plexus of Raktzik)

Fig. 1. Distribution of emissary veins

Emissary veins connecting the intracranial and extracranial venous system through the bone are distributed in specific parts of the vault or base of the skull[9]. They are usually accompanied by and penetrate together through the same foramen with emissary arteries (transosseous perforating arteries) (Fig. 2A). Fig. 2 shows the scheme of this process in the DAVF at SSS (a representative of sinus type DAVF). First, some inflammatory reaction occurs at the penetrating site of EV. It may be reasonable to consider the cause of inflammation to the infection of adjacent tissue such as sinusitis and mechanical inflammation after trauma (including catheter intervention). Sinus thrombosis is occasionally observed before the occurrence of DAVF[7], however, such thrombosis might be the result of focal inflammation. In most cases with DAVF, inflammation will develop undetected or as an autoimmune allergic reaction. Local inflammation may expand with expression of various cytokines, cause vessel dilatation, and open the physiological AV shunt at the level of capillary vessels (Fig. 2B).

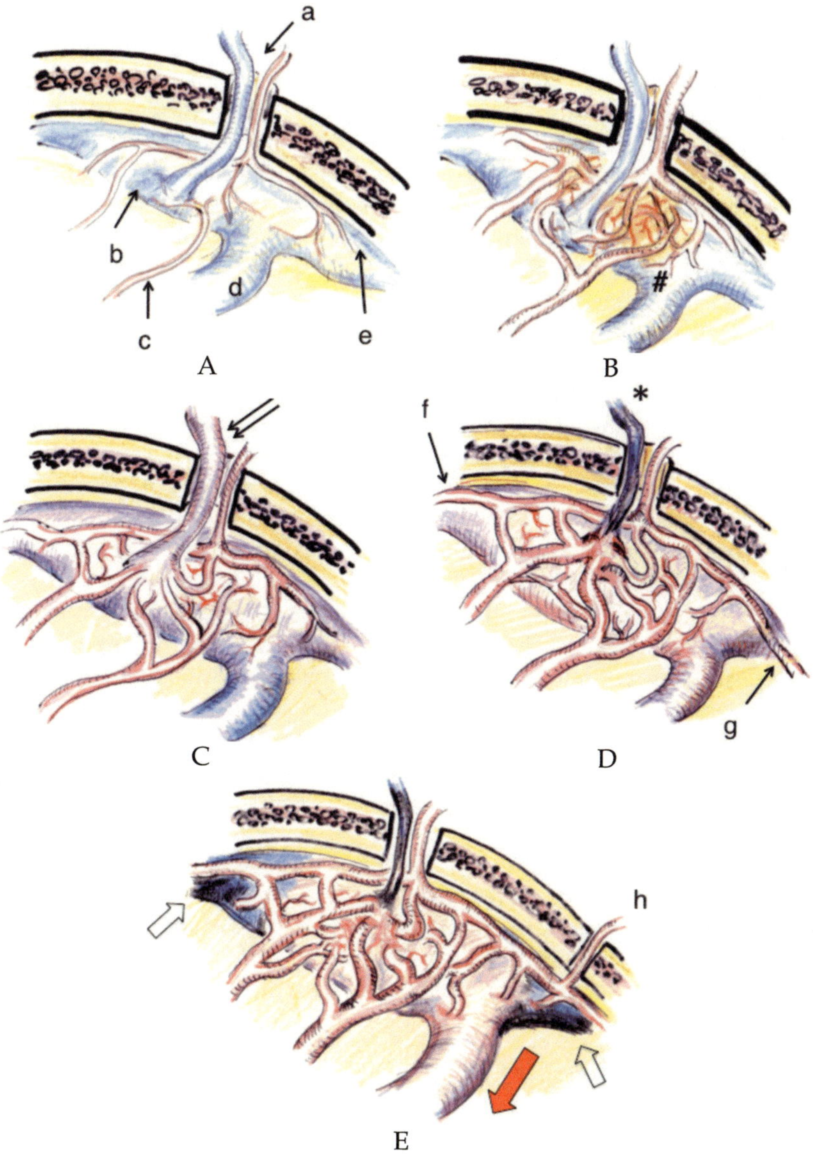

A Normal site. Emissary vein (EV) and artery (a) is penetrating through a foramen of the parasagittal skull. EV is connected with the venous lacunae (b). Meningeal arteries (c) have no connection with SSS (d) and cortical vein (e).
B Neovascularization (arrow) and vessel dilatation induced by dural inflammation
C AV shunt formation at the level of dural arteriole and penetration into the sinus (initial stage of DAVF). Note the shunt flow draining into the sinus as well as EV (double arrow).
D. Shunt development with thrombosis of an emissary vein (asterisk) and recruitment of distal arteries from anterior falx artery (f) and posterior meningeal arteries (g).
E. Maturation of DAVF with the reflux to cortical veins (red arrow) due to sinus occlusion (white arrow). Note the further recruitment of feeders from the other side or transosseous branches (h).

Fig. 2. Mechanism of development of the DAVF at the superior sagittal sinus (SSS) as a representative of the sinus type DAVF.

In sinus type DAVF, a micro AV shunt between the emissary artery and vein will enlarge to the adjacent sinus wall. The increase in shunt flow triggers drainage into the sinus, and subsequently changes the main drainage route from the EV to the sinus. As a result, the sinus will be occupied by the shunt flow more than the normal intracranial venous outflow pathway (Fig. 2C). While this shift in shunt flow direction decreases the role of EV as the drainage pathway, the developed and swollen emissary artery compresses the accompanied EV and impairs the drainage flow. This results in occlusion of the EV (Fig. 2D).

This degeneration of the EV is an important process in the formation of a well-known style of sinus type of DAVF. However, in some cases of DAVF at CS and SSS the EV may remain patent and serve as a drainage route to the pterygoid plexus or parietal vault. Also an EV that connects with diploic veins can form an enlarged intraosseus venous lake, and appear as a new channel of sinus or duplication. The shunt recruits other dural feeders from the distant and contralateral parts due to angiogenetic and hemodynamic factors, and forms the extended vascular network as a new DAVF[10]. Extracranial arteries on the skull or under the skull base are often mobilized through the bone. Such active recruitment of feeders is considered to be due to angiogenesis enhanced by the expression of vasculogenetic factors at the affected dura (including vascular endothelial growth factor (VEGF)) [11-16].

The next key process in maturation of the DAVF is the occlusive change of the draining system. Although draining pathway may finally occlude due to intrasinus thrombosis associated with hypercoagulopathy, the essence of the occlusive mechanism should be hypertrophy of the sinus wall[12]. This occlusive process is typical in the DAVF at CS[17]. Its drainage route gradually occludes from the inferior petrosal sinus and superior ophthalmic vein[11], and occasionally causes a paradoxical worsening of visual acuity and chemosis with ocular hypertension following occlusion of the anterior drainage route. During this progression, the thrombophilic abnormalities characteristic of DAVF are also reported[18-22]. In some cases such thrombotic change of drainage route may occur in the initial stage preceding the development of the shunt.

Next, the same process progresses in the upstream side because the remaining upstream drainage with more hemodynamic stress may yield the hypertrophic change of sinus wall[12, 23]. As a result, the meeting point of the shunt flow will be isolated, and shunt flow without exit to the sinus may reflux into cortical veins (Fig. 2E). Such a matured and aggressive type of DAVF with an affected isolated sinus or dural vein[24] (Fig. 3), may be the final expression

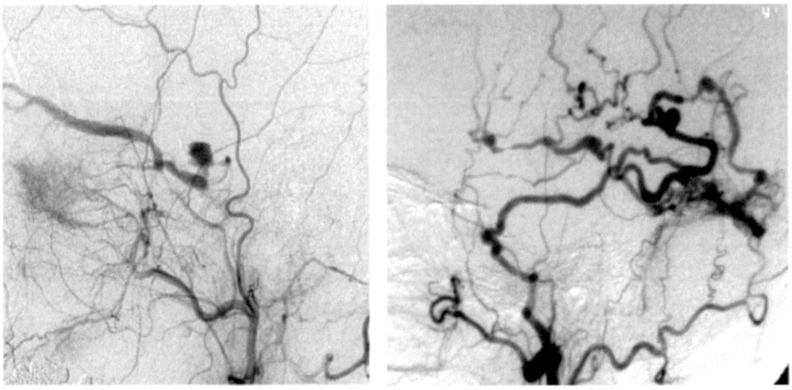

A B

A. DAVF at cavernous sinus, B. DAVF at transvers-sigmoid sinus

Fig. 3. Examples of matured sinus type DAVF

of this process. However, this final isolated part of the DAVF will not be always consistent with the first trigger point of a micro AV shunt, because the inflammatory extension and recruitment of many dural arteries will easily cause the movement of the main shunt point.
It is quite easy to adopt this mechanistic hypothesis to non-sinus type DAVF. Fig. 4 demonstrates the scheme of the development of ethmoidal (anterior skull base) DAVF as a representative of non-sinus type DAVF.

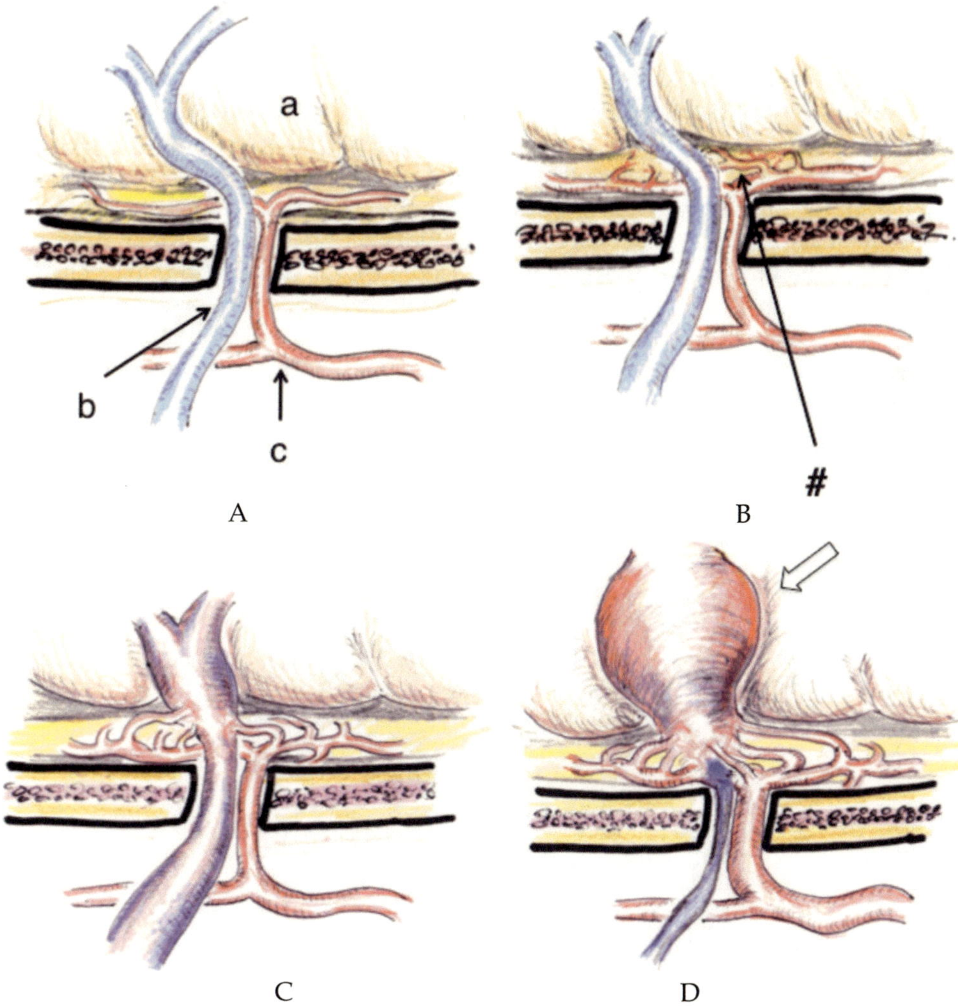

A. Normal state. a; frontal cortex, b; frontal emissary vein, c; dural branches from anterior ethmoidal artery
B. Neovascularization and dilatation induced with dural inflammation (#)
C. AV shunt formation at the level of dural arteriole and reflux into an EV (initial stage of DAVF)
D. Shunt development and increased reflux into the varicose cortical vein (white arrow) following the occlusion of an emissary vein

Fig. 4. Mechanism of development of the DAVF: an ethmoidal (anterior skull base) DAVF as a representative of the non-sinus type DAVF.

EV at the anterior skull base (Fig. 4A) connecting with the cortical vein will create, secondary to the ethmoidal inflammation, a micro AV shunt at the skull base dura (Fig. 4B). Subsequently the EV will occlude according to the same process as described above (Fig. 4C, D). As a result, all the shunt flow supplied from ethmoidal arteries drains into the cortical veins, which is the common style encountered in the clinical setting. The pathological process at the spine or craniocervical junction DAVF can be explained by the same mechanism.

4. Atypical DAVF

1. Tentorial DAVF It is true that there is no EV on the tent. The name of this type of DAVF may come from the participation of tentorial artery, however the main shunt point is not on the tent but at the clival dura (Fig. 5). The tentorial artery as the feeder usually creates the AV shunt just posterior to its origin, and the shunt flow immediately drains into the subtentorial venous complex. Although there are some classifications of various type of tentorial DAVF25, the most common type of tentorial DAVF at the clivus may be caused by the pathological process of a concerned EV, petrosal bridging vein 26, that connects between the ventral venous system in the posterior fossa and the basilar plexus. The exceptional tentorial DAVFs affecting the posterior tentorial sinus or the confluence are considered to be variants of TS-DAVF with the influence of EV at the petrous and occipital skull.

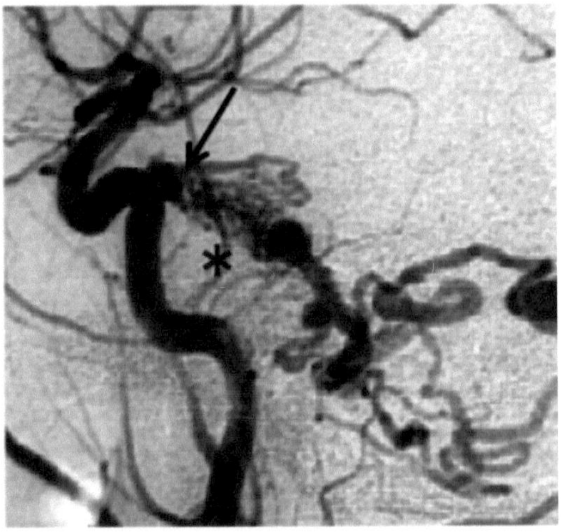

Fig. 5. Tentorial DAVF. The lateral view of the left carotid angiogram showing the dilated feeder from the tentorial artery (arrow) and AV shunt at the clival portion (asterisk) immediately draining into the prepontine venous network.

2. DAVF at the anterior condylor confluence DAVF at the anterior condylor confluence has been newly defined as the generic clinical entity24, and includes DAVF of the inferior petrosal sinus, DAVF of the marginal sinus, hypoglossal DAVF, DAVF of the anterior condylor vein within the hypoglossal canal, and jugular foramen DAVF27. Anterior condylor confluence (ACC) is extracranially located, and is a major venous crossroad at the posterior base of the skull. Tributaries from the hypoglossal canal, petroclival fissure, and the vertebral venous plexus meet together at the ACC and drain into the jugular bulb

through multiple channels28. As seen in previous nomenclature, one of the important drainage routes is the anterior condylor vein is the EV passing though the hypoglossal canal. However, in most cases, the anterior condylor vein has been already occluded, and other venous systems (including the lateral condylor vein, inferior petroclival vein, and inferior petrosal sinus) may function as a drainage route via ACC. Specific characteristics of this type of DAVF include patients suffering from strong tinnitus just when the DAVF is initially formed. Hypoglossal palsy develops in some cases. DAVF at the ACC tends to be diagnosed in the early stages. Therefore, as the original drainage route, the anterior condylor vein occasionally remains one of the draining veins.

3. Vault DAVF This rare type of DAVF is located at the temporal or occipital convexity, and is a non-sinus type DAVF. An aggressive feature of this type of DAVF is that it directly drains into cerebral cortical veins. According to our theory, it may be caused by the focal inflammation around the atypically located EV, or due to the congenital focal connection between pial and dural veins.
4. Multiple, de novo, recurrent DAVF. These clinical features cannot be explained with the single inflammation theory, and spreading or multifocal inflammation should be considered (Fig. 6). Although recurrence of the same lesion can be due to incomplete occlusion of the shunt29, de novo creation of DAVF independent from the previous ones may follow the newly developing process, possibly be promoted with constitutional factors.

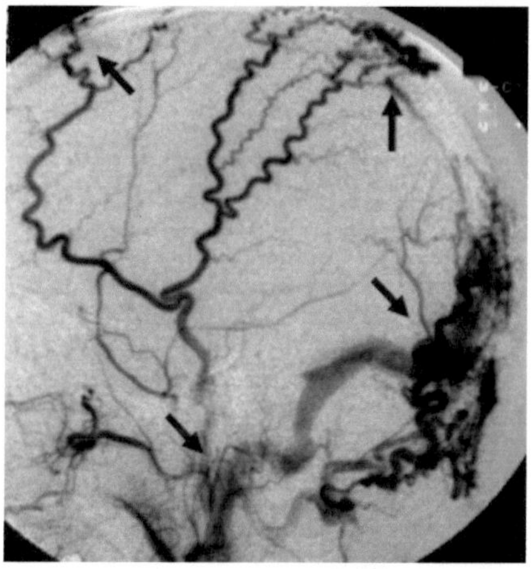

Fig. 6. Mulitple DAVF Multiple DAVF at superior sagittal, tranevers and sigmoid sinus (arrows)

5. Supporting clinical situation

This hypothesis is supported by some familiar features encountered in clinical cases. First, in the case of mature SSS-DAVF, shunt flow usually drains into the cortical vein through an isolated sinus with the particular congestion of pial veins. However, in spite of such an aggressive type with reflux to the cortical vein, SSS is still patent in some particular cases. This unusual situation suggests the influence of EV at the initial location of the micro AV shunt. As seen in Fig. 7, the parasagittal (parietal) EV has no direct connection with SSS itself and drains from venous lacunae. The abnormal state mentioned above can be interpreted as follows; the occlusive change of drainage site might occur at the channel between venous lacunae and SSS after the formation of AV shunt, therefore SSS as the normal cortical drainage route is independent from DAVF and can be preserved. It may suggest that the shunt point is located not the sinus wall of SSS but venous lacunae, exit of EV. In the early stage of CS-DAVF without ocular symptoms there are various drainage routes into the pterygoid plexus as well as the superior ophthalmic vein and inferior petrosal sinus. Similarly, the anterior condylor vein is patent in the initial stage of ACC-DAVF. In such young DAVF, EV of the foramen ovale or foramen lacerum and hypoglossal EV still remain as the original drainage pathway. This fact suggests the possibility that the EV plays an important role in the initial stages of newly developed DAVF.

One often encounters a multiplicity about the location or TS-SS-DAVF. This fact is also explainable using the present hypothesis. At the confluence, the lateral side and the sigmoid junction, the initially affected EVs: may be torcular, petrosquamosal and mastoid EVs, respectively.

Unfortunately, our hypothesis has not yet been proven in a pathological specimen of clinical cases as well as from the animal experiments. Further, it is difficult to explain the etiology of DAVF in locations without emissary veins or those without arterial supply coming from emissary arteries with the exception of osteodural AV shunts. Although our theory was not based on the anatomical, physiopathological or clinical observational convincing background, if the very early stage of DAVF is incidentally found, inflammatory investigation into the inflammation and meticulous observation of the flow change will be helpful to predict the development of DAVF and also to support this theory.

6. Conclusion

According to previous theories concerning the mechanism of DAVF, it is very important to consider the occlusive pathway and hypertension of the affected sinus. However, previous theories did not indicate an initiation of this pathological situation which can explain both sinus and non-sinus type DAVF and the promoting factors to develop the extension of DAVF. We propose a new theory: the inflammatory vascular network at the penetration site of emissary veins may induce local shunt formation. Subsequent occlusion of the affected EV completes the usual figure of DAVF, and, the sinus (venous) occlusive pathway and arterial recruitment are important steps in the maturation of the DAVF. Previous mechanistic hypotheses focusing on sinus hypertension and sinus thromboses cannot explain the pathogenesis of non-sinus type of DAVF. Although the etiology of DAVF may be concerned by the thrombo-occlusive change of sinus, and our theory is only a speculation without the base of experimental study, it may enable to understanding the common etiology of the two (sinus & non-sinus) types of DAVF, and is not contradictory to the previous sinus-oriented theory. Pathological proof of the initial stage of DAVF will be mandatory.

Abbreviations: DAVF: dural arteriovenous fistula, EV: emissary vein, CS: cavernous sinus, SSS: superior sagittal sinus, TS: transvers sinus, SS: sigmoid sinus, ACC: anterior condylor confluence, CCJ: craniocervical junction

7. References

[1] Hamada Y, Goto K, Inoue T, et al. Histopathological aspects of dural arteriovenous fistulas in the transverse-sigmoid sinus region in nine patients. *Neurosurgery.* 1997; 40:452–458

[2] Herman JM, Spetzler RF, Bederson JB, et al: Genesis of a dural arteriovenous malformation in a rat model. *J Neurosurg.* 1995; 83:539–545
[3] Nishijima M, Takaku A, Endo S, et al. Etiological evaluation of dural arteriovenous malformations of the lateral and sigmoid sinuses based on histopathological examinations. *J Neurosurg.* 1992;76:600–606
[4] Terada T, Higashida RT, Halbach VV, et al. Development of acquired arteriovenous fistulas in rats due to venous hypertension. *J Neurosurg.* 1994; 80:884–889
[5] Houser OW, Baker HL Jr, Rhoton AL Jr, Okazaki H: Intracranial dural arteriovenous malformations. Radiology 105:55-64, 1972
[6] Kusaka N, Sugiu K, Katsumata A, et al. The importance of venous hypertension in the formation of dural arteriovenous fistulas: a case report of multiple fistulas remote from sinus thrombosis, *Neuroradiology.* 2001;43: 980–984
[7] Vilela P, Willinsky R, terBrugge K.: Dural arteriovenous fistula associated with neoplastic dural sinus thrombosis: two cases. *Neuroradiology.* 2001;43:816-820
[8] Witt O, Pereira PL, Tillmann W: Severe cerebral venous sinus thrombosis and dural arteriovenous fistula in an infant with protein S deficiency. Childs Nerv Syst 15:128-130, 1999
[9] Lasjaunias P, Berenstein A, Surgical Neuroangiography I, Berlin: Springer-Verlag; 1987; 675-678.
[10] Lawton MT, Jacobowitz R, Spetzler RF. Redefined role of angiogenesis in the pathogenesis of dural arteriovenous malformations. *J Neurosurg.* 1987;87:267–274
[11] Klisch J, Kubalek R, Scheufler KM, et al. Plasma vascular endothelial growth factor and serum soluble angiopoietin receptor sTIE-2 in patients with dural arteriovenous fistulas: a pilot study. *Neuroradiology.* 2005; 47:10-17
[12] Kojima T, Miyachi S, Sahara Y, et al. The relationship between venous hypertension and expression of vascular endothelial growth factor: Hemodynamic and immunohistochemical examinations in a rat venous hypertension model. *Surgical Neurol.* 2007; 68: 277-284
[13] Tirakotai W, Bertalanffy H, Liu-Guan B, et al. Immunohistochemical study in dural arteriovenous fistulas and possible role of local hypoxia for the de novo formation of dural arteriovenous fistulas. *Clinical Neurology and Neurosurgery.* 2005; 107: 455-460
[14] Terada T, Tsuura M, Komai N, et al. The role of angiogenic factor bFGF in the development of dural AVFs. *Acta Neurochir. (Wien)*1996;138:877–883
[15] Uranishi R, Nakase H, Sakaki T. Expression of angiogenic growth factors in dural arteriovenous fistula, *J Neurosurg.* 1999;91:781–786.
[16] Zhu Y, Lawton MT, Du R, et al. Expression of hypoxia-inducible factor-1 and vascular endothelial growth factor in response to venous hypertension. *Neurosurgery.* 2006;59:687-696
[17] Satomi J, Satoh K, Matsubara S, et al.: Angiographic changes in venous drainage of cavernous sinus dural arteriovenous fistulae after palliative transarterial embolization or observational management: A proposed stage classification. *Neurosurgery.* 2005; 56:494–502

[18] Gerlach R, Boehm-Weigert M, Berkefeld J et al. Thrombophilic risk factors in patients with cranial and spinal dural arteriovenous fistulae. *Neurosurgery.* 2008;63:693-698
[19] Gerlach R, Yahya H, Rohde S, et al. Increased incidence of thrombophilic abnormalities in patients with cranial dural arteriovenous fistulae. *Neurol Res.* 2003; 25:745–748
[20] Izumi T, Miyachi S, Hattori K, et al. Thrombophilic abnormalities among patients with cranial dural arteriovenous fistulas *Neurosurgery.* 2007; 61: 262-269
[21] Kraus JA, Stuper BK, Muller J, et al. Molecular analysis of thrombophilic risk factors in patients with dural arteriovenous fistulas. *J Neurol.* 2002; 249:680–682
[22] Safavi-Abbasi S, Di Rocco F, Nakaji P, Feigl GC, Gharabaghi A, Samii M, et al: Thrombophilia due to Factor V and Factor II mutations and formation of a dural arteriovenous fistula: case report and review of a rare entity. Skull Base 18:135-143, 2008
[23] Sahara Y, Miyachi S, Nagasaka T, et al. Radiological and pathological changes in the sinus of an experimental arteriovenous fistula of the rat. *Interv Neuroradiol.* 2003; 9(Suppl 1):101-105
[24] Miyachi S. Endovascular treatment for dural arteriovenous fistula. [in Japanese] *No to Shinkei.* 2008; 60: 907-914
[25] Lawton MT, Sanchez-Mejia RO, Pham D, et al. Tentorial dural arteriovenous fistulae: operative strategies and microsurgical results for six types. *Neurosurgery.* 2008;62(3 Suppl 1):110-124
[26] Mitsuhashi Y, Aurboomyawat T, Pereira VM, Geubprasert S, Toulgoat F, Ozanne A, Lasjaunias P. Dural arteriovenous fistulas draining into the petrosal vein or bridging vein of the medulla: possible homologs of spinal dural arteriovenous fistulas. Clinical article. J Neurosurg. 2009 ;111: 889-99
[27] Miyachi S, Kojima T, Ohshima T, Izumi T, Yoshida J. Dural arteriovenous fistula at the anterior condylor confluence. *Interv Neuroradiol.* 2008;14:303-311
[28] San Millán Ruíz D, Gailloud P, Rüfenacht DA, Delavelle J, Henry F, Fasel JH. The craniocervical venous system in relation to cerebral venous drainage. *AJNR Am J Neuroradiol.* 2002;23:1500-1508.
[29] Ushikoshi S, Kikuchi Y, Houkin K, et al. Multiple dural arteriovenous fistulas. *Neurol Med Chir (Tokyo).* 1998;38:478-484.